MEDICAL AND
PSYCHOLOGICAL ASPECTS
OF SPORT AND EXERCISE

Medical and Psychological Aspects of Sport and Exercise

David I. Mostofsky, Ph.D.

Leonard D. Zaichkowsky, Ph.D.

— Boston University —

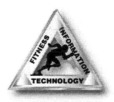

Fitness Information Technology, Inc. • P.O. Box 4425 •
Morgantown, WV 26504-4425 • USA

Library of Congress Card Catalog Number: 01-132722

ISBN: 1-885693-29-X

Copyeditor: Sandra Woods
Cover Design: Jessica Stewart
Managing Editor: Geoffrey C. Fuller
Production Editor: Craig Hines
Proofreader: Maria denBoer
Indexer: Maria denBoer
Printed by Graphic Image Group

10 9 8 7 6 5 4 3 2 1

Fitness Information Technology, Inc.
P.O. Box 4425, University Avenue
Morgantown, WV 26504 USA
800.477.4348
304.599.3483 phone
304.599.3482 fax
Email: fit@fitinfotech.com
Website: www.fitinfotech.com

Contents

Preface

Sport and exercise have generally been associated with amateur or professional athletics, and with enhancing the physical development of the young child. The title to this book, however, has been carefully chosen to reflect the profound changes that are now generally accepted, namely that there are significant implications in exercise and sport that affect medical and psychological functions. Only relatively recently have such activities been recognized as an important adjunct to the maintenance of health, in otherwise healthy individuals and as serving a valuable therapeutic element in treatment and rehabilitative settings. Chronic disorders, in particular, have shown themselves responsive to well designed programs of sport and exercise; a development that is of critical concern with a population whose aging citizens are increasing and in a climate where health costs dominate much of the deliberations surrounding health service delivery. Both the efficiency and cost effectiveness of introducing sport and exercise in medical practice has been recognized by many disciplines, although training and program development has been hampered by the lack of appropriate instructional materials. It is particularly noteworthy that a major portion of an issue of the esteemed *Journal of the American Medical Association* was dedicated to fitness, exercise, and related considerations as they apply to the physicians' concern with cardiorespiratory status and mortality, obesity, and the need to increase physical activity.

Historically, academic programs in both medicine and physical education have largely neglected considerations concerning the contribution of exercise and sport in the modulation of physiological processes. Physicians and other primary health care professionals have failed to communicate the many practical realizations that would allow such activities to provide relief for physical discomforts and dysfunctions as well as for restoring an improved psychological status and an enhanced quality of life. Psychologists and other behavioral and social science clinicians and researchers have not shared the medical literature, nor have physicians visited the libraries of psychology. In part, the response to such a failing energized the increased attention paid to Behavioral Medicine that has emphasized the interdisciplinary nature of health-psychology-medicine and the activities of sport and exercise. It has also drawn attention to the role of patient involvement in optimizing the quality and efficiency of health care services, and the heretofore anecdotal truths concerning the clinically significant interactions between psychological and physiological systems. Such interactions have since been reliably demonstrated to operate on the organic and disease processes, and hence the interest in exercise and sport in dealing with cardiac, respiratory, and sundry nervous system, immune system, and endocrine disorders. Other interactions may be less direct but hardly less important, hence the interest in compliance, stress reduction, and the special needs of the young, the aged, and the developmentally disabled. Finally, there are considerations that focus on issues of wellness, prevention and prophylaxis, and changes in life style.

The pages that follow respond to the need expressed by many primary care physicians, health psychologists, sport psychologists, and other educators and clinicians in medicine and allied health specialties. The literature in these areas has grown enormously over the recent decade and has matched the explosion of journals and monographs. Few professionals in either medicine, physical education, allied health, or sports medicine can afford the luxury of efficiently tracking the reports and innovations in research and clinical practice that has taken place during this period in this multidisciplinary and variegated field of science, scholarship, and clinical practice. This book is the first to address the multifaceted issues that are defined by the title. Training programs, advanced seminars, and reference libraries do not yet enjoy the benefit of a single volume that can begin to direct the reader or serious student to the salient issues and source reports where the relevant methodologies and findings are discussed. This has been our primary goal as we undertook to design the current volume.

We believe that the present book fills an important place in the education of professionals whose teaching or practice intersects with health and exercise. It is more than simply an issue of creating some sense of "well being" for the client or patient. Rather, we expect that the collection of chapters will sensitize the respective professionals to the role that sport and exercise can play in modulating medical problems and the considerations needed for implementing rehabilitation or prevention programs in such areas. "Sensitizing" is to be understood not only as an aesthetic quality, but rather as a motivation and stimulation to incorporate such thinking in curriculum design and in the conduct of programmatic research. While the volume does not represent itself as the definitive word on the topic nor does it claim to provide a complete solution for all professionals, it is hoped that the writings will offer practical guidelines and examples of models that have been shown to succeed, so that the professional will be able to envision how such efforts can be integrated in the course of providing clinical services. Clearly, the material offers more

than simply information transfer. The intent is to convey a cutting-edge message, specifically, that medical management extends beyond the office of the medical specialist and involves the professionals in all areas of medicine as well as psychology and education, social work, and others. In an attempt to capture the exciting developments of this interdisciplinary network of interests with respect to the topics we selected, we were successful to win the participation of truly eminent authors for the respective areas. The selection of chapters and their organization in the volume were largely decided by several key factors: the extent to which a problem area is already being addressed in the professional literature and meetings; the availability of a healthy literature in an area (such that a discussion of sport and exercise with multiple sclerosis, however important and promising, has not received as much attention from the specialists in these areas as is the case with pain, or eating disorders) as well as the availability of an author of excellence to whom to assign the topic; and the generalizability of the issues to more than a single sample or disorder.

We trust that medical and psychiatric/ psychological professionals, including (but not limited to) to those physicians in general and family practice, orthopedics, pediatrics, and geriatrics as well as specialists in sports medicine, rehabilitation, sports psychologists, athletic directors and coaches, allied health and rehabilitation professionals, as well as graduate students and academics, will all benefit from having this work available.

David I. Mostofsky, Ph.D.
Leonard D. Zaichkowsky, Ph.D.
Boston University

Reference

Journal of the American Medical Association (1999). *282*(16), October 27. Washington, DC: American Medical Association.

1
Importance of Sport and Exercise to Quality of Life and Longevity

Roy J. Shephard

Summary

Concepts and methods of measurement of quality-adjusted life expectancy are discussed. It is argued that an improvement in the quality-adjusted life expectancy is a stronger argument for exercising than is a mere increase of life span. A physically active lifestyle probably increases quality-adjusted life years more than it augments total life span, although techniques to estimate the likely impact of exercise need refinement. Gains in the quality of life seem more likely to motivate a young person to exercise than does a promise of increased longevity because an increase in the quality of life provides an immediate reward, rather than one that occurs at some time in the distant future. Some benefits are obtained from a reduced probability of acute and chronic disease, but the main bases for improvement in the quality of life lie in an immediate enhancement of mood state and a greatly reduced likelihood of disability and dependency in old age. Given the importance of quality of life to both motivation of the exerciser and overall population health, this topic deserves greater attention on the part of exercise scientists and practitioners.

Introduction

The past 20 years have seen the emergence of a strong belief that sport and exercise are effective means of increasing both the quantity and the quality of a person's life. Moreover, this belief is increasingly emphasized in efforts to promote an increase of physical activity among the general public.

Epidemiologists who have sought to summarize the health benefits of regular physical activity, sport, and exercise have commonly focused their attention on the quantity of life, or reductions in the relative risk of death, rather than on the quality of survival, probably because indices of mortality are easily measured and seem relatively incontrovertible statistics (see, for example, the review of Paffenbarger, Hyde, Wing, Min-Lee, & Kampert, 1994). Nevertheless, there is growing recognition of the need to assess treatment-related changes in the quality of a patient's life (Kaplan, Anderson, & Wingard, 1989; Rejeski, Brawley, & Shumaker, 1996), and indeed the U.S. National Institutes of Health now requires some assessment of quality of life in most clinical trials of new medications.

The present chapter discusses issues of terminology and the nature of available evidence before evaluating critically the respective impacts of sport, exercise, and regular physical activity on the span of life and its quality. A final section looks briefly at implications for public policy.

Issues of Terminology

Sport, Exercise, snd Physical Activity

Various consensus statements have drawn clear distinctions among sport, exercise, and physical activity (see, for example, Bouchard & Shephard, 1994). Clarification of terminology not only has theoretical interest, but is also of some practical importance in our present context.

Sport. In many European countries, the term sport is used to describe various forms of voluntary physical activity, both recreational and competitive, but in North America, the same word usually implies participation in competitive activity, whether voluntary or professional in type. There is often a strong selection of competitive athletes in terms of their body build, and this immediately has important practical implications when comparisons of mortality experience are made between athletes and the general public (Sarna, Sahi, Koskenvuo, & Kaprio, 1993). Athletic selection is also favored by personality traits that increase the risk of an early and violent death, and this trend can offset possible favorable effects of regular, vigorous physical activity on susceptibility to various chronic diseases (Polednak, 1978). Comparisons with the sedentary population are further complicated because a proportion of athletes are health-conscious individuals who seek to extend their life span by such practices as eating a prudent diet, consuming mega-doses of vitamins, and abstaining from cigarette smoking (Shephard, 1989). In terms of the health impact of the sport itself, there are often benefits from regular, intensive

physical activity. However, the "weekend athlete" may engage in occasional bouts of strenuous competitive activity for which he or she is poorly prepared; the combination of an excessive intensity of effort and the emotional excitement of competition may then precipitate rather than postpone a heart attack (Shephard, 1995; Vuori, 1995). Particularly for teenagers, the impact of sport on the participant's quality of life is augmented by peer adulation of sports teams. Many sports participants also value the excitement of competition, and for such individuals, a closely competed game may do more to enhance their quality of life than an equivalent expenditure of energy on a laboratory treadmill. Nevertheless, this again is partly a question of self-selection, and those who do not engage in competitive activities may find little attraction in the bonhomie and group mores of an exercise class.

Exercise. Exercise may be defined as any form of leisure activity that is undertaken for a specific purpose, such as the improvement of health, the increase of physical fitness, or the extension of life span. Often, a physician or exercise specialist prescribes a clearly specified mode of activity, together with an appropriate intensity, frequency and duration of individual sessions (American College of Sports Medicine, 1995; Shephard, 1994). In theory, such exercise is the most effective method of enhancing health because the dose is carefully regulated to optimize its conditioning effect. However, in practice, the actual dose of physical activity may be less than adequate, because of poor attendance at exercise sessions or fears to implement the prescription on the part of the individual or those supervising exercise classes. Moreover, the "sameness" of a prescribed activity may limit its contribution to the quality of life. Sometimes, a person feels compelled to conform to the recommendations of the health specialist and may even suffer from feelings of guilt if for any reason the exercise prescription cannot be filled.

Physical activity. Physical activity is a much broader rubric than either sport or exercise. It encompasses both of these items, but it also includes vigorous occupational activity, domestic chores, energy spent in commuting to and from work, and active leisure pursuits other than sport and exercise.

Automation has greatly reduced the energy cost of much traditional "heavy work," to the point that now such employment usually has little impact on either health or longevity. Nevertheless, there are still a few occupations that demand a substantial daily energy expenditure. For example, the postal carrier must each day carry a heavy bag of mail over a substantial distance, climbing a flight of steps to the front door of most houses (Shephard, 1983). Walking and cycling are the commonest forms of active leisure for most city-dwellers. In young adults, the chosen speed of walking is often too low for this activity to have any beneficial influence on health, but in older adults, brisk walking can demand a large fraction of the individual's maximal oxygen intake (Shephard, 1997a).

Leisure activities may contribute more to the quality of life than an equivalent investment of time in a regimented program of exercise classes. Spontaneous leisure avoids the unpleasant coercion of a formal exercise class, and what for some people is the "stress" of meeting preassigned targets. The activities that are selected can be varied in type, and they can be built into the normal daily schedule, thus overcoming one common excuse for inactivity ("a lack of time"). Moreover, some leisure pursuits such as fast walking can be pursued in a pleasant recreational environment; conversation with a companion is possible, and other interesting pursuits such as the study of urban architecture or the fauna and flora of various habitats can be integrated

into exercise sessions. Such secondary interests boost the impact of a given activity session on the individual's quality of life. The main practical limitation of spontaneous leisure activity from a public health point of view is that the intensity of effort is unregulated, and particularly in a young adult, the chosen intensity of effort may be insufficient to have a conditioning effect.

Quality of life. The overall quality of life is influenced by personal perceptions of a wide variety of factors that include physical functions such as mobility and the capacity for self-care; a reasonable level of intellectual and emotional function; social dimensions such as opportunities for intimacy and social contact; opportunities for appropriate role performance within the family, the community, and the workplace; feelings of comfort, well-being, and self-efficacy; and the extent of any pain or other symptoms (Rejeski et al., 1996; Wenger & Furberg, 1990).

An individual's quality of life on any given day is located somewhere along a continuum. At one end of the scale lies an optimal quality of life. This can be assigned an arbitrary multiplier of 1.00. If a person were to enjoy such a quality of life on a continuing basis throughout a calendar year, this would give that individual one quality-adjusted life-year (QALY) of survival. At the other end of the scale, the quality of life has dropped to near zero. The individual concerned loses the will to survive, refusing to eat or pressing for euthanasia. Such a state can be assigned an arbitrary multiplier of zero. Too often, a doctor who is faced with this circumstance attempts to extend life span by drastic and/or costly measures, ranging from forced or intravenous feeding to heart/lung transplants. Such an approach may increase longevity, but it does nothing to augment the individual's QALY.

Some authors (for example, Fries & Spitz, 1990, and Kaplan & Bush, 1982) have attempted to distinguish what they term a health-related quality of life from the social and environmental factors that influence the total quality of the life experience, but it is plain that patients do not draw such a nice distinction. Social and environmental factors (including the availability of aids for daily living and the support of family, friends, and caregivers) exert a strong influence upon an individual's perceptions of the quality of life and health status (Hart, Bowling, Ellis, & Silman, 1990; Vetter, Lewis, & Llewellyn, 1992). Moreover, some interventions (for example, involvement in a group exercise program) can have an impact (usually favorable) on the social and psychological dimensions of quality of life, as well as influence medical outcomes for the individual (Fisher et al., 1993). It thus seems best to regard quality of life as a gestalt that integrates the individual's instantaneous appraisal of all factors influencing the life experience, ranging from ill health and physical disability to a sense of self-efficacy and pride in performance, and embracing also such psychosocial influences as the extent of independence and opportunities for contacts with friends and relations.

Some authors speak also of healthy life expectancy (Robine & Ritchie, 1991), active life expectancy (Kinsella, 1992) or quality-adjusted life-expectancy (Butler, 1992; Fitzpatrick et al., 1992; R. Kaplan, 1985; Shephard, 1982; Wood-Dauphinee & Küchler, 1992). These terms integrate an individual's experience over the entire life-course, in effect discounting the observed longevity for periods when health or physical activity is impaired or the individual's quality of life is less than ideal.

Available Evidence

Longevity

Studies of longevity may count the actual ages of death in active and inactive populations. or the likelihood of death can be predicted from instruments such as the Health Hazard Appraisal Questionnaire (Shephard et al., 1982a). The latter approach looks at an individual's lifestyle and uses this information to compute the likelihood of death from each of the 12 most commonly fatal conditions over the next 10 years; pooling of this information yields an appraised age, which exceeds the individual's calendar age by a margin that depends on the extent of risk-taking behavior (including a lack of regular exercise).

Plainly, the weightings adopted when evaluating responses to the Health Hazard Appraisal Questionnaire are arbitrary and apply with varying degrees of precision to different populations. The counting of deaths might thus seem a more secure method of investigating the impact of regular physical activity upon life span. However, the observed mortality rate is a complex number, determined by both the positive and the negative effects of exercise. Moreover, an accurate determination of survival rates depends on the investigator's success in tracing all members of a given cohort; this can be quite a difficult task in the very mobile society of North America. Finally, the death of an athlete may receive more publicity than that of a sedentary person, so that the counting of deaths may be more complete for athletes than for any comparison group that has been chosen.

If a study lasts no more than a few months, it may be possible to assign people to exercise programs on a random basis. Such an approach can yield useful data to examine the impact of regular physical activity on Health Hazard Appraisal scores (Shephard et al., 1982a). However, the calculation of survival curves requires that large cohorts be followed over periods of 10 years or longer. It is then necessary to accept a nonrandom assignment of subjects. Comparisons can be drawn between athletes and nonathletes, heavy workers and those holding sedentary jobs, those with active vs. sedentary leisure pursuits, or those who enter a study with high vs. low levels of aerobic fitness. One somewhat more sophisticated variant of this approach is to compare those who adopt exercise over a period of 10 years or more with those who cease exercising over the same interval (Paffenbarger & Lee, 1996). Plainly, there are many differences between those who choose or maintain physical activity and those who are sedentary or drop out of exercise programs. Although the analysts may attempt to control for these extraneous factors by the use of covariance techniques, it is likely that such adjustments will be incomplete. For example, some studies have merely distinguished smokers vs. nonsmokers, ignoring possible differences in patterns of smoking between those who are active and those who are sedentary. Given the major influence of smoking on longevity, this is an important criticism. A further difficulty is that the initial categorization of habitual physical activity does not always persist; those who were involved in university sports teams may become inactive in middle age (Montoye, Van Huss, Olson, Pierson, & Hudec, 1957), and seniority rules may allow those who were classed as heavy workers to gain physically easier employment as they become older (Shephard, 1997b).

Quality of Life

Assessment of the quality of life holds even greater challenge than the determination of average survival prospects. The investigator needs a measuring technique that is reliable and valid within a given cultural setting, yet responds well to subtle differences in a person's quality of life. There are many possible instruments, but few are widely accepted. Moreover, alternative approaches may yield widely differing estimates of a person's qual-

ity of life (Spiegelhalter et al., 1992). Options include the interpretation of the quality of life as a gestalt, use of detailed generic questionnaires, disease-specific instruments, and function-specific assessments.

Gestalt approach. Early measures such as the Karnofsky Index (Karnofsky & Burchenal, 1949) represented the quality of life as a single number. Although reasonably reliable and valid relative to other assessments, the Karnofsky Index has been criticized as failing to capture the conceptual domain of quality of life (Grieco & Long, 1984). Other options within the gestalt rubric include a category rating, a magnitude estimation, a health utility measure, a time trade-off, and a "standard gamble" (Feeny, Furlong, & Torrance, 1996; Guyatt, Dego, Charlson, Levine, & Mitchell, 1989; D. L. Patrick & Erickson, 1993; Spiegelhalter et al., 1992; Torrance, 1987).

In the standard gamble, the individual is asked to imagine that there is now some wonder drug that promises a perfect quality of life, but this new treatment has the disadvantage of carrying a substantial mortality. A computer terminal is used to display the relative likelihoods of cure and death in the form of a pie chart. The probability of the two outcomes is then varied until the person agrees that there is nothing to choose between acceptance of his or her current health status and adoption of the proposed new treatment.

A single score of this type is useful when comparing the impact of various types of physical activity on overall population health in order to make recommendations for future resource allocation (Oldridge, 1997). The main disadvantage is that the global score gives no indication which aspects of function have enhanced the quality of life, so that it is difficult to decide *why* one type of physical activity is more effective than another.

Generic instruments. Generic instruments sometimes look at a single concept, such as a person's tendency to report symptoms, the number of bed-rest days that are taken each year, or the demands on health services as seen in medical billings for the individual (Shephard, Corey, Renzland, & Cox, 1982b). More commonly, generic instruments ask the subject to rate many components of health (physical, emotional, and social function), along with items such as role performance, pain, and other symptoms. Examples of generic instruments include the Sickness Impact Profile (Bergner. Bobbit, Carter, & Gilson, 1981), the Nottingham scale (Hunt, McEwen, & McKenna, 1986), the massive 44-scale Index of Health-related Quality of Life (Rosser & Kind, 1978), a 36-item short form of the Rand Corporation questionnaire (Jenkinson, Coulter, & Wright, 1993) and the simple 6-scale "Euroqol" instrument (Williams & Kind, 1992).

Much reliable and detailed information may be obtained, but there are several disadvantages to this type of approach:

1. In order to cover a variety of potential clinical problems, the instrument includes many questions that the individual may perceive as irrelevant. This reduces cooperation, and frequent negative responses limit the overall sensitivity of the instrument (D. Patrick & Deyo, 1989; McHorney, Ware, Rogers, Raczek, & Lu, 1992). Generic questionnaires are often more appropriate to evaluation of a rehabilitation program than to a study of the influence of sport on the quality of life of a young adult.

2. Separate ratings are obtained for such items as mastery, fatigue, and dyspnea. It then becomes difficult to assess the overall quality of life, particularly if different test scales show contradictory trends. Any attempts to select weighting factors that will allow scores to be combined require subjective value judgments, and it seems inherently improbable that a single weight-

ing system will be appropriate and stable in all ages, socioeconomic groups and disease conditions (Fletcher et al., 1992a).

3. Some responses to a generic questionnaire (for example, those covering social relationships) may remain relatively static, resisting improvement from a lifestyle intervention such as an increase of physical activity (Fitzpatrick et al., 1991).

4. Because of the number of functions that must be assessed, only scanty information is collected on the ability to undertake various types of physical activity. For example, the Quality of Well-being Scale of R. M. Kaplan and Bush (1982) examines only the individual's ability to engage in very low levels of physical activity; almost all young and middle-aged adults would engage in a much higher level of physical activity than that which is discussed.

5. Because of the time demanded to complete a detailed questionnaire, people are unwilling to be tested repeatedly. Although information can be obtained about a person's immediate status, it is difficult to administer followup tests to examine changes in the quality of life over a number of years of survival.

Disease-specific instruments. Examples of disease-specific instruments include the arthritis impact scale (Meenan, German, Mason, & Dunaif, 1982), the back pain disability questionnaire (Roland & Morris, 1983), and various indices of cardiac and pulmonary rehabilitation outcome (Oldridge, 1997; Pashkow et al., 1995).

Disease-specific instruments can be quite successful when comparing the impact of various types of physical activity on patients with a specific disease, but they are much less helpful when evaluating population health. It is difficult to compare scores obtained in those with one form of disability with results obtained using a different instrument in people with some other type of disease or disability, and most scales of this type are not suitable for the ostensibly healthy adult.

Function-specific instruments. Function-specific instruments such as the Activities of Daily Living scale, the Profile of Mood States (McNair, Lorr, & Doppleman, 1971), the Psychological General Well-being index (Dupuy, 1984), or the symptom rating test (Kellner & Sheffield, 1973) have been suggested as halfway houses between generic and disease specific instruments (Fletcher et al., 1992b).

Such tests can demonstrate improvements in function, mood state, and well-being in both health and disease, but it is difficult to relate any gains in score that result from an increase in habitual physical activity to alterations in life expectancy or QALY.

General limitations of current methodology. None of the currently available methods is ideal, and whichever method is chosen, quality-of-life scores remain relatively crude. Results may be biased by response acquiescence, particularly in elderly individuals (Moum, 1988). It also remains unclear whether an increase in quality-of-life multiplier from 0.1 to 0.2 units has the same significance as an increase from 0.9 to 1.0 units. Indeed, Wagstaff (1991) has advanced equity arguments for the development of a nonlinear quality-of-life scale; from the public health point of view, we should be more concerned about moving people off the lower end of the scale than in making minor improvements to the well-being of those for whom life is already relatively satisfactory.

If an exerciser feels better, but the quality-of-life score remains unchanged, it is possible that activity has boosted some aspect of function that is important to the individual, yet cannot be detected by what is a rather crude measuring instrument (Deyo & Inui, 1984). Gains in some aspect of the quality of life that is of particular importance to the individual may develop more quickly than gains in other areas, and this response may be masked by calculating a global score (Rejeski et al., 1996). Moreover, we are looking at perceptions of function and the patient's coping strategies, rather than some objective index of performance. Thus, changes in the quality of life may correlate quite weakly with gains in physical fitness (Jasnoski, Holmes, Solomon, & Aguiar, 1981; Rejeski et al., 1996; Woodruff & Conway, 1992).

There is sometimes a conflict between an anticipated shortening of life span and an expected increase in the quality-adjusted life span (for instance, regular bouts of vigorous sport or exercise may enhance the quality of life for a 90-year-old who enjoys physical activity, but at this age such a lifestyle may also shorten calendar survival). It is important that any conflict between the two outcomes not be obscured by calculations that combine duration and quality of life (Fletcher et al., 1992a, b).

It is generally agreed that young adults do not value late health benefits as much as do older individuals because the rewards are much more distant; nevertheless, there is still considerable controversy concerning an appropriate discounting of QALY to allow for what are termed age-related time preferences (Spiegelhalter et al., 1992). Age affects not only the responses of the subjects, but also the approach adopted by the investigators; young researchers do not always make a correct assessment of what is important to older people. Quality-of-life instruments have now been developed specifically for the testing of elderly people (Fletcher et al., 1992b; George & Bearon, 1980; Kane & Kane, 1981). Analysis of the results is further complicated because certain benefits such as an extension of life span diminish as a person becomes older. This inevitably makes the use of simple QALYs an ageist instrument of public policy (Busschback, Hessing, & de Charro, 1993; Harris, 1991); when measured in such units, the dividends will almost always be greater if resources are allocated to the young rather than to the elderly. One possible alternative is to express treatment-related gains in QALY as a percentage of the individual's anticipated residual life span (Spiegelhalter et al., 1992).

Finally, any change in an individual's perceived quality of life does not reflect simply the response to a given program of physical activity. The reported score depends on a wide range of perceptions of health, function, and mood state. Particularly during the final years of life, there is a strong interaction between the quality of a person's life and the immediate physical and social environment (Birren, 1983; Golant, 1985; Mor-Barak, Miller, & Syme, 1991; Pearlman & Uhlmann, 1988; Sherbourne, Meredith, Rogers, & Ware, 1992). The availability of adapted housing and simple aids to daily living do much to enhance the quality of life at this stage (Hart et al., 1990); other positive factors include the survival of a spouse (Latten, 1989; Moore, Stambrook, Gill, & Lubusko, 1992, Sherbourne et al., 1992), a secure financial status (Pearlman & Uhlmann, 1991), a well-developed spirituality and/or religious beliefs (Oldridge, 1997), and the opportunity to make a productive contribution to the community (Birren, 1983).

Impact of an Increase in Physical Activity

Most developed nations have experienced substantial reductions in mortality from cardiovascular disease, with associated gains in average life expectancy over the past 30 years. These changes reflect advances in medical and surgical treatment, combined with changes in personal lifestyle (the greater prevalence of regular physical activity, a prudent diet, and abstinence from cigarette smoking). Changes in smoking patterns have been particularly important. A young man who stops smoking can extend his life span by an average of 8 years. There is also some cross-sectional evidence that longevity can be increased by 1 to 2 years if regular exercise is begun at the age of 35 years (Paffenbarger & Lee, 1996; Paffenbarger et al., 1994). However, any such extensions in life span raise an important and challenging question. If preventive measures such as stopping smoking and exercising regularly avert a sudden and premature death from cardiac arrest, will the individual who has adopted a prudent lifestyle merely survive to endure an extended period of ill health as one of the growing population of frail elderly individuals?

Fries (1989) has hypothesized that preventive measures reduce the prevalence of ill health and disability and thus yield not only an extension of life span, but also a compression of the final years of morbidity, when the quality of life becomes poor. More pessimistically, Kramer (1980) and Gruenberg (1977) have argued that medical technology is merely prolonging the survival of those who are already in poor health. In support of the latter view, Robine and Ritchie (1991) noted that the average life expectancy in the United States had increased by 3.1 years in men, and 3.0 years in women between 1970 and 1980. Over this same interval, however, disability-free life expectancy had shown no change in women, and a gain of only 0.7 years in men.

In the remainder of the present chapter, we will argue that habitual physical activity can increase not only life span, but also the quality of life. Indeed, the benefits associated with an enhanced mood state, reduced dependency, and reductions in the incidence of acute and chronic illness seem to offer the regular exerciser a larger and more persuasive reward than a mere extension of life span.

Longevity

Evidence concerning the impact of habitual physical activity upon longevity is conflicting, in part because sport, exercise, and even heavy work are largely self-selected. On one hand, studies of those who were athletes as young adults in general have found no advantage of longevity relative to sedentary controls (Montoye et al., 1957; Polednak, 1978). On the other hand, substantial prolongation of survival has been described in endurance athletes (Sarna et al., 1994) such as cross-country ski champions (Karvonen, Klemola, Virkajarvi, & Kekkonen, 1974), but much of this advantage may reflect a combination of a favorable body build and lifelong abstinence from cigarettes. Perhaps the most convincing evidence that regular exercise *causes* an extension of life span has been drawn from a longitudinal study of Harvard alumni (Paffenbarger & Lee, 1996). Individuals from this well-educated group who had adopted regular physical activity (estimated at about 8 MJ/week, 2000 kcal/week) by the age of 35 to 44 years lived 1–2 years longer than those who spent less than 2 MJ/week (500 kcal/week) on deliberate leisure activity. Benefit was still seen after statistical adjustment of the data for age, cigarette smoking, hypertension, overweight-for-height, alcohol consumption, early parental death, and chronic disease at entry to the study. The extension of life span appeared to be somewhat greater for those who engaged in sports or other activities with an intensity greater than 4.5 METS (25 kJ/min, 6 kcal/min) than for more moderate activities such as walking. Benefit was also seen in those who had adopted physical activity over an average 12-year followup, but not in those who had ceased exercising over the same interval. The potential for extension of life span diminished progressively as the age of the individual increased, and in those who did not begin exercising until the age of 75 to 84 years, the benefit was only a 2 month increase in survivorship.

A study by Pekkanen et al. (1987) reported a substantial difference in cumulative mortality curves between active and inactive segments of the Finnish population. However, the survival curves for the two segments of the Finnish population came together around the age of 80 years, so that the

Table 1. Relationship Between Reported Level of Physical Activity at Age 50 Years and Level of Institutional Support as a Senior Citizen

Activity at age 50 years (arbitrary units, Mean + SD)	Level of disability
9.3 ± 9.8 (n=286)	None
8.1 ± 8.9 (n=126)	Minor
7.7 ± 9.4 (n=173)	Major
4.1 ± 6.6 (n=25)	Institutionalized

From "Geriatric Benefits of Exercise as an Adult." by R. J. Shephard and W. M. Montelpare, 1998, *Journal of Gerontology*, 43, pp. M86–M90.

oldest subjects did not extend their survivorship by exercising regularly.

In support of a differential effect of age on the benefits of exercise, Linsted, Tonstad, and Kuzma (1991) reported that whereas the all-cause mortality of highly active Seventh Day Adventists aged 50–59 years was only 63% of that for their inactive peers, by the age of 80 to 89 years, the highly active subjects had a 10% greater risk of death than did their sedentary contemporaries.

It might be questioned whether the reason for this reversal of benefit is that age increases the risk that exercise will precipitate sudden death (Vuori, 1995). This could be true for that minority of old people who engage in very intensive activity although the observations of Vuori (1995) suggest that on a population-wide basis, the risk of death per exercise session actually diminishes with age, probably because most older people are quite cautious about exercising too vigorously.

Quality of Life

Most people have some scope to enhance the quality of their life, even as young adults. This potential increases with age, as disability and resulting dependency increase. R. M. Kaplan et al. (1991) estimated that the total discrepancy between life expectancy and well-life expectancy was 11.5 years for men and 15.6 years for women. Likewise, in a survey of several different countries, Robine and Ritchie (1991) noted that relative to calendar age, there was a loss of 8.8 to 14.6 well years in men and 10.8 to 17.0 well years in women.

The exact quality of life multipliers for each age category have yet to be determined, but the principles of analysis have been discussed in a previous review (Shephard, 1996).

Healthy Middle-Aged Adults

Most healthy middle-aged adults live at some intermediate point between the two poles on the quality-of-life scale. Their quality of life is not Utopian, and the multiplier may be 0.9 rather than 1.0. Thus, each calendar year of survival gives them 0.9 rather than 1.0 QALY. This implies that they have the potential to enhance their multiplier by 0.1 units, and if this potential were to be realized, they would gain (0.1 × 35), or 3.5 QALY, between the ages of 30 and 65 years.

Mood state. The main problem for the young and middle-aged adult is a less than optimal mood state. Many people indicate that the reason they exercise is because it "makes them feel better." A reduction of fatigue and an increased energy level are commonly reported immediate dividends of physical activity (Thayer, 1989). It has thus been suggested that regular physical activity can counter depression and enhance mood state. However, randomized controlled trials of exercise and mood state are rare, particularly in the general, nondepressed population, and it would be dangerous to conclude that an increase of physical activity will always enhance mood state and thus improve quality of life. Even if current exercisers are correct in their perception of benefit, they are a self-selected group, and there may be at least an equally large group of nonexercisers (who are not usually seen by sports medicine experts) who find that exercise causes a deterioration in their mood state.

There is some empirical evidence that exercise can improve mood state in young and middle-aged individuals although the benefit seems greater in those who are initially depressed than in those who are initially in at least moderate mental health (North, McCullagh, & Tran, 1990). A moderate association between physical activity and mood state is also found in the elderly although there is as yet little experimental evidence that the association is a causal one (Brown, 1992; Gauvin & Spence, 1996; O'Connor, Aenchbacher, & Dishman, 1993). Where data are cross-sectional in type, it is at least equally plausible that a sense of well-being encourages a person to exercise. McNeil, LeBlanc, and Joyner (1991) established that in moderately depressed elderly subjects, programs of experimenter-accompanied exercise reduced moderate depression, but the researchers concluded that any benefit was largely a placebo effect or a consequence of group membership, because it was also found with increased social contact alone. Nieman, Warren, Dotson, Butterworth, and Henson (1993) and Emery and Gatz (1990) reached essentially similar conclusions after exercising women aged 65 to 84 years for periods of 12 weeks.

It remains conceivable that the instruments that were used in these experiments failed to detect gains of mood because they were designed for clinical purposes, and the experimental subjects generally entered the studies in good initial psychological health. Moreover, even a small gain in quality of life could have a large and immediate effect on overall population health.

One crude objective measure of any improvement in mood state is a decrease in the demand for medical services. Several studies have suggested that individuals who begin an exercise program make a 20–30% smaller demand for physician consultations and hospital services (Bly, Jones, & Richardson, 1986; Shephard et al., 1982b). Putting the potential benefit from an optimization of mood throughout adult life at a gain of 3.5 QALY, a 25% improvement in mood would yield almost 0.9 QALY.

Acute illness. The influence of regular physical activity on susceptibility to acute and chronic illness also yields some gains in QALY, but the population impact is much smaller than that from an exercise-induced enhancement of mood state because only a small proportion of the population is affected by either acute or chronic disease at any one time.

Adults sustain 1–2 episodes of acute illnesses such as upper respiratory infections over the course of a year. Let us suppose that each episode reduces the quality of life by a factor of 0.1 for 10 to 20 days. When data are averaged over the entire year, acute illness thus leads to a loss of $(0.1 \times 2 \times 15/365)$, or 0.008 QALY per year of adult life. Moderate physical activity may shorten the duration of symptoms and/or reduce the number of infections, possibly by increasing the number of natural killer cells and enhancing resting immune function (Brenner, Shek, & Shephard, 1994; Nieman, 1995). Even if the impact of acute infections were to be reduced by 30%, the benefit relative to a sedentary person would amount to only about 0.008×0.3 QALY per year, or a *total* gain of 0.084 QALY over the period between 30 and 65 years of age. Moreover, an appropriate choice of exercise intensity would be vital to assure even this small gain; an excessive volume of physical activity could actually increase both the incidence and the duration of infections (Brenner et al., 1994; Nieman, 1995).

Chronic illness. Ischemic heart disease is a major cause of chronic illness between the ages of 30 and 65 years. The incidence of nonfatal episodes is about 2/1,000 per year in men, and 1/1,000/year in women. In other words, a total of $(1.5 \times 35)/1,000$, or about 5% of the population, are likely to be personally affected by a clinical manifestation of ischemic heart disease before they reach the age of 65 years. For the purpose of calculation, we may suggest that each episode causes an immediate 50% reduction in the quality of life, with progressive recovery to a loss of perhaps 10% over the first 3 months of recovery. The average impact would then be (0.3×0.25) QALY per episode, or (when averaged across the entire working population) $(0.3 \times 0.25 \times 0.05)$, a loss of 0.004 QALY per episode. The affected individual will also have a continuing concern about the heart for the remainder of his or her working life; we may arbitrarily suggest that this causes a continuing 10% deterioration in the quality of life. When we allow also for a substantial shortening of average life span following a first episode of myocardial infarction, the chronic effects of the infarct will have an impact of (0.1 × 20), or 2 QALY, on the individuals who are affected, and the impact will drop to 0.1 QALY when averaged across the entire population. Adding together the short- and long-term effects of ischemic heart disease, we have a total impact of 0.104 QALY. An optimal program of physical activity is likely to halve both the incidence of first nonfatal heart attacks (Powell, Thompson, Caspersen, & Kendrick, 1987; Shephard, 1981) and the resultant deterioration in quality of life, for a gain of some 0.052 QALY.

Older Individuals

During the final 8–10 years of life, most people develop some type of chronic disability that reduces the quality of their life (Health and Welfare, Canada, 1982). Problems range from arthritis to a stroke, poorly compensated congestive cardiac failure, a deterioration in sight or hearing, or a loss of cerebral function. Independence and thus the quality of life are progressively threatened by the loss of mobility (Grieco & Long, 1984; Osberg, McGinnis, DeJong, & Seward, 1987).

Scope to augment QALY. Statistics Canada (1986) found that 83% of seniors aged 75 to 84 years and 89% of those over 85 years had disabilities that limited their mobility and agility. In the 1991 survey, 25% of seniors over the age of 85 years classed their disability as moderate, but 64% considered it severe (Health and Welfare Canada, 1993). Likewise, in Britain, a survey of seniors found that 2.1 million men and 5.2 million women could not walk at 4.8 km/h even on a level surface, and the number who could not

maintain this speed on a moderate slope rose to 5.6 million men and 11.7 million women, including 81% of all men and 92% of all women aged 65–74 years (Sports Council and the Health Education Authority, 1992).

Over the age-range 65 to 75 years of age, such disabilities progressively reduce the quality-of-life multiplier from 0.9 to somewhere in the range 0.5–0.8; this offers the prospect of gaining a further [(0.2–0.5) × 10], or 2–5 QALY. In the final year of life, the average person is liable to develop frequent pain (Moss, Lawton, & Glicksman, 1991) and near total dependency. The quality-of-life multiplier thus decreases still further, perhaps to 0.2–0.5. In this final year of life, there is thus a potential to enhance the quality of life by 0.5 to 0.8 units, yielding a final dividend of [(0.5–0.8) × 1.0], or 0.5 to 0.8 QALY, for the final year of survival.

Functional loss and dependency. Many of the problems that limit the quality of the life experience for seniors are due to an age-related loss of function. Already, by the age of 65 years, many women and some men find difficulty in performing some normal daily activities. In the succeeding years, further losses in aerobic power, muscle strength, and flexibility cause dependency to become complete (Guralnik et al., 1993). One 6-year followup noted that about a quarter of seniors who were initially independent had become dependent by the end of the study (Strawbridge, Kaplan, Camacho, & Cohen, 1992).

Prolonged aerobic activity is fatiguing if the task demands more than 40% of aerobic power (Shephard, 1994), and effort at more than 70% of aerobic power is rapidly exhausting. Thus, the cumulative loss of aerobic power with aging (5ml/[kg.min] per decade, beginning around the age of 25 years) leaves many senior citizens with inadequate oxygen transport to undertake everyday activities. Likewise, a progressive deterioration in muscle strength causes problems in opening jars, carrying parcels, and lifting the body mass from a chair, toilet seat, or bed (Bassey et al., 1992). Statistics Canada (1985) found that by the age of 55 years, some 10% of women and 2% of men were unable to carry out their shopping alone, and in those aged 80 years and older, the prevalence of this limitation had risen to near 30% of women and 20% of men. In similar fashion, a progressive loss of joint flexibility can restrict such daily activities as climbing steps, entering a bath, climbing into a car, or even dressing unaided.

The immediate causes of institutionalization include difficulty in ambulation or transfer, falling, failure to eat or drink adequately, incontinence, loss of manual dexterity, loss of self-esteem, and intellectual deterioration (Mathews, 1989). It is difficult to distinguish losses of function due to sedentary living from the cumulative impact of chronic disease in the elderly, and some authors (for example, Robine & Ritchie, 1991) have attributed all of the loss in disability-free life expectancy to the effects of specific diseases (Table 2). Nevertheless, in their analysis, the main causes of loss in QALY are cardiovascular, locomotor, and respiratory problems. Whether disability is blamed on general aging or some specific pathology, there is plainly a large burden of disability that can be corrected, and from the nature of the conditions listed, exercise seems likely to have a beneficial influence.

Impact of regular physical activity. Both retrospective (Shephard & Montelpare, 1988) and prospective data (Bokovoy & Blair, 1994; LaCroix, Guralnik, Berkman, Wallace, & Satterfield, 1993; Morey et al., 1991) suggest that people who are active and fit in later middle age are less likely to develop problems of mobility as they become older. Despite the likelihood that physical condition will decline as age advances, a program of regular physical activity can maintain or even enhance functional capacity in many elderly people (Manton, 1988). Aerobic power, muscle strength, flexibility, and balance can be increased by as much as 10–20%, and this represents the equivalent of a 10- to 20-year reversal of aging (Fiatarone et al., 1988; Lord & Castell, 1994; Morey et al.,

Table 2. Gain of Life Expectancy and of Disability-Free Years If Different Causes of Ill Health Were to Be Eliminated (Based on Data of Robine & Ritchie, 1991)

Cause	Life expectancy	Disability-free life expectancy	Total life expectancy
Circulatory diseases	4.1 years	4.2 years	8.3 years
Locomotor disorders	0.2	5.1	5.3
Respiratory disorders	0.5	2.2	2.7
Malignant neoplasms	1.7	0.3	2.0
Injuries	1.5	0.4	1.9
Visual & hearing impairments	1.1	1.1	
Mental disorders	0.4	0.6	1.0
Diabetes	0.2	0.7	0.9
Perinatal mortality	0.7		0.7
Infectious diseases	0.1	0.2	0.3

1991; Shephard, 1994; Sipilä, Viitasalo, Era, & Suominen, 1991). Given that exercise does little to extend life expectancy beyond the age of 80 years, the active individual thus tends to avoid the period of impaired function that a sedentary person encounters during the final 10 years of life, but remains independent until close to the time of death.

The quality of an individual's life depends on perceived rather than actual function, so that there is no direct relationship between physiological gains and the quality-of-life multiplier. Nevertheless, enhanced physiological function usually increases a person's sense of self-efficacy, and this, in turn, leads to a greater mobility and a willingness to undertake the activities of daily living (McAuley, 1994; Rejeski et al., 1996).

Much of the information linking regular physical activity to continuing independence has been obtained from cross-sectional surveys. Cunningham, Paterson, Himann, and Rechnitzer (1994) found that some 40% of the variance in an incapacity index was associated with participation in vigorous outdoor activities; scores were also correlated with flexibility and with choice of walking speed. However, it was unclear from this investigation whether institutional dependency was a cause or a consequence of lack of habitual physical activity. Moreover, members of the dependent group were some 5 years older than those who were independent, and it is unclear how far the authors were successful in using covariance techniques to allow for the age difference between their two groups of subjects. Hawkins and Duncan (1991) attempted to disentangle the various possible causes of an enhanced life quality by application of structural equation analysis (Lisrel VII). They concluded that regular exercise was associated with greater life satisfaction, less depression, fewer physical disabilities, greater self-esteem, and a more internal locus of control. Shephard and Montelpare (1988)

made a retrospective evaluation of lifestyle among a substantial sample of senior citizens. They found that a high perceived level of physical activity at age 50 years was associated with a greater likelihood of current independence. A prospective study by LaCroix et al. (1993) noted that over a 4-year followup, the loss of function among 6,981 men and women over the age of 65 years who initially had intact mobility was related to cigarette smoking, alcohol consumption, a large body mass index, and a low level of habitual physical activity.

Resulting change in QALY. If half of any dependency and resultant deterioration in the quality of life is directly attributable to a progressive, age-related decrease in functional capacity, there is scope for regular physical activity to reverse this and to prevent the loss of 0.5 (2.5 to 5.8) QALY. Even this may be a conservative estimate of benefit because the function of a more active person is favored by a greater sense of self-efficacy (McAuley et al., 1994), and regular physical activity may cause some enhancement of cognitive function (seen by Dustman, Emmerson, & Shearer, 1994; and Rikli & Edwards, 1991, but not by Blumenthal et al., 1991). Moreover, as in younger individuals, the active person delays the likely time to onset of various cardiovascular diagnoses (Posner et al., 1990).

Implications for Health Policy

Plainly, the scope to increase QALY is large. The potential benefits suggested for both working life (up to 3.5 years) and the period of retirement (up to 5.8 years) far outweigh the 1–2 year increase in calendar life span promised for those who exercise regularly (Paffenbarger & Lee, 1996; Paffenbarger et al., 1994). The actual benefit resulting from regular physical activity is unlikely to exceed a half of the potential gain, but this could still amount to as much as 4 QALY over the span of adult life. Moreover, and in strong contrast to the promise of increased longevity, the increase in the quality of life begins immediately; thus, it can have a much greater influence on motivation. Those developing mass-media campaigns to encourage regular exercise should emphasize improvements in the quality of life rather than the extension of life span.

Future research should focus on the ability of various types of physical activity to increase the quality of life, rather than its quantity. This should be the determining factor in the allocation of health-care dollars, both for research and for the treatment of the individual patient. In order to adopt such a public policy, however, it will also be necessary to develop more precise tools to assess the quality of life at various life stages.

Conclusion

Regular physical activity can increase both longevity and quality of life. However, an increase in quality-adjusted life expectancy seems more important than any extension of life both in justifying the expenditure of public funds on exercise programs and in motivating people to engage in regular physical activity. Techniques to measure the quality of life are only just merging, and estimates of the likely benefits from enhanced physical activity are correspondingly crude. Nevertheless, it seems that there may be substantial gains in quality-adjusted life years both from "feeling better" during middle-age and from the control of the terminal dependency that reflects the loss of cardiovascular, locomotor, and respiratory function in the sedentary elderly person.

Acknowledgment. Dr. Shephard's research has been supported in part by a research grant from Canadian Tire Acceptance Limited.

References

American College of Sports Medicine. (2000). *Guidelines for graded exercise testing and prescription* (6th ed). Philadelphia: Williams & Wilkins.

Bassey, E. J., Fiatarone, M., O'Neill, E. F., Kelly, M., Evans, W. J., & Lipsitz, L. A. (1992). Leg extensor power and functional performance in very old men and women. *Clinical Science, 82,* 321–327.

Bergner, M., Bobbitt, R., Carter, W., & Gilson, B. (1981). The sickness impact profile: Development and final revision of a health status measure. *Medical Care, 19,* 787–805.

Birren, J. E. (1983). Aging in America: Roles of psychology. *American Psychologist, 38,* 298–299.

Blumenthal, J. A., Emery, C. F., Madden, D. J., Schniebolk, S., Walsh-Riddle, M., George, L. K., McKee, D. C., Higginbotham, M. B., Cobb, F. R., & Coleman, R. E. (1991). Long-term effects of exercise on psychological functioning in older men and women. *Journal of Gerontology, 46,* P352–P361.

Bly, J. L., Jones, R. C., & Richardson, J. E. (1986). Impact of worksite health promotion on health care costs and utilization: Evaluation of Johnson & Johnson's Live for Life Program. *Journal of the American Medical Association, 256,* 3235–3240.

Bokovoy, J. L., & Blair, S. N. (1994). Aging and exercise: A health perspective. *Journal of Aging and Physical Activity, 2,* 243–260.

Bouchard, C., & Shephard, R. J. (1994). Physical activity, fitness and health. The model and key concepts. In C. Bouchard, R. J. Shephard, & T. Stephens (Eds.), *Physical activity, fitness and health* (pp. 77–88). Champaign, IL: Human Kinetics Publishers.

Brenner, I. K. M., Shek, P. N., & Shephard, R. J. (1994). Infection in athletes. *Sports Medicine, 17,* 86–107.

Brown, D. R. (1992). Physical activity, ageing, and psychological well-being: An overview of the research. *Canadian Journal of Sport Sciences, 17,* 185–193.

Busschback, J. J., Hessing, D. J., & de Charro, F. T. (1993). The utility of health at different stages in life: A quantitative approach. *Social Science and Medicine, 37,* 153–158.

Butler, R. N. (1992). Quality of life: Can it be an endpoint? How can it be measured? *American Journal of Clinical Nutrition, 55,* 1267S–1270S.

Cunningham, D., Paterson, D. H., Himann, J. E., & Rechnitzer, P. A. (1994). Determinants of independence in the elderly. *Canadian Journal of Applied Physiology, 18,* 243–254.

Deyo, R., & Inui, T. (1984). Toward clinical application of health status measures: Sensitivity of scales to clinically important changes. *Health Services Research, 19,* 275–289.

Dupuy, H. J. (1984). The psychological well-being (PGWB) index. In N. K. Wenger, M. E. Mattson, C. D. Furberg, & J. Eliason (Eds.), *Assessment of quality of life in clinical trials of cardiovascular therapy* (pp. 170–183). New York: Le Jacq.

Dustman, R. E., Emmerson, R., & Shearer, D. (1994). Physical activity, age and cognitive-neuropsychological function. *Journal of Aging and Physical Activity*, *2*, 143–181.

Emery, C. F., & Gatz, M. (1990). Psychological and cognitive effects of an exercise program for community-residing older adults. *Gerontologist*, *30*, 184–188.

Feeny, D. H., Furlong, W. J., & Torrance, G. W. (1996). Health utilities index. In B. Spilker (Ed.), *Quality of life and pharmacoeconomics in clinical trials* (pp. 253–265). Philadelphia: Lippincott-Raven.

Fiatarone, M. A., Marks, E. C., Ryan, N. D., Meredith, C. N., Lipsitz, L. A., & Evans, W. J. (1990). High-intensity strength training in nonagenarians. *Journal of the American Medical Association*, *263*, 3029–3034.

Fisher, N. M., Gresham, G. E., Abrams, M., Hicks, J., Horrigan, D., & Pendergast, D. R. (1993). Quantitative effects of physical therapy on muscular and functional performance in patients with osteoarthritis of the knee. *Archives of Physical Medicine and Rehabilitation*, *74*, 840–847.

Fitzpatrick, R., Fletcher, A., Gore, S., Jones, D., Spiegelhalter, D., & Cox, D. (1992). Quality of life measures in health care: 1. Applications and issues in assessment. *British Medical Journal 305*, 1074–1077.

Fletcher, A., Gore, S., Jones, D., Fitzpatrick, R., Spiegelhalter, D., & Cox, D. (1992a). II. Design, analysis and interpretation. *British Medical Journal, 305*, 1145–1148.

Fletcher, A. E., Dickinson, E., & Philp, I. (1992b). Review: Audit measure: Quality of life instruments for everyday use with elderly patients. *Age and Ageing*, *21*, 142–150.

Fries, J. F. (1989). Compression of morbidity near or far? *Millbank Memorial Quarterly*, *67*, 208–232.

Fries. J. F., & Spitz, P. W. (1990). The hierarchy of patient outcomes. In B. Spilker (Ed.), *Quality of life assessments in clinical trials* (pp. 25–35). New York: Lippencott-Raven Press.

Gauvin, L., & Spence, J. C. (1996). Physical activity and psychological well-being: Knowledge base, current issues and caveats. *Nutrition Reviews*, *54*, S53–S65.

George, L. K., & Bearon, L. B. (1980). *Quality of life in older persons: Meaning and measurement*. New York: Human Sciences Press.

Golant, S. M. (1985). The influence of the experienced residential environment on old people's life satisfaction. *Journal of Housing for the Elderly*, *3*, 23–49.

Grieco, A., & Long C. J. (1984). Investigation of the Karnofsky Performance Status as a measure of quality of life. *Health Psychology*, *3*, 129–142.

Gruenberg, E. M. (1977). The failures of success. *Millbank Memorial Fund Quarterly*, *55*, 3–24.

Guralnik, J. M., LaCroix, A. Z., Abbott, R. D., Berkman, L. F., Satterfield, S., Evans, D. A., & Wallace, R. B. (1993). Maintaining mobility in late life. *American Journal of Epidemiology*, *137*, 845–857.

Guyatt, G. H., Dego, R. A., Charlson, M., Levine, M. N., & Mitchell, A. (1989). Responsiveness and validity in health status measurement: A clarification. *Journal of Clinical Epidemiology*, *42*, 403–408.

Harris, J. (1991). Unprincipled QALYs. *Journal of Medical Ethics*, *17*, 185–188.

Hart, D., Bowling, A., Ellis, M., & Silman, A. (1990). Locomotor disability in very elderly people: Value of a programme for screening and provision of aids for daily living. *British Medical Journal, 301*, 216–220.

Hawkins, W. E., & Duncan, T. (1991). Structural equation analysis of an exercise/sleep health practices model on quality of life of elderly persons. *Perceptual and Motor Skills*, *72*, 831–836.

Health and Welfare Canada. (1993). *Aging and independence: Overview of a national survey*. Ottawa: Health and Welfare, Canada.

Hunt, S., McEwen, J., & McKenna, S. (1986). *Measuring health status*. London: Croom Helm.

Jasnoski, M. L., Holmes, D. S., Solomon, S., & Aguiar, C. (1981). Exercise, changes in aerobic capacity, and changes in self-perceptions: An experimental investigation. *Journal of Research in Personality*, *15*, 460–466.

Jenkinson, C., Coulter, A., & Wright, L. (1993). Short form 36 (SF 36) health survey questionnaire: Normative data for adults of working age. *British Medical Journal, 306*, 1437–1440.

Kane, R. A., & Kane, R. L. (1981). *Assessing the elderly: A practical guide to measurement*. Lexington, MA: Lexington Books.

Kaplan, R. (1985). Quantification of health outcomes for policy studies in behavioral epidemiology. In R. Kaplan & M. H. Criqui (Eds.), *Behavioral epidemiology and disease prevention* (pp. 31–56). New York: Plenum Press.

Kaplan, R. M., Anderson, J. P., & Wingard, D. L. (1991). Gender differences in health-related quality of life. *Health Psychology*, *10*, 86–93.

Kaplan, R. M., & Bush, J. W. (1982). Health-related quality of life measurement for research and policy analysis. *Health Psychology*, *1*, 61–68.

Karnofsky, D., & Burchenal, J. (1949). The clinical evaluation of chemotherapeutic agents in cancer. In C. Macleod (Ed.), *Evaluation of chemotherapeutic agents* (pp. 191–205). New York: Columbia University Press.

Karvonen, M. J., Klemola, H., Virkajarvi, J., & Kekkonen, A. (1974). Longevity of endurance skiers. *Medicine and Science in Sports*, *6*, 49–51.

Kellner, R., & Sheffield, B. F. (1973). A self-rating scale of distress. *Psychological Medicine, 3*, 88–100.

Kinsella, K. G. (1992). Changes in life expectancy. *American Journal of Clinical Nutrition*, *55*, 1196S–1202S.

Kramer, M. (1980). The rising pandemic of mental disorders and associated chronic diseases and disabilities. *Acta Psychiatrica Scandinavica*, *62*, 282–297.

LaCroix, A. Z., Guralnik, J. M., Berkman, L. F., Wallace, R. B., & Satterfield, S. (1993). Maintaining mobility in late life. II. Smoking, alcohol consumption, physical activity, and body mass index. *American Journal of Epidemiology*, *137*, 858–869.

Latten, J. J. (1989). Life course and satisfaction, equal for everyone? *Social Indicators Research*, *21*, 599–610.

Linsted, K. D., Tonstad, S., & Kuzma, J. W. (1991). Self-report on physical activity and patterns of mortality in Seventh Day Adventist men. *Journal of Clinical Epidemiology*, *44*, 355–364.

Lord, S. R., & Castell, S. (1994). Physical activity program for older persons: Effect on balance, strength, neuromuscular control and reaction time. *Archives of Physical Medicine and Rehabilitation*, *75*, 648–652.

Manton, K. G. (1988). A longitudinal study of functional change and mortality in the United States. *Journal of Gerontology*, *43*, S153–S161.

Mathews, A. M. (1989). *Contributors to the loss of independence and the promotion of independence among seniors* [Report to Seniors Independence Research Programme, Community Health Division, Health and Welfare Canada]. Ottawa: Health & Welfare, Canada.

McAuley, E. (1994). Physical activity and psychosocial outcomes. In C. Bouchard, R. J. Shephard, & T. Stephens (Eds.), *Physical activity, fitness and health* (pp. 851–867). Champaign, IL.: Human Kinetics Publishers.

McHorney, C. A., Ware, J. E., Rogers, W., Raczek, A. E., & Lu, J. F. R. (1992). The validity and relative precision of MOS short- and long-form health status scales and Dartmouth COOP charts: Results from the medical outcomes study. *Medical Care*, *30* (Suppl.), 253–265.

McNair, D. M., Lorr, M., & Doppleman, L. F. (1971). *Manual for the profile of mood states*. San Diego: San Diego Educational and Industrial Testing Service, 1971.

McNeil, J. K., LeBlanc, E. M., & Joyner, M. (1991). The effect of exercise on depressive symptoms in the moderately depressed elderly. *Psychology and Aging*, *6*, 487 488.

Meenan, R., Gertman, P., Mason, J., & Dunaif, R. (1982). The arthritis impact measurement scales: Further investigation of a health status instrument. *Arthritis and Rheumatism*, *25*, 1048–1053.

Montoye, H. J., Van Huss, W. D., Olson, H. W., Pierson, W. O., & Hudec, A. J. (1957). *The longevity and morbidity of college athletes*. Lansing, MI: Michigan State University, Phi Epsilon Kappa Fraternity.

Moore, A. D., Stambrook, M., Gill, D. D., & Lubusko, A. A. (1992). Differences in long-term quality of life in married and single traumatic brain injury patients. *Canadian Journal of Rehabilitation*, *6*, 89–98.

Mor-Barak, M. E., Miller, L. S., & Syme, L. S. (1991). Social networks, life events, and health of the poor, frail elderly: A longitudinal study of the buffering versus the direct effect. *Family and Community Health*, *14*, 1–13.

Morey, M. C., Cowper, P. A., Feussner, J. R., DiPasquale, R. C., Crowley, G. M., Samsa, G. P., & Sullivan, R. J. (1991). Two-year trends in physical performance following super-

vised exercise among community-dwelling older veterans. *Journal of the American Geriatric Society*, *39*, 986–992.

Moss, M. S., Lawton, M. P., & Glicksman, A. (1991). The role of pain in the last year of life of older persons. *Journal of Gerontology*, *46*, P51–P57.

Moum, T. (1988). Yea-saying and mood-of-the-day effects in self-reported quality of life. *Social Indicators Research*, *20*, 117–139.

Nieman, D. C. (1995). Exercise and infection. In J. Torg & R. J. Shephard (Eds.), *Current therapy in sports medicine 3*. Philadelphia: Mosby/Yearbook.

Nieman, D. C., Warren, B. J., Dotson, R. G., Butterworth, D. E., & Henson, D. A. (1993). Physical activity, psychological well-being, and mood state in elderly women. *Journal of Aging and Physical Activity*, *1*, 22–33.

North, T. C., McCullagh, P., & Tran, Z. V. (1994). Effect of exercise on depression. *Exercise and Sport Sciences Reviews*, *18*, 379–415.

O'Connor, P. J., Aenchbacher, L. E., & Dishman, R. K. (1993). Physical activity and depression in the elderly. *Journal of Aging and Physical Activity*, *1*, 34–58

Oldridge, N. (1997). Outcome assessment in cardiac rehabilitation. Health-related quality of life and economic evaluation. *Journal of Cardiopulmary Rehabilitation*, *17*, 179–194.

Osberg, J. S., McGinnis, G. E., DeJong, G., & Seward, M. L. (1987). Life satisfaction and quality of life among disabled elderly adults. *Journal of Gerontology*, *42*, 228–230.

Paffenbarger, R. S., & Lee, I-M. (1996). Physical activity and fitness for health and longevity. *Research Quarterly*, *67*, 11–28.

Paffenbarger, R. S., Hyde, R. T., Wing, A. L., Min-Lee, I., & Kampert, J. B. (1994). Some inter-relations of physical activity, physiological fitness, health and longevity. In C. Bouchard, R. J. Shephard, & T. Stephens (Eds.), *Physical activity, fitness and health* (pp. 119–133). Champaign, IL: Human Kinetics Publishers.

Pashkow, P., Ades, P. A., Emery, C. F., Frid, D. J., Miller, N. H., Peske, G., Reardon, J. Z., Schiffert, J. H., Southard, D., & Zuwallack, R. L.(1995). Outcome measurement in cardiac and pulmonary rehabilitation. *Journal of Cardiopulmonary Rehabilitation*, *15*, 394–405.

Patrick, D., & Deyo, R. (1989). Generic and disease-specific measures in assessing health status and quality of life. *Medical Care*, *27*, S217–232.

Patrick, D. L., & Erickson, P. (1993). *Health status and health policy. Quality of life in health care evaluation and resource allocation*. New York: Oxford University Press.

Pearlman, R. A., & Uhlmann, R. F. (1988). Quality of life in the elderly: Comparisons between nursing home and community residents. *Journal of Applied Gerontology*, *7*, 316–330.

Pearlman, R. A., & Uhlmann, R. F. (1991). Quality of life in elderly, chronically ill outpatients. *Journal of Gerontology*, *46*, M31–M38.

Pekkanen, J., Marti, B., Nissinen, A., Tuomilehto, J.,

Punsar, S., & Karvonen, M. J. (1987). Reduction of premature mortality by high physical activity: A 20-year followup of middle-aged Finnish men. *Lancet, 1*, 1473–1477.

Polednak, A. P. (1978). *The longevity of athletes.* Springfield, IL: C. C. Thomas.

Posner, J. D., Gorman, K. M., Gitlin, L. N., Sands, L. P., Kleban, M., Windsor, L., & Shaw, C. (1990). Effects of exercise training in the elderly on the occurrence and time to onset of cardiovascular diagnoses. *Journal of the American Geriatric Society, 38*, 205–210.

Powell, K. E., Thompson, P. D., Caspersen, C. J., & Kendrick, J. S. (1987). Physical activity and the incidence of coronary heart disease. *Annual Reviews of Public Health, 8*, 253–287.

Rejeski, W. J., Brawley, L. R., & Shumaker, S. A. (1996). Physical activity and health-related quality of life. *Exercise and Sport Sciences Reviews, 24*, 71–108.

Rikli, R., & Edwards, D. J. (1991). Effects of a three-year exercise program on motor function and cognitive processing speed in older women. *Research Quarterly, 62*, 61–67.

Robine, J-M., & Ritchie, K. (1991). Healthy life expectancy: Evaluation of global indicator of change in population health. *British Medical Journal, 302*, 457–460.

Roland, M., & Morris, R. (1983). A study of the natural history of back pain. 1. Development of a reliable and sensitive measure of disability in low back pain. *Spine, 8*, 141–144.

Rosser, R., & Kind, P. (1978). A scale of valuations of states of illness: Is there a social consensus? *International Journal of Epidemiology, 7*, 347–358.

Sarna, S., Sahi, T., Koskenvuo, M., & Kaprio, J. (1993). Increased life expectancy of world class male athletes. *Medicine and Science in Sports and Exercise, 25*, 237–244.

Shephard, R. J. (1981). *Ischemic heart disease and exercise.* London: Croom Helm.

Shephard, R. J. (1982). Are we asking the right questions? *Journal of Cardiac Rehabilitation, 2*, 21–26.

Shephard, R. J. (1983). The workload of the postal carrier. *Journal of Human Ergology, 11*, 151–164.

Shephard, R. J. (1989). Exercise and lifestyle change. *British Journal of Sports Medicine, 23*, 11–22.

Shephard, R. J. (1994). *Aerobic fitness and health.* Champaign, IL: Human Kinetics Publishers.

Shephard, R. J. (1995). Exercise and sudden death. *Sport Sciences Review, 4*(2), 1–11.

Shephard, R. J. (1996). Habitual physical activity and the quality of life. *Quest, 48*, 354–365.

Shephard, R. J. (1997a). *Aging, physical activity and health.* Champaign, IL: Human Kinetics Publishers.

Shephard, R. J. (1997b). What is the optimal type of physical activity to enhance health? *British Journal of Sports Medicine, 31*, 277–284.

Shephard, R. J., Corey, P., & Cox, M. (1982a). Health hazard appraisal: The influence of an employee fitness programme. *Canadian Journal of Public Health, 73*, 183–187.

Shephard, R. J., Corey, P., Renzland, P., & Cox, M. (1982b). The influence of an industrial fitness programme upon medical care costs. *Canadian Journal of Public Health, 73*, 259–263.

Shephard, R. J., & Montelpare, W. M. (1988). Geriatric benefits of exercise as an adult. *Journal of Gerontology, 43*, M86–M90.

Sherbourne, C. D., Meredith, L. S., Rogers, W., & Ware, J. E. (1992). *Quality of life research, 1*, 235–246.

Sipilä, S., Viitasalo, J., Era, P., & Suominen, H. (1991). Muscle strength in male athletes aged 70–81 years. *European Journal of Applied Physiology, 63*, 399–403.

Spiegelhalter, D. J., Gore, S. M., Fitzpatrick, R., Fletcher, A. E., Jones, D. R., & Cox, D. R. (1992). Quality of life measures in health care: III. Resource allocation. *British Medical Journal, 305*, 1205–1209.

Sports Council and the Health Education Authority. (1992). *The Allied Dunbar National Fitness Survey: The main findings: summary report.* London: Author.

Statistics Canada (1985). *General social survey.* Ottawa: Statistics Canada.

Statistics Canada (1986). *Health and activity limitations survey.* Ottawa: Statistics Canada.

Strawbridge, W. J., Kaplan, G. A., Camacho, T., & Cohen, R. D. (1992). The dynamics of disability and functional change in an elderly cohort: Results from the Alameda County study. *Journal of the American Gerontological Society, 40*, 799–806.

Thayer, R. E. (1989). *The biopsychology of mood and arousal.* New York: Oxford University Press.

Torrance, G. W. (1987). Utility approach to measuring health-related quality of life. *Journal of Chronic Diseases, 40*, 593–600.

Vetter, N. J., Lewis, P. A., & Llewellyn, L. (1992). Supporting elderly dependent people at home. *British Medical Journal, 304*, 1290–1292.

Vuori, I. (1995). Sudden death and exercise: Effects of age and type of activity. *Sport Sciences Reviews, 4*(2), 46–84.

Wagstaff, A. (1991). QALYs and the equity-efficiency trade-off. *Journal of Health Economics, 5*, 1–30.

Wenger, N. K., & Furberg, C. D. (1990). Cardiovascular disorders. In B. Spilker (Ed.), *Quality of life assessments in clinical trials* (pp. 335–345). New York: Raven Press.

Williams, A., & Kind, P. (1992). The present state of play about QALYs. In A. Hopkins (Ed.), *Measures of quality of life* (pp. 21–34). London: Royal College of Physicians.

Wood-Dauphinee, S., & Küchler, T. (1992). Quality of life as a rehabilitation outcome: Are we missing the boat? *Canadian Journal of Rehabilitation, 6*, 3–12.

Woodruff, S. I., & T. L. Conway. (1992). Impact of health and fitness-related behavior on quality of life. *Social Indicators Research, 25*, 391–405.

2

Working Out Those Tensions: Exercise and the Reduction of Stress

Mark B. Andersen

Georgina Sutherland

In popular, or "naive" stress management psychology, vigorous physical activity represents an avenue for dealing with stressful situations that bring about uncomfortable levels of frustration, anxiety, or anger. Taking time for a run, going several rounds with a punching bag, or attending an aerobics class are all, at least in moderation, relatively more salubrious methods of dealing with stress than, say, kicking the dog (and definitely more healthy from the dog's point of view). The emotional and physiological sequelae that often accompany acute stress responses, for many, seem to attenuate after a bout of exercise. Also, exercise enthusiasts often report that regular exercise is what keeps their stress levels under control, which suggests that regular exercise is useful for managing chronic stress. The common vernacular for the effects of exercise on the "stressed" individual alludes to a pneumatic model of stress management in that exercise helps one "blow off steam." Stress causes a buildup of some sort of dangerous (read: unhealthy, damaging) internal pressure that if not relieved will be turned inward, resulting in a variety of harmful or even fatal mal-

adies. "Calm down! You're going to give yourself a heart attack!" Exercise, in this "popular" pneumatic model acts, in some way, as a release valve, venting the pressure and helping bring things back to "normal," the common understanding of Bernardian homeostasis.

Given the popular wisdom, the questions for this chapter are

1. Does exercise reduce acute, and possibly chronic, stress responses as a naive stress management psychology viewpoint would suggest?
2. For individuals with substantial stresses in their lives, what are the medical outcomes, and more important, the quality-of-life issues connected with exercising and stress reduction?
3. If exercise reduces the negative effects of stress, how does it do so, and what are the pathways (psychological, physiological, neurological, endocrinological) of its effectiveness?

To answer these questions we need first some definitions of what it is we are trying to reduce; that is *stress*, or probably more precisely, chronic and acute stress responsivity. We then need essentially three intertwined reviews of literature: (a) the evidence of exercise's reducing stress from experimental clinical trials, correlational studies, and other methods (e.g., case studies); (b) the methods by which stress, and changes in stress, have been measured; and (c) the various models and theories, based on experimental and clinical evidence, built to explain how exercise helps reduce stress responsivity and the negative effects of prolonged exposure to stressors. The evidence for (a), that exercise is helpful in reducing stress, is substantial. Several meta-analyses have borne out that exercise can play an important role in the modification of acute and chronic stress (Crews & Landers, 1987; Long & Van Stavel,1995; Petruzzello, Landers, Hatfield, Kubitz, & Salazar, 1991). The strength of association between stress reduction and exercise varies from study to study and is tied to the choice of dependent variables. The literature has been repeatedly reviewed, and the reader is directed to the reference section of this chapter for relevant readings. This well-established literature will be reviewed only in the context of examining the support for the different models of how exercise acts to reduce stress. We will start with the problem of defining stress and stress responsivity.

The Stress of Everyday Life

The title of this section was chosen with a nod to a classic text by Freud (1901/1960) because stress, like Freud's everyday "psychopathology," appears to be an inescapable and ubiquitous phenomenon. Stresses, also like Freud's minor pathologies (e.g., "forgetting," slips of the tongue), in many cases are rather innocuous and generally manageable. It is when stresses begin to dominate parts of one's life that they become, like overused defense mechanisms, serious concerns.

Stress, stressors, arousal, anxiety, and so forth are common terms for well-known, but often loosely defined, concepts related to various psychophysiological phenomena. What is stress? Going back to the font of stress research, Selye (1956, 1974, 1976) defined stress as the body's nonspecific response to any demand placed upon it, a definition rather global and "nonspecific" itself. Selye went on, however, to describe three stages of stress: acute stress (his alarm stage), corresponding to sympathetic nervous system mobilization; chronic stress (his resistance stage), in which relatively long-term physiological (e.g., increased blood pressure) and biochemical (e.g., increased serum glucocorticoids) changes increase wear and tear on organ systems; and stress-related disease outcome (his exhaustion stage). Lazarus and Folkman (1984) offered a more narrow definition of stress as "a particular relationship between a person and the environment that is appraised by the person as taxing or exceeding his or her resources and endangering his or her well-being" (p. 19). This definition emphasizes the negative aspect of stress, and although it is the part of stress that is probably of most interest to many medical practitioners, it is a limited view of stress and stressors.

Selye (1974, 1976) also made a distinction between what he called *distress* and *eustress*. Stresses come in a variety of flavors, with the major distinction being between stresses that make us feel good and stresses that make us feel bad. There are many stress situations that bring about acute stress responses (e.g., increased heart rate, blood pressure, respiration). Making love, emotionally (and "sympathetically"), is highly arousing; riding a rollercoaster can give one a serious "adrenaline rush," and going for a strenuous run can really tax many organ systems. In general, however, we usually feel good after such experiences, and it is these stress experiences that Selye (1974) calls *eustress*, or positive stress.

On the darker side of stress lie experiences that bring similar initial sympathetic responses but that are accompanied by the emotions and cognitions of fear, dread, anger, confusion, or worry. These stresses Selye (1974) labeled *distress*. Eustress, in general, produces feelings of exhilaration (common responses to both sex and rollercoasters) and ultimately, in many cases, relaxed lassitude (that post-10K comfortably "spent" feeling). Distress, in general, often produces one of a variety of "anxious" states. The aftermath of an acute distressing incident is often not relief, but continued worry and anxiety. For example, a dressing down by one's boss may bring about an acute stress response, but it also may result in days or weeks of lost sleep and worry over one's job security. Long-term distress has been intimately connected to a host of biological and psychological disorders that are way beyond the scope of this chapter to document, but that include most major medical (e.g., heart disease, pulmonary disease, alcoholism) and many psychological disorders (e.g., depression, anxiety, PTSD).

For this chapter, we will first concentrate on indices and measures of stress. If one believes exercise reduces stress, then some measure, or marker, of stress needs to be the yardstick to determine if exercise has indeed reduced stress levels. We will concentrate primarily on psychological measures of stress, but will also note physiological/biochemical ones.

We will next examine some current models explaining why, in many (but not all) instances, exercise has a stress-reducing effect and the research that supports (and fails to support) the models. In conclusion, we will offer some caveats about the choice of dependent variables in exercise and stress research.

Measuring Stress

A psychologist examining stress might be most interested in behavioral or emotional symptoms that a person is under stress such as agitation or anxiety. An exercise physiologist might be more interested in biochemical responses such as changes in cortisol levels, and a radical behaviorist might wish to focus on the contingencies of reinforcement and punishment in the environment that are maintaining "stress" behavior (e.g., insomnia, overeating). Because stress can be viewed from many perspectives, the way researchers measure stress also varies considerably.

Psychological Measures

The number of psychometric instruments used in stress research is legion, and measures of psychological traits such as hardiness, hostility, and Type A behavior are central to understanding stress responsivity. A review, however, of such instruments is beyond the scope of this chapter, and we will examine only a few of the most common instruments directly involved in measuring stress and anxiety in exercise research. By far the most common psychometric instruments used in the exercise and stress reduction literature are measures of anxiety. Not all stress is anxiety provoking, but it is probably safe to say that most anxiety is, at least, somewhat stressful. The instrument of choice in this field of research has been the *State-Trait Anxiety Inventory* (STAI: Spielberger, Gorsuch, & Lushene, 1970; Spielberger, Gorsuch, Lushene, Vagg, & Jacobs, 1983). This instrument has two scales, one to measure dispositional anxiety (A-trait) and one to measure current situational anxiety (A-state). It is thus well suited for examining changes in trait anxiety due to exercise interventions conducted over relatively long periods of time and to explore the short-term psychological and stress responses to acute bouts of exercise.

Other instruments have been used to measure other aspects of psychological responses to stress and exercise. The *Profile of Mood States* (POMS; McNair, Lorr, & Doppelman, 1971) assesses a variety of moods (e.g., anger, tension) that could be considered to measure stress indirectly and is the second most commonly used psychological measure in exercise and stress research. Two other instruments have been used to a lesser extent, the *Hopkins Symptom Check List-90* (SCL-90; Derogatis, 1980) and the Multiple Affect Adjective Checklist (MAACL; Zuckerman & Lubin, 1965). For more information on measuring mood and affect, and the relationship of mood and affect to exercise, please see the chapter by Gavin in this volume.

Biochemical Measures

The primary biochemical measures of stress in the stress and exercise literature include cortisol, catecholamines, and endorphins. Research has shown that regular exercise attenuates stress responsivity as measured by lower cortisol and catecholamine responses to exercise (e.g., Rudolph & McAuley, 1995, Sothmann, 1991). Research has also shown that plasma beta-endorphin levels respond to the duration and intensity of exercise (Goldfarb, Hatfield, Armstrong, & Potts, 1990; Goldfarb, Hatfield, Potts, & Armstrong, 1991).

Physiological Measures

Systolic and diastolic blood pressure, heart rate, electroencephalography, electromyography, and skin temperature all have been physiological measures used in the exercise and stress-reduction literature. In general, the cardiovascular measures have not shown as large a stress-reduction change due to exercise as have other measures such as EEG (see Petruzzello et al., 1991).

Models of Exercise and Stress Reduction

The relationship between exercise and psychological and physiological symptoms of stress has been widely researched, and there seems little doubt that exercise is an effective means of reducing anxiety and stress. How exercise acts to attenuate stress and how stress responsivity occurs have been explained in a variety of neurophysiological, biochemical, and psychological models. Although it is not possible in this chapter to examine all the proposed mediating mechanisms of exercise-induced stress reduction, we will describe a number of hypothesized models grounded in empirical scientific investigation.

Thermogenic Model

The essence of the thermogenic model is recognizable to anyone who, after a stressful day, has taken a long, hot bath. Elevating core body temperature, through a variety of methods, has been used for centuries for therapeutic benefits, and research has shown that saunas and warm showers can reduce muscle tension (Kuusinen & Heinonen, 1972) and self-reported levels of state anxiety (Raglin & Morgan, 1987). Based on research into passive heating, deVries (1987) proposed that the stress-reducing benefits of exercise may also be related to elevations in body temperature. This mechanism of exercise-induced psychological benefits is based on a neurophysiological model. Originally developed by von Euler and Soderberg (1957) and based on research with animals, this model hypothesized that elevation in core body temperature, mediated by the hypothalamic influence on the thalamus, promoted EEG alpha activity and reduced gamma motor neuron activity, which led to "relaxing" changes in peripheral musculature and CNS activity associated with relaxation. Although during exercise the physical demand on the muscles would seem to negate the reduction in afference, the main period of research focus has been on postexercise when temperature remains elevated for some time after the termination of physical activity.

Researchers have employed passive body-temperature manipulation strategies in order to quantify the relationship between anxiety and body temperature. It appears that the relationship between body temperature and stress reduction (or relaxation) is curvilinear, with moderate increases in temperature reducing stress and anxiety and larger changes in temperature increasing stress responses (Koltyn, 1997). Although a number of studies have demonstrated an association between exercise-induced elevated core temperature and decreases in state anxiety levels (Petruzzello, Landers, & Salazar, 1993), there appears to be limited evidence supporting this hypothesis. Moreover, research has demonstrated decreases in anxiety following exercise at an intensity, or under environmental conditions, that do not elicit body temperature rises (Koltyn & Morgan, 1993; Reeves, Levison, Justesen, & Lubin, 1985). Although the thermogenic hypothesis of exercise-induced anxiety reduction remains tenable, there are methodological and measurement considerations that need addressing before it can be discounted. Esophageal or rectal temperature measures may not reflect physiological changes mediated by the hypothalamus. Future research adopting new technology examining tympanic temperatures may be able to measure brain warming more accurately. In addition, elevated body temperature may affect other physiological mechanisms, such as changes in cellular structures, enzyme systems, and temperature-dependent chemical reactions that occur during exercise as a result of elevated temperatures. It may be that these other temperature-induced changes are actually more closely connected to stress reduction.

Opponent-Process Model

The opponent-process model explains psychological changes due to exercise (feelings of relief or relaxation) primarily in terms of physiological mechanisms (central nervous system [CNS] and sympathetic nervous system [SNS] activation, endorphin release). In contrast to the thermogenic hypothesis, this model attempts to explain the stress-reducing benefits in terms of acute and habitual physical activity. The model's theoretical basis assumes a rebound effect of the central nervous system (CNS) to a given stressor. (Solomon & Corbit, 1973). That is, arousal of the sympathetic nervous system (SNS) during engagement in a stressful activity, such as exercise, is followed by an opposing process and affective state (e.g., relaxation, feelings of pleasantness) upon cessation of exercise. A central feature of this hypothesis is that with habitual physical activity, the arousal level of the SNS does not change but remains the same, whereas the opposing process and perception of anxiety reduction become enhanced. In a recent meta-analysis, Petruzzello et al. (1991) supported the model, in that postexercise state anxiety was significantly reduced in most of the studies examined. The researchers did state, however, the difficulty in adequately assessing the model in terms of acute exercise only. Boutcher and Landers (1988) also supported the model in their research using acute exercise with trained and untrained runners. The results indicated that the runners who were more fit had significantly greater opponent processes (i.e., significantly reduced self-reported state anxiety) after ceasing exercise than did the untrained runners.

Although it is possible that a number of physiological mechanisms may act as mediators of the opponent-process sequence, the focus has often been on endorphin release. A number of studies have demonstrated decreased state anxiety and a feeling of pleasantness, together with an increase in peripheral plasma beta-endorphin levels in the postexercise period (Goldfarb et al., 1990, 1991; Wildman, Kruger, Schmole, Niemann, & Matthaei, 1986). Endorphins are the body's natural, endogenously produced, opioid peptides and tend to remain "silent" unless a challenging stressor, such as vigorous exercise, appears or is initiated (Hatfield, 1991; Hoffman, 1997). With regard to the opponent-process model, Solomon (1980) proposed that endorphins may be the biochemical initiators of the opposing process following exercise, resulting in reduced feelings of anxiety. The issue, however, has been debated because increases in peripheral plasma beta-endorphins do not necessarily reflect changes in CNS opioid activity. Actually, the influence of peripheral endorphins on the brain is questionable considering the blood brain barrier to peptides (Dishman, 1994). Although experimental data indicate activation of endorphins by exercise, their role in reducing anxiety is questionable. Research has suggested that endorphins may act to promote positive psychological affect by simply reducing discomfort during exercise (Morgan, 1985). Although it seems that endorphins may explain some of the stress and anxiety reduction associated with exercise, it must be considered that other physiological and psychological adaptations to physical activity are involved.

Neurotransmitter Model

Finally, in terms of physiological models, recent evidence supports the role of neuroendocrine responses as possible mediators of the reductions in anxiety observed following physical activity. The model relates to changes in monoamine activity in response to exercise, which are thought to reflect sympathoadrenal activity (Crews & Landers, 1987; Dishman, 1997; Mazzeo, 1991; Sothmann, 1991). The sympathoadrenal system

has been the focus of many studies because of its ability to mediate a host of physiological adjustments to physical, environmental, and psychological stressors. Attempts to test the model have involved the measurement of peripheral monoamines, which are principally secreted from the sympathetic nervous system and adrenal gland (Sothmann, Hart, & Horn, 1991). The amines are some of the most common CNS and SNS neurotransmitter substances, and thus, any change in activity could have an influence on central brain processes (Simono, 1991). Although few studies in the physical activity literature have focused specifically on brain monoamine activity and anxiety, there is evidence that exercise-induced changes in neurotransmitters and hormones, such as norepinephrine, may act as neuromodulators of anxiety. A number of studies have shown aerobic exercise reduces levels of plasma norepinephrine in response to endurance training for a given submaximal workload (Galbo, Kjaer, Richter, Sonne, & Mikines, 1986).

Research has also shown that exercise may reduce levels of sympathoadrenal responses to psychological stress (Blumenthal et al., 1990). In addition, a number of studies have indicated elevated levels of norepinephrine in response to an acute psychological stressor in untrained individuals relative to trained counterparts (Light, Orbist, James, & Strogatz, 1987; Sothmann, Horn, Hart, & Gustafson, 1987). From such findings, researchers have suggested that exercise training may modify psychological stress reactivity (LaPerriere et al., 1994). Yet, there is also a large number of studies failing to observe any association between exercise and indicators of change in sympathoadrenal activity (Brooks & Long, 1987; Hull, Young, & Ziegler, 1984).

The relationship between exercise, aminergic activity, and psychological stress is complex. It is important to note that research has generally employed either plasma catecholamine measures or urinary metabolites of norepinephrine as quantitative indices of the relationship between exercise, aminergic responses, and stress reactivity. Interpretation of these indices, therefore, must be viewed with caution because such peripheral measures may not necessarily originate from brain locations (Dishman, 1997). In addition, exercise-induced changes in psychological stress reactivity may depend on interactions between neurotransmitters, as opposed to any singular influence promoted by them (Hatfield, 1991). Although the neurotransmitter model for exercise-induced anxiety reduction remains questionable, it may provide an important component, in conjunction with other psychophysiological adaptations to exercise, that can result in positive affective change.

Distraction Hypothesis

Although the previous theories have suggested that exercise-induced anxiety reduction is primarily physiological in nature, Bahrke and Morgan's (1978) distraction hypothesis proposes a psychological mechanism. The hypothesis proposes that cognitive diversion is the agent responsible for stress reduction seen with exercise. Exercise may act as a temporary distraction from immediate emotional concerns or as a time-out from stressful stimuli. The premise of the hypothesis, however, leads to the possibility that exercise may not be the critical variable in alleviating anxiety. In formulating the distraction hypothesis, Bahrke and Morgan contrasted an equal amount of treadmill running, at 70% VO_2 max, with meditation and reading. They found that physical activity was as effective in reducing state anxiety as the other cognitively based distraction therapies. In a recent meta-analysis, Petruzzello et al. (1991) also supported the finding that exercise and cognitive interventions such as quiet rest, meditation, and relaxation are equally effective for reducing state anxiety.

For trait anxiety, however, Petruzzello et al. (1991) found that the anxiolytic properties of exercise were superior to other cognitive strategies. Research has also revealed that exercise-induced anxiety reduction lasts significantly longer than other cognitive interventions when outcome measures are assessed over prolonged periods (Raglin & Morgan, 1987). Such research has suggested that, although exercise and other cognitively based interventions may provide similar anxiety reduction benefits, the processes by which they achieve this end may be substantially different. Based on the research, it appears that exercise as a time-out from emotional concerns positively affects anxiety, but it may only represent one possible factor in exercise-induced anxiety reduction. Morgan and O'Connor (1989) concluded that the distraction theory complements, rather than contradicts, other psychological and physiological mechanisms.

Self-Efficacy and Mastery Theory

Several other cognitively based mechanisms have also been proposed to explain how the psychological benefits of exercise are mediated. Research has suggested that exercise influences a variety of personality variables that may be related to anxiety and stress reactivity (Sime, 1996). In particular, exercise-induced reductions in anxiety appear associated with increases in self-efficacy. Bandura (1991) has proposed that the positive psychological influence of physical activity may be an outcome of increases in, or the restoration of, self-efficacy. Broadly defined, self-efficacy concerns the convictions that one has the capabilities to engage successfully in a course of action required to satisfy situational demands. Bandura (1977, 1986) emphasized that self-efficacy is not directly concerned with ability, but with perception or belief in those abilities. Efficacy cognitions influence not only behavior, but also thought patterns and affective reactions to anticipatory and actual stressors.

Research investigating self-efficacy and physical activity has consistently demonstrated that both chronic and acute exercise produces increases in self-efficacy (McAuley & Courneya, 1992; McAuley, Courneya, & Lettunich, 1991; Rudolph & McAuley, 1995). Research, however, has also shown that exercise itself may not be as important as mastery experiences that occur as an outcome of physical activity (Norris, Carroll, & Cochrane, 1992). For example, Dzewaltowski, Acevedo, and Pettay (1992) found that exercise participants who did not achieve their fitness goals had lower self-efficacy than that of those who did achieve their goals. Self-efficacy theory also acknowledges the psychological strengthening effects of mastery experiences gained through habitual physical activity, which can lead to increased efficacy cognitions and reduced physiological stress reactions (Bandura, 1991). This concept complements Dienstbier's (1989, 1991) model of active toughening in the form of regular exercise, which postulates that mastery experiences affect physiological and psychological functioning.

Interestingly, recent evidence supports the relationship between exercise and efficacy cognitions in the regulation of psychobiological functioning. A number of studies have demonstrated that increases in self-efficacy may be related to the regulation of endocrine, catecholamine, and endogenous opioid systems (Bandura, Cioffi, Taylor, & Brouillard, 1988; Weidenfeld et al., 1990). As noted above, such neurophysiological systems are thought to be integrally linked to exercise-induced reductions in anxiety. Moreover, exercise and self-efficacy studies have supported the notion that habitual physical activity acts to "toughen" physiological functioning, which

in turn may enhance the perception of anxiety reduction (Mathur, Toriola, & Dada, 1986; Rudolph & McAuley, 1995).

It is important to note the suggestion that the effectiveness of exercise to reduce anxiety may be a result of a placebo effect (Sime, 1996). Exercise is a prominent feature in mental health-related information, and partaking in exercise may carry with it an expectancy of psychological benefits. Studies focusing specifically on the placebo effect have concluded that exercise does indeed carry an expectancy for affective change (McCann & Holmes, 1984). Although participation in an exercise program may give rise to an expectancy effect, particularly for clinical populations, the placebo effect does not appear to be as influential as the other psychological and physiological mechanisms discussed.

From the preponderance of literature available, there seems little doubt that both acute and chronic exercise represents effective means of reducing stress. Understanding the mechanisms of exercise-induced stress and anxiety reduction will, more than likely, contribute to the development of efficacious treatments. Although much of the research has attempted to isolate and explore a single mechanism, it is far more likely that different mechanisms work in concert with one another, possibly in an interactive manner. It is possible that some of the physiological models are interrelated. For example, elevated body temperature may influence the release and function of monoamines (Morgan, 1985). In addition, evidence supports the interrelationship between endocrine function and monoamine and endorphin release (Smith & Curzner, 1994). It is also likely that cognitive mechanisms are intimately associated and that both physiological and psychological factors mediate the decreases in anxiety observed with physical activity (Dienstbier, 1991). It is also possible that any one mechanism, or the interactive effect of mechanisms mediating the exercise-induced reduction in anxiety, may work differently for different people (Martinsen & Morgan, 1997). Although the exact process by which exercise promotes changes in psychological affect is uncertain, the value of exercise in reducing stress and anxiety is clear.

Choosing Good Dependent Variables

Whether one measures psychological variables using questionnaires, examines blood chemistry, or monitors psychophysiological indices (e.g., EMG, HR), there is relatively solid evidence, despite studies with non-significant results, that exercise can have an effect on stress (however it is measured) and stress responsivity (Berger, 1994, 1996; Berger, Friedmann, & Eaton, 1988; Berger & Owen, 1987, 1988; Biddle, 1995; J. D. Brown, 1991; Brown, Heberman, & Cohen, 1995; Kleine, 1994; Roth & Holmes, 1987; Shephard, 1995; Spielberger, 1987; Steptoe, Moses, Edwards, & Mathews, 1993). The magnitude of those effects, however, varies considerably from variable to variable and study to study. Studies showing "no differences" between exercise and control groups could benefit from power analyses and estimation of effect sizes. Stress management programs may actually be more effective than some studies suggest because of sample-size issues and problems with power (cf., Andersen & Stoové, 1998). Average and individual study effects reported in meta-analyses have ranged from small to moderate to large, but what exactly are these effects and what do they mean? It is here that the vital question of the choice of dependent variable emerges. In stress research, as in most all health and medical research, what are the outcome variables of interest?

Kaplan (1990) reported on a reanalysis of a study of the effectiveness of the drug gem-fibrozil (Frick et al., 1987) in preventing a second, and possibly fatal, myocardial infarction (MI). The longitudinal study did show that patients on gemfibrozil were indeed less likely to die of an MI than were those in the placebo group, and that is where the study stopped. Further analysis revealed, however, that the death rates for the experimental and control groups were the same. The gemfibrozil group died from MIs (the chosen D.V.) less often than the control group, but they still died at the same rates. Thus, the drug had no effect on the ultimate dependent variable, mortality—a good example of a trees-versus-forest problem in choosing a good dependent variable.

What guidelines should we use for choosing dependent variables? Kaplan (1990, 1994) has convincingly argued that the final and most important outcome in health research is behavior (not blood chemistry and not necessarily scores on paper-and-pencil tests). Do the interventions prescribed actually change behavior in such a way that people function better, can engage in more activities and, in general, have a better quality of life? To the medical practitioner, whose goal is to improve quality of life, blood chemistry changes due to exercise are of interest only if they are connected to behavior and quality of life. We have several different "maps" for looking at stress and exercise (psychological, biochemical, and psychophysiological measures), and the "territory" of interest is behavior and the quality of life. Unfortunately, as in all cases, the map is not the territory. Another problem for many of the maps is that we have only a vague idea about what the different "scales" are for the various maps we use.

Sechrest, McKnight, and McKnight (1996) have presented a cogent warning about maps and territories in psychotherapy outcome research that has relevance for stress and exercise research. For example, in psychotherapy research on depression, researchers may administer a Beck's Depression Inventory (BDI; Beck, Ward, Mendelson, Mock, & Erbaugh, 1961) at pretreatment, deliver a psychotherapeutic intervention, and use the BDI again at the end of treatment. If the BDI scores drop significantly, then the treatment was successful. That is an oversimplified example, but something similar happens in stress and exercise research. By far, the most common "maps" used to chart changes in stress and exercise research are paper-and-pencil tests that measure some psychological aspect of stress (e.g., STAI, POMS). Measures are taken preintervention, an exercise bout or regimen is introduced, and then measures are taken again. Changes in "stress" scores are then compared between experimental and control groups. *Mirabile dictu*, stress scores on the "map" have gone down for the experimental group, but not for the control group. What do changes in POMS, or STAI, or BDI scores, or drops in cortisol for that matter, actually mean? For example, if some study reported "There was an average 5.6 drop in A-trait scores over six weeks and the effect size was .48," then what would that mean? By convention (Cohen, 1988), we know that this is a medium-size effect, but what does it really mean? How does it translate into behavior? Is it a big enough change to have a noticeable impact on someone's life? Is it a change worth paying for? Sechrest et al.'s point is that we have no real solid calibration of the instruments we use in psychotherapy research, which are some of the same ones used in stress and exercise research such as the POMS and the anxiety scales. We do not know what changes in POMS actually mean in terms of behavior or functioning. Thus, research has produced significant findings and generally small, but occasionally medium and large effect sizes in psychological, biochemical, and psychophysiological variables as a result of acute, or more long-term, exercise interventions. What it all means in terms of behavior and quality of life is still not firmly established. Making closer ties of these changes in the maps (STAI, POMS) to the actual territories (behavior and the quality of life) should be the goal of exercise scientists.

One final point is that doing more exercise may improve one's quality of life, and it may not (see Shephard's chapter on quality of life in this volume). Exercise can be an aversive event for some, but familial, social, and medical pressures may coerce some individuals to engage in exercise even though, from their point of view, it is an onerous undertaking (and actually stressful). We do not want the equivalent of the medical joke "the operation was successful, but the patient died" in exercise and stress research (e.g., "after an exercise regimen the patient's cortisol levels dropped significantly, but he hated the exercise and was miserable the whole time and yelled a lot at his children"). What we use as a map to measure the effects of exercise on stress may be quite far removed from the actual territory of interest.

References

Andersen, M. B., & Stoové, M. A. (1998). The sanctity of *p* < .05 obfuscates good stuff: A comment on Kerr and Goss. *Journal of Applied Sport Psychology, 10,* 168–173.

Bahrke, M. S., & Morgan, W. P. (1978). Anxiety reduction following exercise and meditation. *Cognitive Therapy and Research, 2,* 323–333.

Bandura, A. (1977). Self-efficacy: Toward a unifying theory of behavioral change. *Psychological Review, 84,* 191–215.

Bandura, A. (1986). *Social foundations of thought and action.* Englewood Cliffs, NJ: Prentice-Hall.

Bandura, A. (1991). Self-efficacy mechanisms in physiological activation and health promoting behavior. In J. Madden (Ed.), *Neurobiology of learning, emotion, and affect* (pp. 229–269). New York: Raven Press.

Bandura, A., Cioffi, D., Taylor, C. B., & Brouillard, M. E. (1988). Perceived self-efficacy in coping with cognitive stressors and opioid activation. *Journal of Consulting and Clinical Psychology, 53,* 406–414.

Beck, A. T., Ward, C. H., Mendelson, M., Mock, J., & Erbaugh, J. (1961). An inventory for measuring depression. *Archives of General Psychiatry, 4*, 561–571.

Berger, B. G. (1994). Coping with stress: The effectiveness of exercise and other techniques. *Quest, 47*, 100–119.

Berger, B. G. (1996). Psychological benefits of an active lifestyle: What we know and what we need to know. *Quest, 48*, 330–353.

Berger, B. G., Friedmann, & Eaton, M. (1988). Comparison of jogging, the relaxation response, and group interaction for stress reduction. *Journal of Sport and Exercise Psychology, 10*, 431–447.

Berger, B. G., & Owen, D. R. (1987). Anxiety reduction with swimming: Relationships between exercise and state, trait, and somatic anxiety. *International Journal of Sport Psychology, 18*, 286–302.

Berger, B. G., & Owen, D. R. (1988). Stress reduction and mood enhancement in four exercise modes: Swimming, body conditioning, hatha yoga, and fencing. *Research Quarterly for Exercise and Sport, 59*, 148–159.

Biddle, S. (1995). Exercise and psychosocial health. *Research Quarterly for Exercise and Sport, 66*, 292–297.

Blumenthal, J., Fredrikson, M., Kuhn, R., Ulmer, M., Walsh-Riddle, M., & Appelbaum, M. (1990). Aerobic exercise reduces levels of sympathoadrenal responses to mental stress in subjects without prior evidence of myocardial ischemia. *American Journal of Cardiology, 65*, 93–98.

Boutcher, S. H., & Landers, D. M. (1988). The effects of vigorous running on anxiety, heart rate, and alpha activity of runners and nonrunners. *Psychophysiology, 25*, 696–702.

Brooks, S., & Long, B. (1987). Efficiency of coping with a real life stressor: A multimodal comparison of aerobic exercise. *Psychophysiology, 24*, 173–180.

Brown, A., Herberman, H., & Cohen, L. (1995). Managing stress and managing illness: Survival and quality of life in chronic disease. *Journal of Clinical Psychology in Medical Settings, 2*, 309–333.

Brown, J. D. (1991). Staying fit and staying well: Physical fitness as a moderator of life stress. *Journal of Personality and Social Psychology, 60*, 555–561.

Cohen, J. (1988). *Statistical power analysis for the behavioral sciences* (2nd ed.). Hillsdale, NJ: Erlbaum.

Crews, D. J., & Landers, D. M. (1987). A meta-analytic review of aerobic fitness and reactivity to psychosocial stressors. *Medicine and Science in Sports and Exercise, 19*, S114–S120.

Derogatis, L. S. (1980). *SCL-90: Administration, scoring, and interpretation manual* (rev. ed.). Baltimore: Clinical Psychometrics Research Unit, Johns Hopkins University School of Medicine.

deVries, H. A. (1987). Tension reduction with exercise. In W. P. Morgan & S. E. Goldston (Eds.), *Exercise and mental health* (pp. 99–104). Washington, DC: Hemisphere.

Dienstbier, R. A. (1989). Arousal and physiological toughness: Implications for mental and physical health. *Psychological Review, 96*, 84–100.

Dienstbier, R. A. (1991). Behavioral correlates of sympathoadrenal reactivity: The toughness model. *Medicine and Science in Sports and Exercise, 23*, 846–852.

Dishman, R. K. (1994). Biological psychology, exercise, and stress. *Quest, 64*, 28–59.

Dishman, R. K. (1997). The norepinephrine hypothesis. In W. P. Morgan (Ed.), *Physical activity and mental health* (pp. 199–212). Washington, DC: Taylor & Francis.

Dzewaltowski, D., Acevedo, E., & Pettay, R. (1992). Influence of cardiorespiratory fitness information on cognitions and physical activity. *Medicine and Science in Sports and Exercise, 24*, S24.

Freud, S. (1960). *Psychopathology of everyday life* (J. Strachey, Trans.). New York: Norton. (Original work published in 1901)

Frick, , M. K., Elo, O., Haapa, K., Heinonen, O. P., Helo, P., Huttunen, J. K., Kaitaniemi, R., Koskinen, P., & Manninen, V. (1987). Helsinki Heart Study: Primary prevention trial with gemfibrozil in middle-aged men with dyslipidemia. *The New England Journal of Medicine, 317*, 1237–1245.

Galbo, H., Kjaer, M., Richter, E., Sonne, B., & Mikines, K. (1986). The effects of exercise on norepinephrine and epinephrine responses with special reference to physical training and metabolism. In N. Christiansen, O. Henriksen, & N. Lassen (Eds.), *The sympathoadrenal system: Physiology and pathophysiology* (pp. 174–184). New York: Raven Press.

Goldfarb, A. H., Hatfield, B. D., Armstrong, D., & Potts, J. (1990). Plasma beta-endorphin concentration: Response to intensity and duration of exercise. *Medicine and Science in Sports and Exercise, 22*, 241–244.

Goldfarb, A. H., Hatfield, B. D., Potts, J., & Armstrong, D. (1991). Beta-endorphin time course response to intensity of exercise. *International Journal of Sports and Medicine, 12*, 264–268.

Hatfield, B. D. (1991). Exercise and mental health: The mechanisms of exercise-induced psychological states. In L. Diamant (Ed.), *Psychology of sport, exercise, and fitness: Social and personal issues* (pp. 17–49). New York: Hemisphere.

Hoffman, P. (1997). The endorphin hypothesis. In W. P. Morgan (Ed.), *Physical activity and mental health* (pp. 163–177). Washington, DC: Taylor & Francis.

Hull, E., Young, S., & Ziegler, M. (1984). Aerobic fitness affects cardiovascular and catecholamine response to stressors. *Psychophysiology, 21*, 353–360.

Kaplan, R. M. (1990). Behavior as the central outcome in health care. *American Psychologist, 45*, 1211–1220.

Kaplan, R. M. (1994). The Ziggy theorem: Toward an outcomes-focused health psychology. *Health Psychology, 13*, 451–460.

Kleine, D. (1994). Sports activity as a means of reducing school stress. *International Journal of Sport Psychology, 22*, 366–380.

Koltyn, K. F. (1997). The thermogenic hypothesis. In

W. P. Morgan (Ed.), *Physical activity and mental health* (pp. 213–232). Washington, DC: Taylor & Francis.

Koltyn, K. F., & Morgan, W. P. (1993). The influence of wearing a wetsuit on core temperature and anxiety responses during underwater exercise. *Medicine and Science in Sports and Exercise, 25,* S45.

Kuusinen, J., & Heinonen, M. (1972). Immediate after effects of the Finnish sauna on psychomotor performance and mood. *Journal of Applied Physiology, 56,* 336–340.

LaPerriere, A., Ironson, G., Antoni, M. H., Schneiderman, N., Klimas, N., & Fletcher, M. A. (1994). Exercise and pychoneuroimmunology. *Medicine and Science in Sports and Exercise, 26,* 182–190.

Lazarus, R. S., & Folkman, S. (1984). *Stress, appraisal, and coping.* New York: Springer.

Light, K., Orbist, P., James, S., & Strogatz, D. (1987). Cardiovascular responses to stress. II. Relationship to aerobic fitness patterns. *Psychophysiology, 24,* 79–86.

Long, B. C., & Van Stavel, R. (1995). Effects of exercise training on anxiety: A meta-analysis. *Journal of Applied Sport Psychology, 7,* 167–189.

Martinsen, E. W., & Morgan, W. P. (1997). Antidepressant effects of physical activity. In W. P. Morgan (Ed.), *Physical activity and mental health* (pp. 93–106). Washington, DC: Taylor & Francis.

Mathur, D., Toriola, A., & Dada, O. (1986). Serum cortisol and testosterone levels in conditioned male distance runners and non-athletes after maximal exercise. *Journal of Sports Medicine, 26,* 245–250.

Mazzeo, R. S. (1991). Catecholamine responses to acute and chronic exercise. *Medicine and Science in Sports and Exercise, 23,* 839–845.

McAuley, E., & Courneya, K. S. (1992). Self-efficacy relationships with affective and exertion responses to exercise. *Journal of Applied Social Psychology, 22,* 312–326.

McAuley, E., Courneya, K. S., & Lettunich, J. (1991). Effects of acute and long-term exercise on self-efficacy responses in sedentary, middle-aged males and females. *The Gerontologist, 31,* 534–542.

McCann, I., & Holmes, D. (1984). The influence of aerobic exercise on depression. *Journal of Personality and Social Psychology, 46,* 1142–1147.

McNair, D. M., Lorr, M., & Doppelman, L. F. (1971). *Profile of Mood States manual.* San Diego, CA: Educational and Industrial Testing Service.

Morgan, W. P. (1985). Affective beneficence of vigorous physical activity. *Medicine and Science in Sports and Exercise, 17,* 94–100.

Morgan, W. P., & O'Connor, R. J. (1989). Psychological effects of exercise and sport. In A. J. Ryan & F. Allman (Eds.), *Sports medicine* (pp. 671–689). Orlando, FL: Academic Press.

Norris, R., Carroll, D., & Cochrane, R. (1992). The effects of physical activity and exercise training on psychological stress and well-being in an adolescent population. *Journal of Psychosomatic Research, 36,* 55–65.

Petruzzello, S. J., Landers, D. M., Hatfield, B. D., Kubitz, K. A., & Salazar, W. (1991). A meta-analysis on the anxiety-reducing effects of acute and chronic exercise. *Sports Medicine, 11,* 143–182.

Petruzzello, S. J., Landers, D. M., & Salazar, W. (1993). Exercise and anxiety reduction: Examination of temperature as an explanation for affective change. *Journal of Sport and Exercise Psychology, 15,* 63–76.

Raglin, J. S., & Morgan, W. P. (1987). Influence of exercise and quiet rest on state anxiety and blood pressure. *Medicine and Science in Sports and Exercise, 19,* 456–463.

Reeves, D. L., Levison, D. M., Justesen, D. R., & Lubin, B. (1985). Endogenous hyperthermia in normal human subjects: Experimental study of emotional states (II). *International Journal of Psychosomatics, 32,* 18–23.

Roth, D. L., & Holmes, D. S. (1987). Influence of aerobic exercise training and relaxation training on physical and psychologic health following stressful life events. *Psychosomatic Medicine, 49,* 355–365.

Rudolph, D. L., & McAuley, E. (1995). Self-efficacy and salivary cortisol responses to acute exercise in physically active and less active adults. *Journal of Sport and Exercise Psychology, 17,* 206–213.

Sechrest, L. B., McKnight, P., & McKnight, K. (1996). Calibration of measures for psychotherapy outcome studies. *American Psychologist, 51,* 1065–1071.

Selye, H. (1956). *The stress of life.* New York: McGraw-Hill.

Selye, H. (1974). *Stress without distress.* Philadelphia: Lippincott.

Selye, H. (1976). *The stress of life* (rev. ed.). New York: McGraw-Hill.

Shephard, R. J. (1995). Physical activity, fitness, and health: The current consensus. *Quest, 47,* 288–303.

Sime, W. (1996). Guidelines for clinical applications of exercise therapy for mental health. In J. L. Van Raalte & B. W. Brewer (Eds.), *Exploring sport and exercise psychology* (pp. 159–187). Washington, DC: American Psychological Association.

Simono, R. B. (1991). Anxiety reduction and stress management through physical fitness. In L. Diamant (Ed.), *Psychology of sport, exercise, and fitness: Social and personal issues* (pp. 17–49). New York: Hemisphere.

Smith, T., & Curzner, M. L. (1994). Neuroendocrine-immune interactions in homeostasis and autoimmunity. *Neuropathological Applied Neurobiology, 20,* 413–422.

Solomon, R. L. (1980). The opponent-process theory of acquired motivation: The costs of pleasure and the benefits of pain. *American Psychologist, 35,* 691–712.

Solomon, R. L., & Corbit, J. D. (1973). An opponent-process theory of motivation: Cigarette addiction. *Journal of Abnormal Psychology, 81,* 158–171.

Sothmann, M. S. (1991). Catecholamines, behavioral stress, and exercise: Introduction to the symposium. *Medicine and Science in Sports and Exercise, 23,* 836–838.

Sothmann, M. S., Hart, B. A., & Horn, T. S. (1991).

Plasma catecholamine response to acute psychological stress in humans: Relation to aerobic fitness and exercise training. *Medicine and Science in Sports and Exercise, 23,* 860–867.

Sothmann, M. S., Horn, T. S., Hart, B. A., & Gustafson, A. (1987). Comparison of discrete cardiovascular fitness groups on plasma catecholamines and selected behavioral responses to psychological stress. *Psychophysiology, 24,* 47–54.

Spielberger, C. D. (1987). Stress, emotions and health. In W. P. Morgan & S. E. Goldston (Eds.), *Exercise and mental health* (pp. 11–16). New York: Taylor & Francis,

Spielberger, C. D., Gorsuch, R. L., & Lushene, R. E. (1970). *STAI manual for the State-Trait Anxiety Inventory.* Palo Alto, CA: Consulting Psychologists Press.

Spielberger, C. D., Gorsuch, R. L., & Lushene, R. E., Vagg, P. R., & Jacobs, G. A. (1983). *Manual for the State-Trait Anxiety Inventory (Form Y).* Palo Alto, CA: Consulting Psychologists Press.

Steptoe, A., Moses, J., Edwards, S., & Mathews, A. (1993). Exercise and responsivity to mental stress: Discrepancies between the subjective and physiological effects of aerobic training. *International Journal of Sport Psychology, 24,* 110–129.

von Euler, C., & Soderberg, V. (1957). The influence of hypothalamic thermoreceptive structures on the electroencephalogram and gamma motor activity. *Electroencephalography and Clinical Neurophysiology, 9,* 391–408.

Weidenfeld, S. A., Bandura, A., Levine, S., O'Leary, A., Brown, S., & Raska, K. (1990). Impact of perceived self-efficacy in coping with stressors on components of the immune system. *Journal of Personality and Social Psychology, 59,* 1082–1094.

Wildman, J., Kruger, A., Schmole, M., Niemann, J., & Matthaei, H. (1986). Increase of circulating beta-endorphin-like immunoreactivity correlates with the change in feeling of pleasantness after running. *Life Sciences, 38,* 997–1003.

Zuckerman, M., & Lubin, B. (1965). *Manual for the Multiple Affect Adjective Check List.* San Diego, CA: Educational and Industrial Testing Service.

3
Injury Prevention

Urho M Kujala

Introduction

The expanding popularity of sports and exercise is focusing concern on the problem of the accompanying injuries, in addition to the health benefits (Helmrich, Ragland, Leung, & Paffenbarger, 1991; Kujala et al., 1995; Kujala, Kaprio, Sarna, & Koskenvuo, 1998; de Loës, 1990; Powell, Thompson, Caspersen, & Kendrick, 1987; Sandelin, Santavirta, Lättilä, Vuolle, & Sarna, 1987). Treating sports injuries is often expensive, so preventive strategies and activities are justified on economic as well as medical grounds (Inklaar, 1994; Kujala et al., 1995; de Loës, 1990; Sandelin et al., 1987; Torg, Vegso, Sennelt, & Das, 1985). Several epidemiological surveys have outlined the frequency and form of injuries in various sports, but study comparisons are complicated by the different injury criteria used as well as inconsistency in data collection and recording (Walter, Sutton, McIntosh, & Connolly, 1985). The risk of acute injury varies enormously: Most endurance sports are extremely safe compared to high-risk disciplines such as Formula 1 car racing, which killed 69 of a small group of drivers between 1950 and 1994 (Kujala, et al., 1995). Injury rates in popular team games such as soccer, volleyball, basketball, and ice hockey lie between these extremities (Kujala et al., 1995; de Loës, 1990). Although endurance sports may involve the highest rates of stress injury, these rarely result in permanent disability. Many new "fashion" modes of sports with high speed and powerful contacts may include high injury risk.

Before embarking on a program for preventing sports injuries, the extent of the problem must first be defined. Second, the mechanisms and factors involved need to be identified. Finally, measures likely to reduce risks are introduced and their effect monitored.

The aim of this chapter is not to review all sports injury prevention studies, but to summarize the different aspects associated with injury surveillance and prevention efforts. Such injuries as falls of elderly people associated with daily physical activity are beyond the focus of this sports-oriented chapter.

Factors Associated With Injury Risk

Sports injuries are multirisk phenomena with various risk factors interacting at a given time. In brief, factors associated with injury proneness can be classified to extrinsic and intrinsic risk factors (Table 1; Lysens, de Weerdt, & Nieuwboer, 1991; Taimela, Kujala, & Österman, 1990). The acute sport injury rate increases with the frequency of violent contacts of the sports event (Backx, Beijer, Bol, & Erich, 1991; Kujala et al., 1995; Watson, 1993), but the use of protective equipment may reduce the difference in injury outcomes between sports. The overall gender difference in the injury risk is small, but the differences by age are clear. In adult team games with various contacts, men probably train more but also tend to have a rougher style of play than women do, which may partly explain the small gender difference in injury risk. Athletes aged 20 to 24 years have the highest annual injury risk, probably because this phase of life tends to involve the most training and highest intensity of competition, injuries in young team players being clearly less frequent than in adults (Baxter-Jones, Maffulli, & Helms, 1993;

Hayes, 1978; Kujala et al., 1995; Nilsson & Rooas, 1978). Athletes usually spend far more time in training than competing. As about half of the injuries to team games athletes occur in competitions (Kujala et al., 1995), it is obvious that competitions involve higher injury risk per hour of activity than training.

The type, frequency, intensity, and duration of training play major roles also in the etiology of stress injuries. Excessive height, weight, and idiopathic or acquired abnormalities in the anatomy or biomechanics in any joint may lead to a local stress injury.

Table 1. Extrinsic and Intrinsic Risk Factors (modified from Lysens et al., 1991; van Mechelen, 1992; and Taimela et al., 1990)

Extrinsic risk factors	Intrinsic risk factors
Exposure	*Physical characteristics*
—type of sports	—age
—exposure time	—sex
—position in the team	—somatotype
—level of competition	—previous injury
—physical fitness	—joint mobility
	—muscle tightness
Training	—ligamentous instability
—type	—motor abilities
—amount	—sports-specific skills
—anatomic abnormalities (malalignments)	
Environment	*Psychological profile*
—type of surface	—motivation
—indoor vs. outdoor	—risk taking
—weather conditions	
—time of the season	
—human factors (team mates, opponent, referee, coach, spectators)	
—stress coping	
Equipment	
—protective equipment	
—instrumental materials (racket, stick, etc.)	
—footwear, clothing	

Recording Injuries and Their Type and Severity

The expression *injury surveillance* means an ongoing collection of data describing the occurrence of, and factors associated with, injury. The success of any sports injury surveillance system and its wide scale applicability are dependent upon valid and reliable definitions of sports injury, injury severity, and sports participation (Finch, 1997). Even though it would be optimal to use the same sports-injury surveillance method in all sports, the method should be tailored to the specific sports situations, if the purpose is to identify the etiology or the effectiveness of preventative measures (van Mechelen, 1997). Overall, sports injury surveillance systems are often unable to identify the exact mechanisms of injury. Unfortunately, comparison of injury rates with different studies is complicated by methodological differences (Kraus & Burg, 1970; Meeuwisse & Love, 1997; Walter et al., 1985), and there may be a need for consensus meetings among those who are responsible for different ongoing injury surveillance systems. Roughly, the studies can be categorized to case-series designs and cohort designs (for different North American experiences, see Meeuwisse & Love). Measurement of the outcome (injury) includes definition of injury, measurement of severity, and method of collecting the information; and measurement of the exposure includes both population-at-risk and time-related exposure (N. Thompson et al., 1987). In more detail, the occurrence of injuries may be calculated (a) per total population when there are also subjects who are not

Table 2. Important Points to Be Considered When Collecting Injury Surveillance Data (modified from Finch, 1997)

1. Clear definition and standardization of what constitutes an injury
2. Sports event and particular activity at the moment of injury
3. Level of sports
4. Place where the injury occurred
5. Injury mechanism, acute or overuse, and identification of malfunction
6. Level of supervision
7. Nature of the injury (sprain, fracture, etc.)
8. Injured body region/s
9. Severity of the injury (activity lost, working time lost, need of treatment, cost of treatment, permanent damage and disability, etc.)
10. Characteristics of the injured person
11. Treatments needed (duration and nature)
12. Use of protective equipment
13. Followup of game rules (foul play and injury)
14. Cost of injury (direct, indirect)
15. Definition of exposure data
16. Estimate of simplicity (vs. education of personnel collecting data) and time needed (is it realistic?) for data collection
17. Acknowledgment of limitations or sources of error—also when reporting results

exposed to sports injury, (b) per active population at risk, or (c) per time unit of exposure (de Loës, 1997). The results should be interpreted accordingly. Time lost from practice is often used as a criterion of injury definition and severity. This seems to be one standard way of reporting injuries, but does not tell about their true medical consequences. High number of medically severe injuries are more easily collected using "passive" methods of data collection, such as review of insurance claims, self-prepared mail-in surveys, and review of medical records. However, these passive methods usually underestimate the true injury incidences. Studies using careful prospective methods initiated by the researcher lead to more valid comparison of injury risk, but they usually are focused on small groups of players at risk, and such studies catch only sporadic severe injuries. Studies using "passive" methods more often cover a high number of severe injuries, and based on these studies, it is possible to define the profiles of severe injuries in different types of sports. So both types of studies, when interpreted correctly, give extremely important data to be used as the basis of prevention and exercise counseling. Table 2 gives a list of information that should be considered when starting to collect injury data.

Injury Prevention Programs May Be Effective, But May Be Ineffective or Have Negative Effects

Research has revealed that strategies designed to prevent sports injuries can be useful and that most interventions effective enough to measurably alter injury profiles in various sports have involved changes in rules or improvements in equipment (Johnson, Ettlinger, & Shealy, 1989; Schieber et al., 1996; Sim, Simonet, Melton, & Lehn, 1987; Torg et al., 1985). It must be noted that some measures may also have negative effects or no effect at all. One often mentioned example of negative effects is the use of improved helmets in American football in the 1960s, which resulted in a reduction in deaths from intercranial haemorrhages and other head injuries, but also resulted in an increase in the number of cervical spine fractures and cases of permanent quadriplegia (Torg et al., 1985). Over 100 severe cervical spine fractures or dislocations were documented annually in American football in the United States in the 1970s. The rule changes banning both spearing and the use of the top of the helmet as the initial point of contact in making a tackle were implemented in 1976. After that, a decrease of these injuries was demonstrated (Torg et al., 1985).

Nonrandom selection of those who use protective equipment and those who do not may cause a bias to some observational studies. However, we are rather convinced that, in terms of relationships, the optimal adjustment of bindings using a testing device is associated with a reduced risk of lower extremity injuries in downhill skiing (Johnson et al., 1989), and that wrist guards and elbow pads are effective in preventing upper extremity injuries in in-line skating (Schieber et al., 1996). In soccer, safety interventions and improved treatment and rehabilitation of injuries may be effective in preventing future injury (Ekstrand & Gillquist,1983; Ekstrand, Gillquist, & Liljedahl, 1983), but the somewhat bothersome programs have not been repeated by other investigators. It should be noted that many measures commonly thought to prevent sports injuries, such as stretching, lack consistent scientific evidence. Of course, there is discrepancy among many studies, and with respect to most problems, the data are too scattered to allow a meta-analysis.

Injury Prevention: How to Go On?

It is clear that there is a need for high-quality scientific studies on the effects of injury prevention programs, and it is important that there be a system of collecting data on injuries occurring in new modes of sports as well as collecting data on catastrophic sports injuries in all sports.

As an example of new modes of sport, the profile of snowboarding injuries differs from the profile of downhill skiing injuries, upper limb fractures being more common in snowboarding (Bladin & McCrody, 1995). The existing data on injury profiles and injury mechanisms in different sports should be used to educate the participators because knowledge of risks has a preventive effect. The injury profiles of the studied sports differed widely (Kujala et al., 1995). To avoid injuries, the preventive measures specific to each sport should be taught to children even though their injury risks are still low. In general, there needs to be greater focus on diminishing rough and violent contacts between athletes. Let us take ice hockey as an example of sports-specific measures: To avoid spinal cord injuries in ice hockey, aggressive checking, particularly from behind the player and near the rink boards, should be minimized by game rules and strict officiating. Aggressive stick use may partly account for the high number of hand and wrist fractures (Kujala et al., 1995) and should be controlled for. Although facial injuries are common, they have declined, thanks to more routine use of helmets and face masks (Sane & Ylipaavalniemi, 1987), which use should be encouraged.

Many sports injuries are unavoidable accidents, but many others could be prevented. Measures such as improved game rules supported by careful officiating should always incorporate the goal of decreasing the number of violent contacts between athletes. Supervision of the rules and the use of protective equipment are important during competitions, and they are also important during training sessions. Existing protective equipment also needs attention because many in-

juries afflict body parts already protected. With respect to the intervention of protective equipment, we too often lack valid pre- and postintervention data. Also, additional information from injury surveillance on such details as the type and condition of protective equipment and a description of the event leading to injury would be most valuable (Hrysomallis & Morrison, 1997). Mouthguard use should be urgently encouraged for many sports, such as ice hockey and karate. No matter which dental treatment alternative is chosen, a young athlete with a fractured tooth will face several treatment periods in years ahead, with each subsequent treatment usually being more costly.

The scientific evidence that bicycle helmets protect against head, brain, and facial injuries has been well established by case-control studies (D. C. Thompson & Patterson, 1998). Also, there are a number of suggested means by which concussions in other sport may be reduced, but the evidence for effect in many cases is theoretical rather than scientifically proven (McCrogy & Berkovic, 1998). These measures include rule changes to avoid head impact, neck-muscle conditioning, and the use of mouth guards, helmets, and head protectors.

Sometimes, it might be a need to change the rules and even the ideology of sports. In karate, the protective padding introduced for hands and feet seems to have reduced severe injuries, but may simultaneously have increased mild injuries (McLatchie, Davies, & Cauley, 1980; McLatchie & Morris, 1977). Thus, the use of more protective padding might be combined with further modification of rules and possibly even changes in the ideology of the sport, which is a difficult task for athletes and sports organizations to accept. Similarly, it would also be difficult to imagine soccer without headings even though heading may predispose to brain damage (Tysvaer, 1992).

It may be difficult to prevent ankle and knee injuries. The options to reduce ankle injuries include ankle-disk training, taping, and bracing (Gauffin, Tropp, & Odenrick, 1988; Rovere, Clarke, Yates, & Burley, 1988). Based on existing literature, Robbins and Waked (1998) have concluded that a sense of foot position in humans is precise when barefoot, but is distorted by athletic footwear, a distinction that accounts for the high frequency of ankle sprains in shod athletes. They suggest that the best solution for reducing ankle sprains in shod athletes is the use of more advanced footwear to retain maximal tactile sensitivity, thereby maintaining an awareness of foot position. Though prophylactic ankle stabilizers seem to prevent ankle injuries, again, further research is required (Sitler & Horodyski, 1995). Trials testing the utility of knee braces in athletes without earlier knee injuries may have shown a decrease in the rate of knee ligament injuries, but not in overall injury rates (Baker, 1990). Knee injuries may also progress to osteoarthritic changes later in life (Kujala, Kaprio, & Sarna, 1994). Preservative surgery for meniscal injuries and reconstructive treatment of knee ligament instabilities should be carried out whenever possible to prevent unnecessary disability or future knee osteoarthritis.

Slow progression of training gives time for adaptive mechanisms of different tissues and is the basis for the prevention of stress injuries. Correction of biomechanical faults using, for example, orthotic devices may prevent some of the injuries, even though sound scientific evidence is lacking.

In summary, based on existing knowledge of the injury profiles and mechanisms, we are able to teach people which sports are high risk and which are not as well as to teach the participants the typical sports-specific injury risks to consider. Cooperation among investigators, clinical physicians, and sports organizations would be most important in this field. Also, there is a continuous need to investigate the possibilities of rule changes and regulations concerning protective and other equipment in the prevention of sports injuries. Scientific prospective studies are needed to test the effectiveness of many means proposed to decrease injuries. New modes of sports need special injury monitoring. In addition to population strategies, trainers, coaches, and team physicians have a challenge to identify injury-prone individuals and tailor their training and rehabilitation programs to prevent their reinjuries and new injuries.

References

Backx, F. J. G., Beijer, H. J. M., Bol, E., & Erich, W. B. M. (1991). Injuries in high-risk persons and high-risk sports. *American Journal of Sports Medicine, 19*, 124–130.

Baker, B. E. (1990). Prevention of ligament injuries to the knee. *Exercise and Sport Sciences Reviews, 18*, 291–305.

Baxter-Jones, A., Maffulli, N., & Helms, P. (1993). Low injury rates in elite athletes. *Archives of Disease in Childhood, 68*, 130–132.

Bladin, C., & McCrory, P. (1995). Snowboarding injuries: An overview. *Sports Medicine, 19*, 358–364.

Ekstrand, J., & Gillquist, J. (1983). The avoidability of soccer injuries. *International Journal of Sports Medicine, 4*, 124–128.

Ekstrand, J., Gillquist, J., & Liljedahl, S. O. (1983). Prevention of soccer injuries: Supervision by doctor and physiotherapist. *American Journal of Sports Medicine, 11*, 116–120.

Finch, C. F. (1997). An overview of some definitional issues for sports injury surveillance. *Sports Medicine, 24*, 157–163.

Gauffin, H., Tropp, H., & Odenrick, P. (1988). Effect of ankle training on postural control in patients with functional instability of the ankle joint. *International Journal of Sports Medicine, 9*, 141–144.

Hayes, D. (1978). An injury profile for hockey. *Canadian Journal of Applied Sport Sciences, 3*, 61–64.

Helmrich, S. P., Ragland, D. R., Leung, R. W., & Paffenbarger, R. S. (1991). Physical activity and reduced occurrence of non-insulin-dependent diabetes mellitus. *New England Journal of Medicine, 325*, 147–152.

Hrysomallis, C., & Morrison, W. E. (1997). Sports injury

surveillance and protective equipment. *Sports Medicine*, *24*, 181–183.

Inklaar, H. (1994). Soccer injuries. Incidence and severity. *Sports Medicine, 18*, 55–73.

Johnson, R. J., Ettlinger, C. F., & Shealy, J. E. (1989). Skier injury trends. In R. J. Johnson, C. D. Mote, & M.-H. (Eds.), *Skiing trauma and safety: Proceedings of the Seventh International Symposium* (pp. 25–31). Philadelphia: American Society For Testing and Materials (ASTM) [ASTM STP, *1022*].

Kujala, U. M., Kaprio, J., & Sarna, S. (1994). Osteoarthritis of the weight bearing joints of the lower limbs in former élite male athletes. *British Medical Journal, 308*, 231–234.

Kujala, U. M., Kaprio, J., Sarna, S., & Koskenvuo, M. (1998). Relationship of leisure-time physical activity and mortality: The Finnish twin cohort. *Journal of the American Medical Association, 279*, 440–444.

Kujala, U. M., Taimela, S., Antti-Poika, I., Orava, S., Tuominen, R., & Myllynen, P. (1995). Acute injuries in soccer, ice hockey, volleyball, basketball, judo, and karate: Analysis of national registry data. *British Medical Journal, 311*, 1465–1468.

Kraus, J. F., & Burg, F. D. (1970). Injury reporting and recording: Some essential elements in the collection and retrieval of sports injury information. *Journal of the American Medical Association, 213*, 438–447.

de Loës, M. (1990). Medical treatment and costs of sports-related injuries in total population. *International Journal of Sports Medicine, 11*, 66–72.

de Loës, M. (1997). Exposure data. Why are they needed? *Sports Medicine, 24*, 172–175.

Lysens, R. J., de Weerdt, W., & Nieuwboer, A. (1991). Factors associated with injury proneness. *Sports Medicine, 12*, 281–289.

McCrogy, P. R., & Berkovic, S. (1988). Concussive convulsions: Incidence in sport and treatment recommendations. *Sports Medicine, 25*, 131–136.

McLatchie, G. R., Davies, J. E., & Caulley, J. H. (1980). Injuries in karate—A case for medical control. *Journal of Trauma, 20*, 956–958.

McLatchie, G. R., & Morris, E. W. (1977). Prevention of karate injuries—A progress report. *British Journal of Sports Medicine, 11*, 78–82.

van Mechelen, W. (1992). *Aetiology and prevention of running injuries*. University of Amsterdam. Amsterdam: The Netherlands.

van Mechelen, W. (1997). Sports injury surveillance systems. 'One size fits all?' *Sports Medicine, 24*, 164–168.

Meeuwisse, W. H., & Love, E. J. (1997). Athletic injury reporting: Development of universal systems. *Sports Medicine, 24*, 184–204.

Nilsson, S., & Rooas, A. (1978). Soccer injuries in adolescents. *American Journal of Sports Medicine, 6*, 358–361.

Powell, K. E., Thompson, P. D., Caspersen, C. J., & Kendrick, J. S. (1987). Physical activity and the incidence of coronary heart disease. *Annual Reviews of Public Health*, *8*, 253–287.

Robbins, S., & Waked, E. (1998). Factors associated with ankle injuries. Preventive measures. *Sports Medicine, 25*, 63–72.

Rovere, G., Clarke, T., Yates, C., & Burley, K. (1988). Retrospective comparison of taping and ankle stabilizers in preventing ankle injuries. *American Journal of Sports Medicine, 16*, 228–233.

Sandelin, J., Santavirta, S., Lättilä, R., Vuolle, P., & Sarna, S. (1987). Sport injuries in a large urban population: Occurrence and epidemiologic aspects. *International Journal of Sports Medicine, 8*, 61–66.

Sane, J., & Ylipaavalniemi, P. (1987). Maxillofacial and dental soccer injuries in Finland. *British Journal of Oral and Maxillofacial Surgery, 25*, 383–390.

Schieber, R. A., Branche-Dorsey, C. M., Ryan, G. W., Rutherford, G. W., Stevens, J. A., & O'Neil, J. (1996). Risk factors for injuries from in-line skating and the effectiveness of safety gear. *New England Journal of Medicine, 335*, 1630–1635.

Sim, F. H., Simonet, W. T., Melton, L. J., & Lehn, T. A. (1987). Ice hockey injuries. *American Journal of Sports Medicine, 15*, 86–96.

Sitler, M. R., & Horodyski, M. B. (1995). Effectiveness of prophylactic ankle stabilizers for prevention of ankle injuries. *Sports Medicine, 20*, 53–57.

Taimela, S., Kujala, U. M., & Österman, K. (1990). Intrinsic risk factors and athletic injuries. *Sports Medicine, 9*, 205–215.

Thompson, D. C., & Patterson, M. Q. (1998). Cycle helmets and the prevention of injuries: Recommendations for competitive sport. *Sports Medicine, 25*, 213–219.

Thompson, N., Halpern, B., Curl, W. W., Andrews, J. R., Hunter, S. C., & McLeod, W. D. (1987). High school football injuries: Evaluation. *American Journal of Sports Medicine, 15*, 117–124.

Torg, J. S., Vegso, J. J., Sennelt, B., & Das, M. (1985). The national football head and neck injury registry. 14-year report on cervical quadriplegia, 1971 through 1984. *Journal of the American Medical Association, 254*, 3439–3443.

Tysvaer, A. T. (1992). Head and neck injuries in soccer: Impact of minor trauma. *Sports Medicine, 14*, 200–213.

Walter, S. D., Sutton, J. R., McIntosh, J. M., & Connolly C. (1985). The aetiology of sport injuries: A review of methodologies. *Sports Medicine, 2*, 47–58.

Watson, A. W. S. (1993). Incidence and nature of sports injuries in Ireland: Analysis of four types of sport. *American Journal of Sports Medicine, 21*, 137–143.

4
Psychological Aspects of Sport Injury Rehabilitation: Toward a Biopsychosocial Approach

Britton W. Brewer

Mark B. Andersen

Judy L. Van Raalte

Abstract

A concise review of the literature on psychological aspects of sport injury rehabilitation is presented. Research on psychological consequences of sport injury and the relationship between psychological factors and sport injury rehabilitation outcomes is discussed. A conceptual framework for investigating biological, psychological, and social influences on the rehabilitation of sport injuries is introduced.

Psychological Aspects of Sport Injury Rehabilitation: Toward a Biopsychosocial Approach

Physical injury occurs commonly in association with involvement in sport and exercise. Consequently, sport injury is recognized as a significant public health issue (Caine, Caine, & Lindner, 1996). The pervasiveness of the problem was recently illustrated by research conducted in the United Kingdom indicating that sport or exercise accounted for approxi-

mately one third of all injuries experienced and was the single leading cause of injury (Uitenbroek, 1996). In the United States, the sheer volume of injuries incurred in association with physical activity is enormous, with an estimated 3 to 17 million sport- and recreation-related injuries occurring annually to adults and children (Bijur et al., 1995; Booth, 1987; Kraus & Conroy, 1984).

Traditionally, sport injury rehabilitation professionals have focused on identifying physical factors that influence the rate and quality of recovery and return to function. Over the past three decades, however, attention to psychological aspects of the rehabilitation process has increased. The purpose of this chapter is to present a concise review of the literature on psychological aspects of sport injury rehabilitation. After research on psychological consequences of sport injury and the relationship between psychological factors and sport injury rehabilitation outcomes has been examined, a conceptual framework for examining biological, psychological, and social influences on the rehabilitation of sport injuries is introduced.

Psychological Consequences of Sport Injury

In addition to the obvious physical effects, sport injury may also affect psychological functioning. Following publication of a seminal article by Little (1969), who documented that injury preceded the onset of neurotic symptoms in athletic men to a greater extent than in nonathletic men, researchers have focused increasingly on the psychological consequences of sport injury. Theoretical and empirical efforts have examined how people respond cognitively, emotionally, and behaviorally to sport injury.

Models of Psychological Response to Sport Injury

In attempting to explain the impact of sport injury on psychological functioning, theoretical frameworks have been borrowed from other domains of psychology and adapted to the sport injury context. Most extant models of psychological response to sport injury can be categorized as either stage models or cognitive appraisal models (Brewer, 1994).

Stage models. Based on the premise that injury-related disability is a form of loss of an aspect of the self (Peretz, 1970), stage models of grief and loss have been used to describe the psychological consequences of sport injury. The core assumption of most stage models is that persons experiencing a sport injury follow a predictable sequence of responses on the way to positive adaptation. The model consisting of sequential denial, anger, bargaining, depression, and acceptance stages developed by Kübler-Ross (1969) to describe the reactions of people with terminal illnesses has been particularly popular with sport injury investigators (e.g., Astle, 1986; Lynch, 1988; B. Rotella, 1985).

Support for some of the claims of stage models has been obtained in research investigations. For example, psychological responses to sport injury generally become more adaptive as time since injury elapses (e.g., McDonald & Hardy, 1990; Smith, Scott, O'Fallon, & Young, 1990; Uemukai, 1993). Nevertheless, no stereotypic, stage-like pattern of psychological reactions to sport injury (Brewer, 1994) and, for that matter, other undesirable life events (Silver & Wortman, 1980) has been identified across studies. Sport injury may elicit a wide variety of psychological responses depending on the characteristics of the person who is injured and the situations in which injury and subsequent rehabilitation occur (Brewer, 1994; Wiese-Bjornstal, Smith, Shaffer, & Morrey, 1998).

Cognitive appraisal models. Stage models tend to ignore individual and contextual differences in the psychological consequences of sport injury. In contrast, cognitive appraisal models underscore the importance of personal and situational factors in determining how sport injury affects people. Based largely on stress and coping theory, cognitive appraisal models are a group of related conceptual frameworks that consider cognition a central determinant of psychological responses to sport injury. Cognitive interpretations of the injury and injury-related sequelae, which themselves are posited to occur as a function of the interaction between personal and situational factors, are thought to influence emotional and behavioral reactions to sport injury (Brewer, 1994; Wiese-Bjornstal et al., 1998). Relationships among cognitive, emotional, and behavioral responses to sport injury in cognitive appraisal models are not purely unidirectional, but may instead be bidirectional or reciprocal in some circumstances (Wiese-Bjornstal et al.), as in the case of dynamic interplay between postinjury cognition (e.g., pessimistic thoughts) and emotion (depressed mood).

In contrast to stage models, cognitive appraisal models have received substantial support in research investigations. Hypothesized relationships among personal characteristics, situational variables, cognition, emotion, and behavior have been obtained consistently in empirical studies (for reviews, see Brewer, 1994, 1998; Wiese-Bjornstal et al., 1998). Evidence for the validity of cognitive appraisal models is summarized in the next section.

Cognitive, Emotional, and Behavioral Responses to Sport Injury

Cognitive responses to sport injury. Sport injury is generally an unexpected event. Consequently, it is not surprising that sport injury stimulates cognitive activity, particularly attributional processes (Wong & Weiner, 1981). Data from three studies have indicated that athletes have no trouble in coming up with causal explanations for their injuries (Brewer, 1991; Laurence, 1997; Tedder & Biddle, 1998). The connection between injury and cognition is further illustrated by the finding that athletes who indicated that they had suffered a major sport injury in the previous year reported experiencing more intrusive thoughts than did athletes who did not indicate that they had had a major sport injury in the previous year (Newcomer, Roh, Perna, & Etzel, 1998).

Changes in self-perception are the type of cognition that has been examined most frequently as a consequence of sport injury in research investigations. Studies of the effects of sport injury on self-referent cognitions have yielded equivocal results, with some studies finding postinjury decrements in self-esteem or self-efficacy and other studies finding no changes in self-perception following injury (Wiese-Bjornstal et al., 1998). Despite the inconsistencies, support for the proposed

role of cognitive appraisals in psychological responses to sport injury is growing.

As postulated in cognitive appraisal models, personal and situational characteristics have been linked to self-perception following injury. In particular, factors such as injury history (Shaffer, 1992), psychological investment in playing sport professionally (Kleiber & Brock, 1992), and surgical intervention (LaMott, 1994) have been associated with postinjury self-referent cognitions. For example, Shaffer found that having experienced previous successful rehabilitation of an ankle injury was associated with greater rehabilitation self-efficacy during ankle-injury rehabilitation. There is also support for the hypothesized relationships of cognitive appraisals to emotional and behavioral responses to sport injury. Causal attributions of injury to global (Brewer, 1991) and internal (Tedder & Biddle, 1998) factors and lower levels of physical self-esteem (Brewer, 1993) have been correlated with emotional distress following sport injury. Cognitive variables such as causal attributions of recovery to stable and personally controllable factors (Laubach, Brewer, Van Raalte, & Petitpas, 1996), appraisals of injury-coping ability (Daly, Brewer, Van Raalte, Petitpas, & Sklar, 1995), rehabilitation self-efficacy (Taylor & May, 1996), and self-esteem certainty (i.e., absence of a perceived threat to self-esteem) (Lampton, Lambert, & Yost, 1993) have been positively associated with sport injury rehabilitation adherence behavior. Thus, current research affirms the plausibility of cognition's occupying a central role in psychological responses to sport injury.

Emotional responses to sport injury. Affective reactions have been a primary focus of scientific inquiry on psychological responses to sport injury. Research findings have suggested that sport injury can be a significant source of stress (Brewer & Petrie,

1995) and can produce emotional disturbance (Brewer & Petrie; Chan & Grossman, 1988; Johnson, 1997, 1998; Leddy, Lambert, & Ogles, 1994; Miller, 1998; Pearson & Jones, 1992; Perna, Roh, Newcomer, & Etzel, 1998; Roh, Newcomer, Perna, & Etzel, 1998; Smith et al., 1993). Although most of the emotional adjustment difficulties experienced by athletes with injuries are likely subclinical in nature (Heil, 1993), an estimated 5–24% of individuals with sport injuries experience clinically meaningful levels of psychological distress (Brewer, Linder, & Phelps, 1995; Brewer, Petitpas, Van Raalte, Sklar, & Ditmar, 1995; Brewer & Petrie; Leddy et al.; Perna et al.).

In addition to the cognitive variables associated with postinjury emotional disturbance described in the previous section, personal factors (e.g., age, psychological investment in sport participation) and situational factors (e.g., injury duration, injury severity, life stress, recovery progress, social support) have also been correlated with mood following sport injury (see Brewer, 1994, for a review). With regard to the hypothesized relationship between emotional and behavioral responses to sport injury, postinjury mood disturbance has been inversely related to adherence to sport injury rehabilitation in three studies (Alzate, Ramirez, & Lazaro, 1998; Brickner, 1997; Daly et al., 1995).

Behavioral responses to sport injury. Adherence to sport injury rehabilitation, which can involve a number of different behaviors (e.g., attending clinic-based rehabilitation sessions, completing home exercises, complying with practitioner instructions), is the behavioral response to sport injury that has garnered the most attention from researchers. Across many studies, which varied considerably in how adherence was measured, sport injury rehabilitation adherence rates ranging from 40% to 91% have been obtained

(Brewer, 1998). Consistent with cognitive appraisal models, variables correlated with adherence to sport injury rehabilitation include personal characteristics (e.g., self-motivation, ego involvement, trait anxiety), situational factors (e.g., social support for rehabilitation, perceived injury severity), cognitive responses (e.g., attributions for recovery, cognitive appraisal of injury-coping ability, rehabilitation self-efficacy), emotional responses (i.e., mood disturbance), and other behavioral responses (i.e., instrumental coping) (see Brewer, 1998 for a review).

Directions for Future Research

Research on the psychological consequences of sport injury has progressed considerably in terms of volume, theory development, and methodological rigor over the past three decades. Nevertheless, there remain many unanswered questions about how people respond psychologically to sport injury. In particular, because few studies have used prospective (i.e., preinjury) repeated-measures designs with adequate controls (i.e., athletes who are not injured), little can be concluded about the process by which psychological adjustment to sport injury occurs (Brewer, 1994; Wiese-Bjornstal et al., 1998). Further, a reliance on correlational designs has made it difficult to draw causal inferences about relationships among components of theoretical frameworks. Accordingly, a clearer picture of the psychological consequences of sport injury will result from use of stronger research designs (including experimental designs) and statistical procedures that enable the disentangling of time-order relationships (Brewer, 1994, 1998; Wiese-Bjornstal et al.). Research on psychological responses to sport injury will also be enhanced by increased attention to definition and measurement of key constructs, such as sport injury, emotional responses, and adherence to rehabilitation

(Brewer, 1998; Flint, 1998; Wiese-Bjornstal et al.).

Psychological Factors and Sport Injury Rehabilitation Outcomes

Despite the advances made in describing and understanding the psychological sequelae of sport injury, psychological practitioners are poorly represented in clinical sports medicine settings (Cerny, Patton, Whieldon, & Roehrig, 1992). This underrepresentation is unlikely to change until research shows a substantial impact of psychological variables (and, ultimately, of psychological interventions) on recovery of physical functioning following sport injury (Brewer, 1994). An emerging body of evidence from case reports, correlational studies, and experimental investigations has indicated that psychological factors may exert an important influence on sport injury rehabilitation outcomes (Cupal, 1998).

Overview of Research Findings

Case reports. Data from several case studies (Nicol, 1993; R.J. Rotella & Campbell, 1983; Sthalekar, 1993) have suggested that psychological interventions such as counseling, imagery, hypnosis, relaxation, and systematic desensitization may have a beneficial effect not only on psychological aspects of rehabilitation (e.g., confidence, pain, reinjury anxiety), but also on physical sport injury rehabilitation parameters (e.g., range of motion). Of course, due to inherent limitations in case study designs, no causal inferences can be drawn about the efficacy of psychological interventions in sport injury rehabilitation from case reports.

Correlational studies. Causation also cannot be inferred from studies using correlational designs. Correlational studies can, however, be useful in identifying psychological factors associated with sport injury

rehabilitation outcomes and, consequently, pinpointing potentially effective intervention strategies. One group of correlational investigations has attempted to identify personal, situational, cognitive, and affective predictors of sport injury rehabilitation outcome. In the first published correlational study on the relationship between psychological factors and sport injury rehabilitation outcome, scores on the MMPI hypochondriasis and hysteria scales (administered presurgically) were inversely related to improvement following knee surgery (Wise, Jackson, & Rocchio, 1979), suggesting that psychological distress may hamper recovery from sport injury. Subsequent studies have been conducted by Shaffer (1992), LaMott (1994), Quinn (1996), Johnson (1996, 1997), Laubach et al. (1996), Grove and Bahnsen (1997), Laurence (1997), Alzate et al. (1998), Niedfeldt (1998), Brewer, Cornelius, et al. (2000), and Brewer, Van Raalte, et al. (2000).

Shaffer (1992) found that rehabilitation self-efficacy was positively correlated with joint functioning over the course of rehabilitation for athletes with ankle sprains. LaMott (1994) documented that a postsurgical rehabilitation outcome (i.e., knee flexion) was positively related to optimism and negatively related to frustration and fear. Using data from four separate phases of rehabilitation, Quinn (1996) obtained significant relationships between recovery time and a host of different variables, including active coping, recovery confidence, vigor, denial, emotion-focused coping, and social support. With the exception of social support, which was associated with slower recovery, all factors mentioned were associated with faster recovery. Johnson (1996, 1997) found that, relative to athletes recovering from injury poorly, athletes recovering adequately or exceptionally tended to be male, have more goals for successful rehabilitation, have more favorable cognitive appraisals of injury situation, show a more positive attitude toward rehabilitation, report greater self-confidence, rely less on social support (as found by Gould, Udry, Bridges, & Beck [1997] in a qualitative study), have less anxiety about injury rehabilitation, and experience greater general well-being. Interestingly, as in a qualitative study conducted by Gould et al., reliance on social support was associated with poor recovery. Across two separate cross-sectional studies (Brewer, Cornelius, et al., 2000; Laubach et al., 1996), attribution of recovery to stable and personally controllable factors was associated with faster perceived recovery from knee surgery.

Grove and Bahnsen (1998) documented significant correlations between self-reported use of several coping strategies and recovery from sport injury. Specifically, use of mental disengagement, positive reinterpretation, emotional focus/venting, and denial were associated with slower recovery and use of instrumental social support was associated with faster recovery. Laurence (1997) found that among physically active individuals with ankle injuries, those who expected to recover quickly actually recovered more quickly than those who expected to recover slowly. Alzate et al. (1998) reported significant inverse relationships between mood disturbances and recovery from sport injury. Niedfeldt (1998) found that cognitive appraisals of one's ability to cope with injury and beliefs about one's ability to recover fully from injury were highly correlated (> .85) with muscular strength during rehabilitation. Most recently, presurgical psychological distress and athletic identity were negatively and positively associated, respectively, with one index of rehabilitation outcome following anterior cruciate ligament reconstruction (Brewer, Van Raalte, et al., 2000).

A second group of correlational studies has assessed the relationship between a behavioral factor, rehabilitation adherence, and sport injury rehabilitation outcome. Positive adherence-outcome correlations have been obtained in five studies (Alzate et al., 1998; Brewer, Van Raalte, et al., 2000; Derscheid & Feiring, 1987; Quinn, 1996; Tuffey, 1991). Other studies, however, have found nonsignificant (Noyes, Matthews, Mooar, & Grood, 1983; Quinn) and inverse (Quinn; Shelbourne & Wilckens, 1990) adherence-outcome correlations. It appears that the relationship between adherence and outcome in sport injury rehabilitation depends, at least in part, on the particular injury, physical therapy protocol, phase of rehabilitation, and adherence index under consideration.

A third group of correlational studies, all of which are hampered by small sample sizes, has assessed the relationship between self-reported use of psychological skills and sport injury rehabilitation outcomes. Ievleva and Orlick (1991) found that athletes whose ankle or knee injuries healed quickly reported using goal setting, positive self-talk, and healing imagery to a greater extent than did those whose injuries healed slowly. Loundagin and Fisher (1993) replicated the findings of Ievleva and Orlick for goal setting and healing imagery and also found that fast slow healers reported having greater attentional focus on healing, relaxation of stress, proportions of positive self-talk, and use of recovery imagery than did slow healers. Tuffey (1991) and Latuda (1995) obtained nonsignificant correlations between self-reported use of psychological skills and sport injury recovery rate, although both studies had fewer than 22 participants and several of the correlations were above .26 in the predicted direction. Tuffey did, however, find (in contrast to the results of Quinn, 1996) that athletes high in social support tended to heal more quickly than those low in social support. Although the findings of this group of correlational studies are inconsistent, they provide at least partial support for the use of psychological skills interventions in sport injury rehabilitation.

Experimental Investigations

The strongest empirical evidence of the impact of psychological factors on sport injury rehabilitation outcomes is provided by studies using experimental designs. Experimental research in the psychological domain of recovery from sport injury has focused exclusively on the effects of psychological interventions presumed to influence mediators of rehabilitation outcomes. The most frequently evaluated psychological intervention in sport injury rehabilitation is biofeedback, which has been generally effective in enhancing rehabilitation outcomes (see Cupal, 1998 for a review). Other psychological interventions that have been effective in enhancing sport injury rehabilitation in experimental investigations include imagery/relaxation (Durso-Cupal, 1996), stress inoculation training (Ross & Berger, 1996), goal setting (Theodorakis, Beneca, Malliou, & Goudas, 1997; Theodorakis, Malliou, Papaioannou, Beneca, & Filactakidou, 1996), and self-talk (Theodorakis, Beneca, Malliou, Antoniou, et al., 1997).

Directions for Future Research

Data from case reports, correlational studies, and experimental investigations have indicated that psychological factors are associated with sport injury rehabilitation outcomes. Although causal relationships have been established between selected psychological interventions and certain rehabilitation outcomes, there is little information available on the mechanisms responsible for the effects of psychological procedures on physical rehabilitation parameters.

Further research, consisting of both experimental and prospective correlational studies, is needed to clarify the role of psychological factors in the rehabilitation process. As a prelude to such research, theoretical models offering plausible explanations for the effects of psychological variables on rehabilitation outcomes should be developed. Psychologically based models (e.g., Brewer, 1994; Wiese-Bjornstal et al., 1998) typically do not specify precise mediators of relationships between psychological factors and physical recovery, and medical models of injury healing generally do not consider the influence of psychological factors (e.g., Leadbetter, 1994). As noted by Flint (1998), "Most psychology of injury research has operated independent of any physiological considerations" (p. 99).

Toward a Biopsychosocial Approach to Sport Injury Rehabilitation

Theoretical advancements are needed to bridge the gap between medical and psychological approaches to sport injury rehabilitation. In particular, it is necessary to develop conceptual frameworks that incorporate the myriad factors that contribute to sport injury rehabilitation outcomes. One such framework, which draws upon existing integrative models of health outcome (Cohen & Rodriguez, 1995; Matthews et al., 1997), is presented in Figure 1. This biopsychosocial model is designed to broaden the scope of sport injury rehabilitation research, augmenting rather than replacing current models of relevance to sport injury rehabilitation (e.g., Flint, 1998; Leadbetter, 1994; Wiese-Bjornstal et al., 1998). Key aspects of the model are reviewed in the following sections.

Components of a Biopsychosocial Model

This rehabilitation model focuses on processes and interrelationships once injury has occurred. We recognize that many of the components of the model may influence the occurrence of injury in the first place (see Williams & Andersen, 1998, for a review).

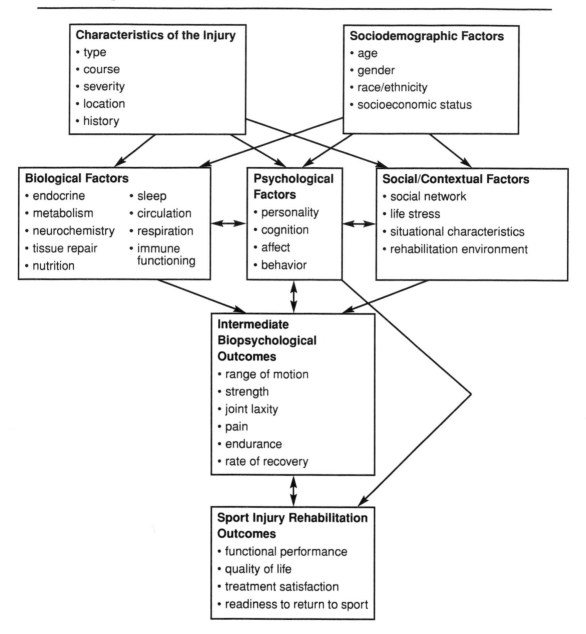

Figure 1
A biopsychosocial model of sport injury rehabilitation

Injury. Injury is an event or process involving physical damage that can lead to the initiation of rehabilitation. Injuries can vary in type (e.g., microtrauma, macrotrauma), cause, severity, and location (Flint, 1998). Injuries may have simple and short histories

(e.g., an acute ankle sprain) or more complex, complicated, and long-term histories (e.g., recurrent rotator-cuff problems).

Sociodemographic factors. Sociodemographic factors provide the personal backdrop against which sport injury rehabilitation occurs. Examples of sociodemographic factors that may be connected to rehabilitation outcome are age, gender, race/ethnicity, and socioeconomic status.

Biological factors. By definition, injury produces damage to biological structures. Biological factors that may be influenced by injury and may affect physical recovery include endocrinological, nutritional, metabolic, neurochemical, and tissue repair processes and functioning of the circulatory, respiratory, and immune systems.

Psychological factors. Individual difference (i.e., personality), cognitive, emotional, and behavioral variables constitute the primary psychological factors associated with sport injury rehabilitation. Relationships among these factors are described in detail by Wiese-Bjornstal et al. (1998).

Social/contextual factors. Sport injury rehabilitation does not occur in a vacuum. Rather, it happens in a particular situational and environmental context that can affect psychological aspects of sport injury rehabilitation. Examples of relevant social/contextual factors include characteristics of the sport situation (e.g., sport type, time of season, team climate, coach/team expectations, level of participation, reliance on sport for monetary income), features of the rehabilitation environment (e.g., accessibility, social skills of rehabilitation professionals), and the athlete's social network and levels of major and minor life stresses (Wiese-Bjornstal et al., 1998).

Intermediate biopsychological outcomes. Intermediate outcomes are factors that may be influenced by the sport injury rehabilitation process and may ultimately contribute to sport injury rehabilitation outcomes. Flexibility (i.e., range of motion), strength, endurance, joint laxity, rate of recovery, and pain are examples of intermediate biopsychological outcomes.

Sport injury rehabilitation outcomes. Sport injury rehabilitation outcomes constitute the end point of the sport injury rehabilitation process and include functional performance, quality of life, treatment satisfaction, and psychological readiness to return to sport participation or life outside of sport. The relative importance of these outcomes may vary across individuals.

Dynamics of a Biopsychosocial Model

As indicated by the bidirectional arrows in Figure 1, a biopsychological model is clearly an interactive approach to conceptualizing sport injury rehabilitation. Interrelationships both between and within key components of the model highlight the complexity of factors influencing rehabilitation outcomes. We will begin at the top of the model and proceed through each "box" and its relationships with the other factors in the model.

Injury is typically considered in terms of its effects on biological functioning, such as inflammatory responses, immune system, mobilization, and tissue repair. Injury may also affect psychological factors (e.g., depressed mood in response to injury). A sport injury can also have an impact on the social environment. For example, if a star player incurs a season-ending injury, the team environment may undergo a negative change.

Similarly, sociodemographic factors may contribute to biological and psychological responses to injury as well as to the context in which rehabilitation occurs. For example, the gender of an athlete with a sport injury may become salient in the rehabilitation process through the influence of biological, psychological, and social characteristics on which gender differences exist, such as hormones, emotional reactions, and societal expectations.

On the next tier of the model, psychological factors hold a central position. They can influence, and in turn be influenced by, biological and social/contextual factors. For example, once one is injured, one's thinking and emotions may influence biological functioning such as appetite and sleep patterns. Disturbed sleep due to the pain and discomfort of an injury can also lead to affective lability. For social/contextual factors, an injured athlete may find herself in an unpleasant rehabilitation environment, which leads to depressed mood (a psychological factor), which leads to social withdrawal, which changes the athlete's social network for the worse.

The connection of biological factors to the next tier of the model, intermediate biopsychological outcomes, is relatively straightforward. Factors such as circulation, rate of tissue repair, and metabolism influence outcomes such as range of motion, pain reduction, and rate of recovery. The import of the bidirectional arrow from psychological factors to intermediate rehabilitation outcomes may not be so readily apparent, but how one approaches rehabilitation, for example, as a challenge or as a repellant chore, may be influenced by personality factors. A positive emotional response may help an athlete complete tedious and painful exercises and thus help improve biopsychological outcomes such as strength and range of motion. Success with intermediate rehabilitation outcomes can also feed back into psychological factors by helping increase positive affect and cognitions.

Social/contextual variables are posited to influence injury rehabilitation outcomes only through the mediating role of psychological factors. For example, disruptive life circumstances may interfere with adherence to a rehabilitation protocol, thereby hampering achievement of favorable intermediate biopsychological outcomes and, ultimately, desired functional performance at the end of rehabilitation.

In addition to its unidirectional relationship with biological factors and its bidirectional relationship with psychological factors,

intermediate biopsychological outcomes are thought to contribute directly to injury rehabilitation outcomes (Cohen & Rodriguez, 1995). Range of motion, strength, and pain, for example, presumably influence functional performance.

Finally, psychological factors are posited to have a bidirectional relationship with sport injury rehabilitation outcomes. For example, irrespective of intermediate biopsychological outcomes, level of motivation may affect both functional performance and readiness to return to sport. Conversely, a positive quality-of-life judgment may increase other positive cognitions and emotions.

Implications of a Biopsychosocial Model for Research and Practice

Adoption of a biopsychosocial perspective on sport injury rehabilitation has important ramifications for both research and practice. For research, acknowledging the influence of the various domains involved in a biopsychosocial approach to sport injury rehabilitation necessitates the inclusion of multiple independent and dependent variables, cutting across disciplines, in scientific investigations. Examination of the interactions between the primary components (in addition to their main effects) is essential. Although the biological, psychological, and social factors relevant to rehabilitation outcomes are likely to vary considerably across diagnoses (an issue that, in itself, merits empirical attention), the biopsychosocial model offered in this chapter has heuristic value in guiding research studies and practical applications.

Traditionally, sport injury rehabilitation practitioners have focused their treatments on biological aspects of injury recovery. In contrast, the main implication of a biopsychosocial approach for applied work in sport injury rehabilitation is that interventions can be directed at any of the malleable components of the model shown in Figure 1 because they all may have a direct or indirect effect on rehabilitation outcomes. For example, altering the social context of rehabilitation may affect an individual's psychological response, which may, in turn, contribute to rehabilitation outcomes directly or through its relationships with biological factors and intermediate biopsychological outcomes. Research support for a biopsychological approach may suggest that the training or qualifications of professionals providing sport injury rehabilitation services should expand to include greater recognition of the psychosocial realm (Gordon, Potter, & Ford, 1998). By developing and implementing theoretically sound and empirically validated interventions that address the full range of biological, psychological, and social influences on sport injury rehabilitation outcomes, practitioners can enhance the quality of care for individuals with sport injuries.

Author Note

Britton W. Brewer and Judy L. Van Raalte, Center for Performance Enhancement and Applied Research, Department of Psychology; Mark B. Andersen, Department of Human Movement, Recreation & Performance and Centre for Rehabilitation, Exercise and Sport Science.

Preparation of this chapter was supported in part by grant number R29 AR44484 from the National Institute of Arthritis and Musculoskeletal and Skin Diseases. Its contents are solely the responsibility of the authors and do not represent the official views of the National Institute of Arthritis and Musculoskeletal and Skin Diseases. We thank Whitney Hartmann for her assistance in preparing Figure 1.

Correspondence concerning this chapter should be addressed to Britton W. Brewer, Center for Performance Enhancement and Applied Research, Department of Psychology, Springfield College, Springfield, Massachusetts 01109. Electronic mail may be sent via Internet to bbrewer@spfldcol.edu.

References

Alzate, R., Ramirez, A., & Lazaro, I. (1998, August). *Psychological aspect of athletic injury.* Paper presented at the 24th International Congress of Applied Psychology, San Francisco, CA.

Astle, S. J. (1986). The experience of loss in athletes. *Journal of Sports Medicine and Physical Fitness, 26,* 279–284.

Bijur, P. E., Trumble, A., Harel, Y., Overpeck, M. D., Jones, D., & Scheidt, P. C. (1995). Sports and recreation injuries in U.S. children and adolescents. *Archives of Pediatric and Adolescent Medicine, 149,* 1009–1016.

Booth, W. (1987). Arthritis Institute tackles sports. *Science, 237,* 846–847.

Brewer, B. W. (1991, June). *Causal attributions and adjustment to athletic injury.* Paper presented at the annual meeting of the North American Society for the Psychology of Sport and Physical Activity, Pacific Grove, CA.

Brewer, B. W. (1993). Self-identity and specific vulnerability to depressed mood. *Journal of Personality, 61,* 343–364.

Brewer, B. W. (1994). Review and critique of models of psychological adjustment to athletic injury. *Journal of Applied Sport Psychology, 6,* 87–100.

Brewer, B. W. (1998). Adherence to sport injury rehabilitation programs. *Journal of Applied Sport Psychology, 10,* 70–82.

Brewer, B. W., Cornelius, A. E., Van Raalte, J. L., Petitpas, A. J., Sklar, J. H., Pohlman, M. H., Krushell, R. J., & Ditmar, T. D. (2000). Attributions for recovery and adherence to rehabilitation following anterior cruciate ligament reconstruction: A prospective analysis. *Psychology and Health, 15,* 283-291.

Brewer, B. W., Linder, D. E., & Phelps, C. M. (1995). Situational correlates of emotional adjustment to athletic injury. *Clinical Journal of Sport Medicine, 5,* 241–245.

Brewer, B. W., Petitpas, A. J., Van Raalte, J. L., Sklar, J. H., & Ditmar, T. D. (1995). Prevalence of psychological distress among patients at a physical therapy clinic specializing in sports medicine. *Sports Medicine, Training and Rehabilitation, 6,* 138–145.

Brewer, B. W., & Petrie, T. A. (1995). A comparison between injured and uninjured football players on selected psychosocial variables. *Academic Athletic Journal, 10,* 11–18.

Brewer, B. W., Van Raalte, J. L., Cornelius, A. E., Petitpas, A. J., Sklar, J. H., Pohlman, M. H., Krushell, R. J., & Ditmar, T. D. (2000). Psychological factors, rehabilitation adherence, and rehabilitation outcome following anterior cruciate ligament reconstruction. *Rehabilitation Psychology, 45*, 20-37.

Brickner, J. C. (1997). *Mood states and compliance of patients with orthopedic rehabilitation.* Unpublished master's thesis, Springfield College, MA.

Caine, D. J., Caine, C. G., & Lindner, K. J. (Eds.). (1996). *Epidemiology of sports injuries.* Champaign, IL: Human Kinetics.

Cerny, F. J., Patton, D. C., Whieldon, T. J., & Roehrig, S. (1992). An organizational model of sports medicine facilities in the United States. *Journal of Orthopaedic and Sports Physical Therapy, 15*, 80–86.

Chan, C. S., & Grossman, H. Y. (1988). Psychological effects of running loss on consistent runners. *Perceptual and Motor Skills, 66*, 875–883.

Cohen, S., & Rodriguez, M. S. (1995). Pathways linking affective disturbance and physical disorders. *Health Psychology, 14*, 374–380.

Cupal, D. D. (1998). Psychological interventions in sport injury prevention and rehabilitation. *Journal of Applied Sport Psychology, 10*, 103–123.

Daly, J. M., Brewer, B. W., Van Raalte, J. L., Petitpas, A. J., & Sklar, J. H. (1995). Cognitive appraisal, emotional adjustment, and adherence to rehabilitation following knee surgery. *Journal of Sport Rehabilitation, 4*, 23–30.

Derscheid, G. L., & Feiring, D. C. (1987). A statistical analysis to characterize treatment adherence of the 18 most common diagnoses seen at a sports medicine clinic. *Journal of Orthopaedic and Sports Physical Therapy, 9*, 40–46.

Durso-Cupal, D. D. (1996). The efficacy of guided imagery for recovery from anterior cruciate ligament (ACL) replacement [Abstract]. *Journal of Applied Sport Psychology, 8*, S56.

Flint, F. A. (1998). Integrating sport psychology and sports medicine in research: The dilemmas. *Journal of Applied Sport Psychology, 10*, 83–102.

Gordon, S., Potter, M., & Ford, I. (1998). Toward a psychoeducational curriculum for training sport-injury rehabilitation personnel. *Journal of Applied Sport Psychology, 10*, 140–156.

Gould, D., Udry, E., Bridges, D., & Beck, L. (1997). Coping with season-ending injuries. *The Sport Psychologist, 11*, 379–399.

Grove, J. R., & Bahnsen, A. (1997). *Personality, injury severity, and coping with rehabilitation.* Unpublished manuscript.

Heil, J. (1993). Sport psychology, the athlete at risk, and the sports medicine team. In J. Heil (Ed.), *Psychology of sport injury* (pp. 1–13). Champaign, IL: Human Kinetics.

Ievleva, L., & Orlick, T. (1991). Mental links to enhanced healing: An exploratory study. *The Sport Psychologist, 5*, 25–40.

Johnson, U. (1996). Quality of experience of long-term injury in athletic sports predicts return after rehabilitation. In G. Patriksson (Ed.), *Aktuell beteendevetenskaplig idrottsforskning* (pp. 110–117). Lund, Sweden: SVEBI.

Johnson, U. (1997). A three-year followup of long-term injured competitive athletes: Influence of psychological risk factors on rehabilitation. *Journal of Sport Rehabilitation, 6*, 256–271.

Johnson, U. (1998). Psychological risk factors during the rehabilitation of competitive male soccer players with serious knee injuries [Abstract]. *Journal of Sports Sciences, 16*, 391–392.

Johnson, U. (1997). Coping strategies among long-term injured competitive athletes: A study of 81 men and women in team and individual sports. *Scandinavian Journal of Medicine & Science in Sports, 7*, 367–372.

Kleiber, D. A., & Brock, S. C. (1992). The effect of career-ending injuries on the subsequent well-being of elite college athletes. *Sociology of Sport Journal, 9*, 70–75.

Kraus, J. F., & Conroy, C. (1984). Mortality and morbidity from injury in sports and recreation. *Annual Review of Public Health, 5*, 163–192.

Kübler-Ross, E. (1969). *On death and dying.* New York: Macmillan.

LaMott, E. E. (1994). *The anterior cruciate ligament injured athlete: The psychological process.* Unpublished doctoral dissertation, University of Minnesota, Minneapolis.

Lampton, C. C., Lambert, M. E., & Yost, R. (1993). The effects of psychological factors in sports medicine rehabilitation adherence. *Journal of Sports Medicine and Physical Fitness, 33*, 292–299.

Latuda, L. (1995). The use of psychological skills in enhancing the rehabilitation of injured athletes. *Journal of Sport & Exercise Psychology, 17*(Suppl.), S70.

Laubach, W. J., Brewer, B. W., Van Raalte, J. L., & Petitpas, A. J. (1996). Attributions for recovery and adherence to sport injury rehabilitation. *Australian Journal of Science and Medicine in Sport, 28*, 30–34.

Laurence, C. (1997, September). *Attributional, affective and perceptual processes during injury and rehabilitation in active people.* Paper presented at the 14th World Congress on Psychosomatic Medicine, Cairns, Australia.

Leadbetter, W. B. (1994). Soft tissue athletic injury. In F. H. Fu & D. A. Stone (Eds.), *Sports injuries: Mechanisms, prevention, and treatment* (pp. 733–780). Baltimore, MD: Williams & Wilkins.

Leddy, M. H., Lambert, M. J., & Ogles, B. M. (1994). Psychological consequences of athletic injury among high-level competitors. *Research Quarterly for Exercise and Sport, 65*, 347–354.

Little, J. C. (1969). The athlete's neurosis—A deprivation crisis. *Acta Psychiatrica Scandinavia, 45*, 187–197.

Loundagin, C., & Fisher, L. (1993, October). *The relationship between mental skills and enhanced athletic injury rehabilitation.* Poster presented at the annual meeting of the Association for the Advancement of Applied Sport Psychology and the Canadian Society for Psychomotor Learning and Sport Psychology, Montreal, Canada.

Lynch, G. P. (1988). Athletic injuries and the practicing

sport psychologist: Practical guidelines for assisting athletes. *The Sport Psychologist, 2,* 161–167.

Matthews, K. A., Shumaker, S. A., Bowen, D. J., Langer, R. D., Hunt, J. R., Kaplan, R. M., Klesges, R. C., & Ritenbaugh, C. (1997). Women's Health Initiative: Why now? What is it? What's new? *American Psychologist, 52,* 101–116.

McDonald, S. A., & Hardy, C. J. (1990). Affective response patterns of the injured athlete: An exploratory analysis. *The Sport Psychologist, 4,* 261–274.

Miller, W. N. (1998). Athletic injury: Mood disturbances and hardiness of intercollegiate athletes [Abstract]. *Journal of Applied Sport Psychology, 10*(Suppl.), S127–S128.

Newcomer, R. R., Roh, J., Perna, F. M., & Etzel, E. F. (1998). Injury as a traumatic experience: Intrusive thoughts and avoidance behavior associated with injury among college student-athletes [Abstract]. *Journal of Applied Sport Psychology, 10*(Suppl.), S54.

Nicol, M. (1993). Hypnosis in the treatment of repetitive strain injury. *Australian Journal of Clinical and Experimental Hypnosis, 21,* 121–126.

Niedfeldt, C. E. (1998). *The integration of physical factors into the cognitive appraisal process of injury rehabilitation.* Unpublished master's thesis, University of New Orleans, LA.

Noyes, F. R., Matthews, D. S., Mooar, P. A., & Grood, E. S. (1983). The symptomatic anterior cruciate-deficient knee. Part II: The results of rehabilitation, activity modification, and counseling on functional disability. *Journal of Bone and Joint Surgery, 65-A,* 163–174.

Pearson, L., & Jones, G. (1992). Emotional effects of sports injuries: Implications for physiotherapists. *Physiotherapy, 78,* 762–770.

Peretz, D. (1970). Development, object-relationships, and loss. In B. Schoenberg, A. C. Carr, D. Peretz, & A. H. Kutscher (Eds.), *Loss and grief: Psychological management in medical practice* (pp. 3–19). New York: Columbia University Press.

Perna, F. M., Roh, J., Newcomer, R. R., & Etzel, E. F. (1998). Clinical depression among injured athletes: An empirical assessment [Abstract]. *Journal of Applied Sport Psychology, 10*(Suppl.), S54–S55.

Quinn, A. M. (1996). *The psychological factors involved in the recovery of elite athletes from long term injuries.* Unpublished doctoral dissertation, University of Melbourne, Australia.

Roh, J., Newcomer, R. R., Perna, F. M., & Etzel, E. F. (1998). Depressive mood states among college athletes: Pre- and post-injury [Abstract]. *Journal of Applied Sport Psychology, 10*(Suppl.), S54.

Ross, M. J., & Berger, R. S. (1996). Effects of stress inoculation on athletes' postsurgical pain and rehabilitation after orthopedic injury. *Journal of Consulting and Clinical Psychology, 64,* 406–410.

Rotella, B. (1985). The psychological care of the injured athlete. In L. K. Bunker, R. J. Rotella, & A. S. Reilly (Eds.),

Sport psychology: Psychological considerations in maximizing sport performance (pp. 273–287). Ann Arbor, MI: Mouvement.

Rotella, R. J., & Campbell, M. S. (1983). Systematic desensitization: Psychological rehabilitation of injured athletes. *Athletic Training, 18,* 140–142, 151.

Shaffer, S. M. (1992). *Attributions and self-efficacy as predictors of rehabilitative success.* Unpublished master's thesis, University of Illinois, Champaign.

Shelbourne, K. D., & Wilckens, J. H. (1990). Current concepts in anterior cruciate ligament rehabilitation. *Orthopaedic Review, 19,* 957–964.

Silver, R. L., & Wortman, C. B. (1980). Coping with undesirable events. In J. Garber & M. E. P. Seligman (Eds.), *Human helplessness: Theory and applications* (pp. 279–375). New York: Academic Press.

Smith, A. M., Scott, S. G., O'Fallon, W. M., & Young, M. L. (1990). Emotional responses of athletes to injury. *Mayo Clinic Proceedings, 65,* 38–50.

Smith, A. M., Stuart, M. J., Wiese-Bjornstal, D. M., Milliner, E. K., O'Fallon, W. M., & Crowson, C. S. (1993). Competitive athletes: Preinjury and postinjury mood state and self-esteem. *Mayo Clinic Proceedings, 68,* 939–947.

Sthalekar, H. A. (1993). Hypnosis for relief of chronic phantom limb pain in a paralysed limb: A case study. *The Australian Journal of Clinical Hypnotherapy and Hypnosis, 14,* 75–80.

Taylor, A. H., & May, S. (1996). Threat and coping appraisal as determinants of compliance to sports injury rehabilitation: An application of protection motivation theory. *Journal of Sports Sciences, 14,* 471–482.

Tedder, S., & Biddle, S. J. H. (1998). Psychological processes involved during sports injury rehabilitation: An attribution-emotion investigation [Abstract]. *Journal of Sports Sciences, 16,* 106–107.

Theodorakis, Y., Beneca, A., Malliou, P., Antoniou, P., Goudas, M., & Laparidis, K. (1997). The effect of a self-talk technique on injury rehabilitation [Abstract]. *Journal of Applied Sport Psychology, 9*(Suppl.), S164.

Theodorakis, Y., Beneca, A., Malliou, P., & Goudas, M. (1997). Examining psychological factors during injury rehabilitation. *Journal of Sport Rehabilitation, 6,* 355–363.

Theodorakis, Y., Malliou, P., Papaioannou, A., Beneca, A., & Filactakidou, A. (1996). The effect of personal goals, self-efficacy, and self-satisfaction on injury rehabilitation. *Journal of Sport Rehabilitation, 5,* 214–223.

Tuffey, S. (1991). *The use of psychological skills to facilitate recovery from athletic injury.* Unpublished master's thesis, University of North Carolina at Greensboro.

Uemukai, K. (1993). Affective responses and the changes in athletes due to injury. In S. Serpa, J. Alves, V. Ferreira, & A. Paula-Brito (Eds.), *Proceedings of the 8th World Congress of Sport Psychology* (pp. 500–503). Lisbon, Portugal: International Society of Sport Psychology.

Uitenbroek, D. G. (1996). Sports, exercise, and other

causes of injuries: Results of a population survey. *Research Quarterly for Exercise and Sport, 67,* 380–385.

Wiese-Bjornstal, D. M., Smith, A. M., Shaffer, S. M., & Morrey, M. A. (1998). An integrated model of response to sport injury: Psychological and sociological dimensions. *Journal of Applied Sport Psychology, 10,* 46–69.

Williams, J. M., & Andersen, M. B. (1998). Psychosocial antecedents of sport injury: Review and critique of the stress and injury model. *Journal of Applied Sport Psychology, 10,* 5–25.

Wise, A., Jackson, D. W., & Rocchio, P. (1979). Preoperative psychologic testing as a predictor of success in knee surgery. *American Journal of Sports Medicine, 7,* 287–292.

Wong, P. T. P., & Weiner, B. (1981). When people ask "why" questions, and the heuristics of attributional search. *Journal of Personality and Social Psychology, 40,* 650–663.

5
Performance-Enhancing Drugs and Ergogenic Aids

J. David Branch

Introduction

Various nutritional supplements, pharmacologic substances, and practices currently used by recreational and elite athletes either are purported to or have been shown to enhance exercise performance. These are known as ergogenic aids. Although some ergogenic aids are unequivocally banned by various national and international governing bodies, use of other aids is banned by some, but not all, governing bodies. Still others await decision concerning legality of use. A separate, but equally important issue is the ethics of ergogenic aid use. This chapter provides a brief introduction to some of the most prevalent ergogenic aids currently in use. The ergogenic agents discussed in this chapter are divided into the following six sections: (a) anabolic agents, (b) energy metabolism, (c) acid/base regulation, (d) oxygen transport/endurance performance, (e) stimulants, and (f) adrenergic blockers/central nervous system depressants. The interested reader who desires information beyond the scope of this chapter is referred to M. H. Williams (1998), a comprehensive text on the subject, as well as recent reviews of each ergogenic aid discussed below.

Anabolic Agents

Anabolic-Androgenic Steroids (AAS)

Cable (1997) and Yesalis and Bahrke (1995) have written summaries of the ergogenic and side effects of AAS. The following section includes key points regarding the biochemistry, mechanism(s) of action, ergogenicity, safety, and legality of AAS use.

Biochemistry. Testosterone was first isolated in the 1930s (Kockakian & Murlin, 1935). Testosterone is produced primarily by the testes and is responsible for masculine features (androgyny) and increased lean body mass (anabolism). Anabolic-androgenic steroids (AAS) are chemically modified analogs of the endogenous steroid hormone testosterone. AAS have been used clinically to treat hypogonadism. Reports of illegal use of AAS by power athletes to increase lean body mass began in the 1950s and continues today. AAS agents are modified on the sterol D ring, either by alkylation at the 17-α position or by carboxylic acid esterification at the 17-β hydroxyl group. The reason for this is that AAS have a longer half-life than does exogenous testosterone, which is rapidly catabolized by the body.

Ergogenic mechanism. AAS are lipid soluble and diffuse across the cell membrane in the same manner as endogenous testosterone. Once across the cell membrane, a receptor-AAS complex is formed on the chromatin of the cell nucleus, which stimulates an increase in mRNA *de novo* biosynthesis and the eventual formation of structural and contractile protein. Other proposed mechanisms of action include a direct stimulation of androgen receptors on α-motor neurons and competitive binding with glucocorticoid receptors. The latter mechanism would inhibit the proteolytic action of cortisol, which is consistent with the anabolic effects of AAS (Cable, 1997).

Evidence of ergogenic effect. AAS are consumed in supraphysiologic (i.e., pharmacologic) doses in injectable and oral forms. Greater gains in muscle strength and body mass have been reported in individuals who undergo regimens of "cycling" (periods of ingesting pharmacologic doses followed by periodic withdrawal) and/or "stacking" (simultaneous use of two or more AAS agents in pharmacologic doses). Much of the knowledge concerning AAS use comes from anecdotal sources and case studies, with evidence of greater ergogenicity in trained compared to untrained individuals (Cable, 1997). Few well-designed clinical trials are found in the literature because of the health-related consequences, discussed below, of AAS use and the resulting reluctance of institutional review boards to approve such studies (Cable). Among studies supporting the efficacy of AAS in improving strength and/or mass, the effects seem to be highly variable and relatively small (Friedl, Dettori, Hannan, Patience, & Plymate, 1991). A meta-analysis by Elashoff, Jacknow, Shain, and Braunstein (1991) reported a median improvement in strength of 5% (range of 1.2 to 18.7) across nine studies of trained subjects, with no change in eight studies of untrained subjects.

The results of these studies may not be generalizable to pharmacologic doses, or "stacking," that more accurately reflect actual AAS use (Elashoff et al.). To illustrate this point, a recent cross-sectional survey of 100 steroid users reported AAS doses ranging from 250 to 3200 mg·wk^{-1} (Evans, 1997). In a double-blind placebo control investigation of 43 males, Bhasin et al. (1996) reported increased strength and muscle size in a group receiving a supraphysiologic AAS dose of testosterone ethanate whereas weight training (600 mg·wk^{-1} IM for 10 wks) compared to placebo only, AAS only, and placebo/weight-training groups.

Safety. Altered lipid metabolism (decreased serum [HDL-C]), hepatic cellular damage, myocardial cellular damage, and cardiomyopathy are well-documented health-related outcomes associated with AAS use in humans and animal models (Cable et al., 1997; Melchert, Herron, & Welder, 1992; Melchert & Welder, 1995; Welder & Melchert, 1993; Welder, Robertson, Fugate, & Melchert, 1995; Welder, Robertson, & Melchert, 1995). AAS agents alter the negative feedback regulation of endogenous testosterone production, resulting in lower [testosterone] and testicular atrophy. There is evidence that the orally ingested 17 α-alkylated AAS agents appear to pose greater health risks than do the injected 17 β-esters, but use of needles increases the risk of HIV/AIDS, hepatitis, and other infections (Welder, Robertson, Fugate, et al., 1995). Male/female reproductive dysfunction, clitoral enlargement, and acne are also associated with AAS use (Lombardo, Hickson, & Lamb, 1991). Due to the ethical difficulties associated with controlled clinical trials using pharmacologic AAS doses, anecdotal reports, clinical case studies, and epidemiologic case-control studies will continue to contribute to the understanding of the health consequences of AAS use. The perception exists that the primary populations to use AAS are power athletes such as American football players and weight lifters (Cable et al., 1997), but other populations such as male high school students also use AAS at an alarming prevalence (Buckley et al., 1988; DuRant, Escobedo, & Heath, 1995; Spence & Gauvin, 1996; Yesalis et al., 1989). AAS use has also been reported to be significantly associated with drinking and driving, nonuse of seat belts, unsafe sexual practices, and suicidal behavior (Middleman et al., 1995). This tends to support reports of increased aggressiveness among chronic AAS users (Cable et al., 1997; Lombardo et al., 1991).

Legality. AAS agents were banned by the International Olympics Committee (IOC) in 1976 and are also prohibited by other governing bodies of amateur and professional sports such as the National Collegiate Athletics Association (NCAA), The Athletics Congress (TAC), and the International Amateur Athletics Federation (IAAF) (Cable et al., 1997).

Human Growth Hormone (hGH)

Compared to AAS, hGH is a relatively recent addition to the list of anabolic ergogenic aids. At one time, the only source of hGH was the pituitary gland of cadavers. In the last decade, hGH has been available through recombinant DNA technology, but it remains prohibitively expensive. For a more thorough discussion of the biochemistry, clinical, and ergogenic potential of hGH, the interested reader is referred to reviews by Bradley and Sodeman (1990), Haupt (1993), Rogol (1989), and D. A. Smith and Perry (1992).

Biochemistry. hGH, also known as somatotrophin, is a 191 residue, 22 kilodalton peptide. hGH is released from the anterior pituitary by such stimuli as sleep, exercise, L-DOPA, and arginine and is regulated by the hypothalamic hormones growth hormone releasing hormone (GHrH) and somatostatin (Lombardo et al., 1991). Metabolic actions

of hGH include increased amino acid uptake, protein synthesis, and the growth of epiphyseal plates of long bones. Although hGH has a short half-life, it stimulates the release of somatomedins (e.g., insulin-like growth factors) that have more prolonged anabolic effects. hGH also stimulates renal and hepatic gluconeogenesis as well as lipolysis (Lombardo et al.).

Ergogenic mechanism and evidence of ergogenic effect. Clinically, hGH is prescribed in cases of pituitary deficiency in children. In adults, hGH has been reported to increase lean body mass and decrease fat mass. The antiaging potential of hGH in increasing lean body mass and bone density, and decreasing fat mass in elderly men has been reported (Rudman et al., 1990). The perception that hGH use may be associated with less risk than AAS, as well as the development of more sophisticated techniques to detect AAS abuse, may prompt some athletes to consider hGH as an anabolic supplement. However, similar increases in strength and lean body mass have been reported following resistance training with and without hGH supplementation, suggesting that hGH-stimulated protein synthesis may be connective tissue instead of contractile muscle (Lombardo et al., 1991; Yarasheski et al. 1992; Yarasheski, Zachwieja, Angelopoulos, & Bier, 1993). According to a recent review of performance-enhancing drugs, no human or animal studies have reported an ergogenic effect of hGH (Smith & Perry, 1992). Additionally, the popular strategy of ingesting commercial amino acid supplements to increase endogenous [hGH] has been reported to have limited effectiveness (Fogelholm, Naveri, Kiilavuori, & Harkonen, 1993; Lambert, Hefer, Millar, & Macfarlane, 1993).

Safety. hGH use by adults can cause acromegaly in adults and gigantism in prepubescent children. Cardiomyopathy is associated with acromegaly. hGH also impairs glucose uptake, predisposing the user to diabetes mellitus. The unsupervised use of hGH is ill-advised (Lombardo et al., 1991; Rogol, 1989).

Legality. The use of hGH is prohibited by various sports-governing bodies. Use of hGH is very difficult to detect.

Other Anabolic Agents— Dehydroepiandrosterone (DHEA), Androstenedione and β-Hydroxy β-Methyl Butyrate (HMB)

DHEA, androstenedione, and HMB are relatively recent additions to the supplement list for individuals seeking to increase mass. Androstenedione received widespread publicity for being used by Mark McGwire of the St. Louis Cardinals during his season home-run record-setting 1998 baseball season. HMB has been reported to increase mass in livestock, but only recently has it been studied in humans. To date, there are no comprehensive reviews on these agents.

Biochemistry and potential ergogenic mechanisms. DHEA and androstenedione are precursors to testosterone. Ingestion of these substances would theoretically increase substrate for testosterone biosynthesis. HMB is a metabolite of leucine, a branched-chain amino acid. In a transaminase reaction, leucine is converted to α-ketoisocaproate, which is then oxidized to β-hydroxy β-methyl butyrate (HMB). Although an understanding of an ergogenic action of HMB is far from complete, the primary mechanism appears to be inhibition of exercise-induced proteolytic activity rather than increased protein synthesis.

Evidence of ergogenic effect. DHEA has been reported to counteract the development of obesity and insulin resistance in rats (Hansen, Han, Nolte, Chen, & Holloszy, 1997). There is evidence that DHEA supplementation may increase muscle mass and

strength and enhance immune function, especially in older individuals (Nestler, Barlascini, Clore, & Blackard, 1988; Yen, Morales, & Khorram, 1995). Nissen et al. (1996) randomly assigned 41 males to one of six groups among three levels of HMB ingestion (0, 1½ or 3 g·d^{-1}) and two levels of protein intake (117 or 175 g·d^{-1}). Subjects lifted weights 12 hr·d^{-1} 3 d·wk^{-1} for 3 weeks. HMB ingestion resulted in decreased proteolysis (measured by urinary [3-methylhistidine], a marker for skeletal muscle breakdown) and increased weight lifted. In a separate group, subjects consumed either 0 or 3 g HMB·d^{-1} and lifted weights 2–3 hr·d^{-1} 6 d·wk^{-1} for 7 wks. An increase in fat-free mass was reported in subjects who consumed HMB. They concluded that consumption of 12 or 3 g of HMB·d^{-1} while weight training can decrease exercise-induced proteolytic activity and increase muscle function. Thus, preliminary evidence tends to support an antiproteolytic action of HMB. A recent report that skeletal muscle protein synthesis was unaffected by a high HMB dose in lambs argues against a significant anabolic aspect to the action of HMB (Papet et al., 1997).

Legality and safety. Androstenedione is banned by most sports-governing bodies. Use of HMB is currently not banned. The effect of long-term use of these supplements remains to be determined.

Energy Metabolism

Creatine Monohydrate

One of the most popular ergogenic aids in current use is creatine monohydrate. Total reported sales of creatine in the United States for 1997 were $3 billion (SKW Trostburg, 1998). Public endorsement of creatine by professional athletes such as Mark McGwire of the St. Louis Cardinals and Greg

Foster of the Utah Jazz contributes to this popularity. Demographic data obtained in a recent cross-sectional survey revealed typical users of creatine to be male weight lifters between the ages of 21 and 35 (Johnson, 1998). Recent reviews by Greenhaff (1995), Balsom, Söderlund, and Ekblom (1994), and M. H. Williams, Kreider, and Branch (1999) are sources for additional information on the biochemistry and ergogenicity of creatine supplementation.

Biochemistry. Creatine is a nitrogenous amine found in animal dietary products. It is also synthesized from the amino acids glycine, arginine, and methionine. Vegetarians rely on *de novo* biosynthesis for their daily needs, which is ~2 $g \cdot d^{-1}$. Ingested creatine crosses the intestinal lumen, enters the bloodstream intact, and is absorbed by various tissues. A 70 kg male has a total creatine content of ~120 g, 95% of which is located in the skeletal muscles, especially the Type IIb fast glycolytic fibers (Casey, Constantin-Teodosiu, Howell, Hultman, & Greenhaff, 1996). Creatine is an osmotically active substance, capable of pulling water into the cell. Once in the cell, ~60–70% of the creatine is phosphorylated and exists as phosphocreatine (PCr), which is unable to exit the cell. PCr, the energy substrate for the ATP-PCr energy system, undergoes rapid dephosphorylation in order to rephosphorylate ADP to generate ATP during high-intensity, short-duration ($\leq$ 10-sec) anaerobic work. Thus, creatine serves an important role as an intracellular "phosphate shuttle" (Balsom et al., 1994; Greenhaff, 1995).

Ergogenic mechanism. Intramuscular [creatine] is ~120 $mmol \cdot kg$ dry mass ^{1} in the average individual. Increases in intramuscular [creatine] of 20 to 35% have been reported following a "loading" phase in which the individual ingests ~20–30 $g \cdot d^{-1}$ (4–6 doses of 5 $g \cdot d^{-1}$), although there is interindividual vari-

ation in response to creatine supplementation (Greenhaff, 1995). Lower dose loading regimens of longer duration (e.g. ~2 $g \cdot d^{-1}$ for ~28-d) have also been reported to increase muscle [creatine] (Hultman, Söderland, Timmons, Cederblad, & Greenhaff, 1996). Creatine ingestion with carbohydrate may facilitate creatine uptake, an observation that supports the involvement of an insulin-mediated mechanism (Green, Hultman, MacDonald, Sewell, & Greenhaff, 1996). There is also evidence that caffeine may inhibit creatine uptake (Vandenberghe et al., 1996). An increase in intramuscular [creatine] following supplementation would provide increased [PCr] as energy substrate for single and repetitive high-intensity, short-duration work tasks.

Evidence of ergogenic effect. Although the existence and ergogenic potential of creatine have long been known, this issue has only recently received scientific study. Although there is much anecdotal and research support for the efficacy of creatine supplementation, the scientific literature is not unanimous, and the issue remains somewhat equivocal. In a recent review of the literature, M. H. Williams, Kreider, and Branch (1999) reported that creatine supplementation improved performance in many, but not all, studies of repetitive cycling tasks of $\leq$ 30-sec in duration and also in many, but not all, studies of isotonic and isokinetic resistive exercise tasks. There is more support for an ergogenic effect following supplementation in laboratory-based performance tasks than in field studies of running and swimming performance. Consistently reported increases in body mass of 1–2 kg (~2.5%) following short-term supplementation are related in part to water retention due to the osmotic effect of creatine. The issue of whether creatine actually stimulates lean tissue growth is still being studied. Increased body mass associated with creatine supplementation may actually impair performance in activities such as swimming (Mujika, Chatard, Lacoste, Barale, & Geyssant, 1996). Increased muscle [PCr] may in theory attenuate the accumulation of lactate, buffer acidity, and decrease reliance on glycolysis. There is some support for improved performance in more prolonged (~30 to 150-sec) anaerobic tasks that rely primarily on glycolysis following creatine supplementation. However, considerably less support exists for improved performance in predominantly aerobic (> 150-sec) tasks into which high-intensity "interval"-type exercise was incorporated. Longer duration tasks have less reliance on the ATP-PCr energy system, thus explaining the diminishing effectiveness for creatine supplementation with tasks of longer duration.

Safety. There have been anecdotal reports of muscle cramping and strains associated with creatine supplementation. Creatine is nonenzymatically converted to creatinine, which is excreted from the body via the kidneys. The effect of chronic use of creatine on renal function remains unknown. Muscle [creatine] and blood [creatine] and [creatinine] return to baseline levels ~4 weeks following cessation of supplementation (Vandenberghe et al., 1997). There are currently no data on health-related outcomes following chronic (months to years) creatine supplementation.

Legality. Creatine can be legally purchased from both health food retailers and mail-order suppliers. In 1999, creatine was determined to be a food by the Medical Commission of the International Olympic Committee. It is commercially available in powder, gel, liquid, pill, or candy form. Although not illegal, the use of creatine is not unanimously endorsed. *USA Today* surveyed 115 professional sports teams regarding creatine use. Of 71 teams responding, 21 officially disapproved of the use of creatine in

their organizations. Sixteen other organizations formally approved of creatine use, with 24 actually providing creatine to their athletes (Strauss, 1998). A similar divergence of opinion exists in collegiate programs.

Acid/Base Regulation

Sodium Bicarbonate (NaHCO₃)

The ingestion of $NaHCO_3$ to control acidity during intense exercise was first studied in the 1930s and has recently received renewed attention by both athletes and researchers as a potential ergogenic mechanism (McNaughton et al., 1999). The following section will summarize the biochemistry, evidence of ergogenicity, safety, and legality of $NaHCO_3$ loading. For a more complete critical review of $NaHCO_3$ loading, the interested reader is referred to the meta-analysis on this topic by Matson and Tran (1993) and the brief review by Linderman and Gosselink (1994).

Biochemistry and ergogenic mechanism. Anaerobic glycolysis is a major source of ATP during intense exercise. The balanced summary equation for glycolysis (with glucose as the substrate) is presented below. The incomplete combustion of the 6-carbon glucose molecule generates two 3-carbon lactate molecules and two protons plus two ATP. Increased reliance on anaerobic glycolysis results in decreased pH due to accumulation of increased H^+ associated with lactate production.

$$C_6H_{12}O_6 \text{ (glucose)} + 2ADP + 2P_i \rightarrow 2C_3H_6O_3 \text{ (lactate)} + 2H^+ + 2ATP + 2H_2O$$

Although the understanding of fatigue mechanisms is not complete, it is known that decreased intracellular pH during intense exercise inhibits the action of key regulatory glycolytic and oxidative enzymes. Furthermore, increased acidity also inhibits both the release of Ca^{++} from the lateral sacs of the sarcoplasmic reticulum and depolarization of α-motor neurons (Hultman & Sahlin, 1980). Under conditions of metabolic acidosis, the bicarbonate (HCO_3^-) anion readily accepts a proton (H^+) to form carbonic acid (H_2CO_3), the weak acid in the carbonic acid/bicarbonate buffer system. H_2CO_3 then dissociates into H_2O and CO_2 to maintain pH within the physiologic range. Theoretically, $NaHCO_3$ 'loading' enhances the capability of this buffer system by providing more HCO_3^- anion to buffer H^+.

$CO_2 + H_2O : H_2CO_3 : H^+ + HCO_3^-$

Evidence of ergogenic effect. According to Matson and Tran (1993), most studies have used a loading dose of 300 mg·kg of body mass^{-1} 1 to 2 hr prior to performance. Their meta-analysis revealed that $NaHCO_3$ ingestion generally improved performance in 19 of 35 studies meeting their inclusion criteria, with a mean effect size 0.44 standard deviation units better than the placebo trial. Linderman and Gosselink (1994) point out that $NaHCO_3$ loading appears to be less effective in improving work or power output. $NaHCO_3$ loading appears to delay the onset of fatigue during exhaustive exercise of ~2 to 5 minutes in duration, but does not appear to be effective in improving performance in tasks that rely on either the ATP-PCr energy system (≤ 1 min) or oxidative phosphorylation (≥ 30 min) (Linderman & Gosselink, 1994; McNaughton, 1992).

Safety. Although a bicarbonate loading dose of 300 mg·kg^{-1} poses no known threat to health, gastrointestinal distress, diarrhea, cramps, and bloating are consistently reported symptoms from both experimental (Linderman & Gosselink, 1994) and anecdotal sources.

Legality. $NaHCO_3$ loading is not banned by the IOC and other sports-governing bodies. However, a highly alkaline urine sample may mask other substances that are banned. Therefore, an athlete who loads with $NaHCO_3$ may be suspected of use of an illegal agent until he or she can produce a normally acidic urine specimen (Linderman & Gosselink, 1994).

Oxygen Transport and Endurance Performance

Blood/Erythropoietin Doping

The practice of increasing circulating mass of red blood cells (blood 'doping') received attention in the 1970s, with rumors of the practice by endurance athletes in the 1972 and 1976 Olympiads. The hormone erythropoietin (Epo), which is secreted by the kidneys in response to hypoxia, stimulates production of red blood cells. Advances in genetic engineering technology have made recombinant human Epo (rHuEpo) available, which is used clinically to treat anemia in hemodialysis patients. Rumors of rHuEpo use by some endurance athletes to increase circulating red cell mass have abounded for the last 10 to 15 years. The recent Tour de France scandal involving rHuEpo possession by worldclass cyclists serves to substantiate these rumors (Abt, 1998). The interested reader is referred to the American College of Sports Medicine position stand on blood doping as an ergogenic aid (Sawka et al., 1996).

Physiologic and ergogenic mechanism. One of the determinants of maximum oxygen consumption (∇O_{2max}) is the transport capacity of oxygen in arterial blood. A gram of hemoglobin (Hb) can bind 1.34 ml of oxygen. Theoretically, an increase in [Hb] and circulating red blood cell mass by doping would increase the content of oxygen in arterial blood and enhance the body's ability to transport oxygen to peripheral exercising muscle. Blood doping is performed by either autologous or homologous infusion of blood. In autologous blood transfusions, several units (~450 ml) of the athlete's own blood are first removed at different times with ~2 months between phlebotomies. Following centrifugation, the red blood cells are harvested, frozen in glycerol, and reinfused at a later date well after the athlete has recovered from the last phlebotomy. Homologous transfusion of another individual's blood is less commonly used. Subcutaneous administration of rHuEpo stimulates a production of red blood cells by the bone marrow, resulting in a gradual increase in total circulating red blood cell mass that is maintained as long as rHuEpo doping continues (Sawka et al., 1996).

Evidence of ergogenic effect. In clinical populations, rHuEpo administration increases cardiorespiratory fitness. Following blood or rHuEpo doping by athletes, which results in an increase in VO_{2max}, a constant rate of power output would result in decreased physiologic stress (i.e., lower [lactate], lower heart rate response, and higher pH). In a study of national class distance runners, Buick, Gledhill, Fronsoe, Spriet, & Meyers (1980) reported a 6.5% increase in VO_{2max} one day following autologous blood reinfusion. The time to exhaustion at 95% of baseline VO_{2max} was increased by 20%. In addition, time to exhaustion remained higher after [Hb] had returned to baseline, an indication that these already conditioned athletes were able to train at a higher intensity following blood doping. There is also evidence that blood doping may improve thermoregulatory function (Sawka et al., 1996).

Safety. Increased hematocrit and viscosity following blood and/or rHuEpo doping may increase the chance of thrombosis formation, which could result in myocardial infarction or stroke. Unsupervised phlebotomy/transfusion may increase the risk of infection.

Legality. Blood and rHuEpo doping are considered unethical by the American College of Sports Medicine (Sawka et al., 1996) and banned by sports-governing bodies. These practices are difficult to detect.

Stimulants

Amphetamines, Ephedrine, and Other Sympathomimetic Agents

Amphetamines are a pharmacologic class whose parent compound is β-phenylethylamine. Amphetamines are chemically related to the catecholamines, but lack the meta- and para-hydroxyl groups on the benzene ring of the catecholamines. Amphetamines do not directly interact with α and β adrenergic receptors, but exert an indirect influence on catecholamine metabolism. Thus, amphetamines are also known as "sympathomimetic amines" (Conlee, 1991). Ephedrine is also a sympathomimetic agent that appears in many over-the-counter products for treating cold symptoms and asthma. Ephedrine is also found in weight-loss medications (e.g., Herbal Phen-Fen) and in herbal supplements (e.g., Chinese Ephedra or Ma Huang).

Biochemistry and ergogenic mechanism. Amphetamines stimulate the release of norepinephrine from sympathetic nerves. Norepinephrine in turn stimulates the α-adrenergic receptors of arterioles, causing vasoconstriction and increased arterial blood pressure. Amphetamines also stimulate the hypothalamus as well as pleasure centers in the brain, elevating mood and increasing resistance to fatigue by either enhancing the release of dopamine and/or inhibiting dopamine uptake or degradation (Conlee, 1991). Effects of amphetamine ingestion include increased alertness, a "masking" of fatigue, and enhanced performance of certain motor tasks.

Evidence of ergogenicity. Little research on the ergogenicity of amphetamines has been reported in recent years, which is consistent with the general decline of amphetamine usage (Conlee, 1991). Two early studies of the effects of amphetamine use on performance reported conflicting findings. G. M. Smith and Beecher (1959) reported in a series of studies that amphetamine sulfate ingestion (0.2 mg·kg^{-1}) improved performance in highly trained swimmers, runners, and discus throwers/shot putters. On the other hand, Karpovich (1959) reported no effect of either 10 mg or 20 mg doses of amphetamine sulfate on various swimming and running tasks in college-aged males. In the 1970s, metamphetamine ingestion (10 mg) was reported to increase time to exhaustion at 90 to 95% of VO_{2max} and blood [lactate] in two champion cyclists (Wyndham, Rogers, Benade, & Strydom, 1971). Chandler and Blair (1980) reported improvements in knee extension strength, acceleration, and anaerobic capacity following Dexedrine ingestion (0.21 mg·kg^{-1}). Time to exhaustion and maximal blood [lactate] were increased, suggesting enhanced resistance to fatigue. They also reported considerable interindividual variation in responsiveness. Amphetamine ingestion has not been reported to increase VO_{2max} (Chandler & Blair, 1980; Wyndham et al., 1971). Ephedrine is reported to exert no effect on such variables as VO_{2max}, ventilation, submaximal or maximal heart rate, blood pressure, or performance time (Clemons & Crosby, 1993; Gillies et al., 1996).

Health concerns. Use of amphetamines has been associated with a host of side effects such as tremors, irritability, formation of ventricular dysrhythmias, hypertension, gastrointestinal distress, and hallucinations. Chronic use may lead to weight loss, addiction, and psychotic behavior (Conlee, 1991). There is also concern that "masking" of fatigue following amphetamine ingestion may predispose athletes to injury in unfavorable conditions such as a hyperthermic environment.

Legality. In 1972, amphetamines were banned by the Medical Commission of the International Olympics Committee. They are considered to be stimulants, and their use is prohibited by the IOC and various other sports-governing bodies. The IOC also prohibits the use of ephedrine. Athletes using over-the-counter cold medications and/or herbal preparations risk disqualification because these agents may contain ephedrine.

Caffeine

Caffeine (1,3,7-trimethylxanthine) is found in coffee, tea, soft drinks, chocolate, and some over-the-counter medications (e.g., Vibram® 200 mg·tablet^{-1}). It is estimated that the average individual consumes ~200 mg of caffeine·d^{-1} (J. H. Williams, 1991; M. H. Williams, 1996). The following section provides an overview of the biochemistry, ergogenic mechanisms, and ergogenic potential of caffeine consumption. For additional information, the reader is referred to reviews by Dodd, Herb, and Powers (1993), Spriet (1995), Tarnopolsky (1994), and J. H. Williams (1991).

Biochemistry and ergogenic mechanism. Caffeine facilitates the release of epinephrine from the adrenal medulla, which stimulates vasodilation, lipolysis, glycogenolysis, and bronchodilation. Increased lipolysis would theoretically increase the availability of free fatty acids as an energy substrate, resulting in a possible "sparing" of muscle glycogen. "Glycogen sparing" is the most studied potential ergogenic mechanism associated with caffeine use. Caffeine inhibits the enzyme phosphodiesterase, which would potentiate the action of 3',5'-cAMP, important in the conversion of phosphorylase and hormone-sensitive lipase to their active forms. Caffeine also facilitates calcium release from the lateral sacs of the sarcoplasmic reticulum and increases myofibrillar and troponin C subunit sensitivity to calcium (Dodd et al., 1993; Nelig & Debry, 1994; Tarnopolsky, 1994; J. H. Williams, 1991). Caffeine increases diuresis due to inhibition of arginine vasopressin (antidiuretic hormone) (J. H. Williams, 1991; M. H. Williams, 1996). Caffeine is a central nervous system stimulant and a competitive antagonist of the receptor for adenosine, a CNS depressant. Recent research attention has turned to the neural effect of caffeine, as well as the direct effect of caffeine in muscle force development, as potential ergogenic mechanisms (Dodd et al.).

Evidence of ergogenicity. Caffeine ingestion of 3–13 mg·kg body mass^{-1} appears to enhance both prolonged endurance performance and high-intensity short-duration exercise performed in a laboratory setting (Spriet, 1995). Improvements in endurance times of 22 to 23% have been reported following ingestion of caffeine doses of 3 to 9 mg·kg^{-1} (Graham & Spriet, 1995; Jackman, Wendling, Friars, & Graham, 1996; Pasman, van Baak, Jeukendrup, & de Haan, 1995). At least one study failed to report dose-response with regard to a higher caffeine dose (Pasman et al.). Although increased [glycerol], [free fatty acids], decreased RER (the ratio of carbon dioxide production—∇CO_2—to oxygen consumption—∇CO_2) have been observed during endurance exercise following caffeine ingestion (all of which are suggestive of increased β-oxidation), paradoxical increases in blood [lactate] (suggestive of increased glycogenolysis) have also been reported (Graham & Spriet; Jackman et al.; Pasman et al.). Thus, the glycogen-sparing mechanism remains to be fully elucidated. A recent report indicated that caffeine did not improve performance in a hyperthermic environment (Cohen et al., 1996). The possibility exists that the diuretic effect of caffeine may adversely affect thermoregulation.

Safety. Controversy exists in the epidemiologic literature concerning the association of caffeine consumption with health-related outcomes. Some studies have reported caffeine consumption to have been associated with many health-related outcomes (e.g., cystic breast tumors, female reproduction dysfunction, hypertension, heart disease, altered lipid metabolism), whereas others report no significant associations. It is generally agreed that moderate caffeine consumption (i.e., 200–300 mg·d^{-1} in 12–18 ounces of coffee) poses no health risks to most individuals and is a dose that should result in urinary [caffeine] excretion below the IOC limit of 12 µg·ml^{-1} (J. H. Williams, Wendling, Friars, & Graham, 1996).

Legality. Caffeine is not a prohibited substance. However, enhanced performance has been observed following caffeine doses that result in urinary [caffeine] excretion below the IOC limit of 12 µg·ml^{-1} (Spriet, 1995).

Ginseng

Many plant extracts are claimed to have medicinal and/or ergogenic properties. Ginseng is one of many commercially available herbal supplements that is purported to have ergogenic potential. Ginseng has been used for thousands of years as a purported ergogenic aid and aphrodisiac. For additional information on ginseng, the interested reader is referred to reviews by Bahrke and Morgan (1994) and Ng and Yeung (1986).

Biochemistry and proposed ergogenic mechanism. According to Ng and Yeung (1986), ginseng is a generic term for many compounds derived from the plant family *Araliaceae*. There are several forms of ginseng available in commercial products including Chinese or Korean (*Panax ginseng*), American (*Panax quinquefolium*), Japanese (*Panax japonicum*), and Russian/Siberian (*Eleutherococcus senticosus*). These compounds may contain specific substances referred to as glycosides, ginseng saponins, or ginsenosides. Ginsenosides are purported to facilitate energy metabolism, prolong performance, delay the onset of fatigue, and increase resistance to stress, possibly via upregulation of the hypothalmic-pituitary-adrenal axis (Brekhman & Dardymov, 1969). It has also been suggested that ginseng may enhance tissue oxygen extraction and utilization, mitochondrial metabolism, and myocardial function (Asano, Takahaski, Kugo, & Kuboyama, 1986).

Evidence of ergogenic effect. The ergogenic benefits of ginseng and ginseng-containing products are extolled in advertisements, but the actual evidence of ergogenicity is largely anecdotal and not supported by research findings. The majority of well-controlled (double-blind placebo-control) studies do not support the ergogenicity of ginseng in improving submaximal or maximal endurance performance (Allen, McLung, Nelson, & Welsch, 1998; Dowling et al., 1996; Engels & Wirth, 1997; Morris et al., 1996).

Safety and legality. Because ginseng is classified by the Food and Drug Administration as a food instead of a drug, it is widely available in health food/nutrition stores. There is evidence that some ginseng products also contain ephedrine, a banned stimulant (Cui, Garle, Eneroth, & Bjorkhem, 1994), which may be related to reports of hypertension, nervousness, and insomnia associated with ginseng consumption (Beltz & Doering, 1993).

Adrenergic Blockers and CNS Depressants

β-*adrenergic Blocking Agents*

β-adrenergic blocking agents, or beta-blockers, are a class of pharmacologic agents developed in the 1960s that compete with norepinephrine and epinephrine for binding at

β_1 and β_2 adrenergic receptors on cell membranes. These agents are clinically prescribed primarily as antihypertensives to reduce myocardial afterload and prophylactically postmyocardial infarction to reduce myocardial oxygen demand. Cardioselective β-blockers preferentially block the β_1 receptor, whereas nonselective agents block either β_1 and β_2 receptors (M. H. Williams, 1991).

Physiology and ergogenic mechanism. β_1 receptors in cardiac tissue are stimulated by norepinephrine, resulting in increased inotropic (force of contraction) and chronotropic (rate of contraction) response. β_1 receptor stimulation in adipose tissue by epinephrine results in increased lipolysis. The β_2 adrenergic receptor is also stimulated by epinephrine and results in increased glycogenolysis, bronchodilation, and vasodilation. Beta-blockers may reduce performance-related anxiety. Therefore, these agents may be ergogenic for certain performers (e.g., golfers, marksmen, archers, musicians, dancers) for whom fine motor control and low state anxiety are essential for success. Early research focused on the theory that beta-blockers would upregulate β_1 and β_2 receptor density, supporting the theory that discontinuation of beta blockade may result in an exaggerated sympathetic response to exercise (Kelly, 1985; Wilmore, Ewy, et al., 1985; Wilmore, Freund, et al., 1985). However, beta-blockers are now considered to be ergolytic for endurance performance tasks due to the well-documented attenuations in cardiorespiratory response (i.e., reduced heart rate, ventilation, peripheral blood flow, and thermoregulation) and impairments in energy substrate availability (i.e., hepatic and muscle glycolysis, lipolysis) (M. H. Williams, 1991).

Evidence of ergogenicity. Beta-blockers do not appear to impair performance of high-intensity, short-duration (<10 sec) activities requiring strength and anaerobic power. However, high-intensity, more prolonged tasks

(~30–60 sec) appear to be negatively affected by beta blockade because there is a greater reliance on glycolysis. Beta-blockers have been shown to decrease tremors and anxiety and are of potential ergogenic value for low-intensity fine-motor precision tasks (e.g., marksmanship, archery). Exercise heart-rate response is decreased during beta blockade, but a compensatory increase in stroke volume maintains cardiac output. Nonselective agents appear to impair $\dot{V}O_{2max}$ and glycolysis to a greater extent than do cardioselective agents, whereas lipolysis is similarly attenuated with use of both types of agents (Jilka et al., 1988). Beta blockade may decrease cutaneous blood flow, which adversely affects thermoregulation. These physiologic consequences of beta blockade, in addition to lethargy associated with the use of some agents, impairs endurance performance (M. H. Williams, 1991).

Safety. Beta-blockers may adversely alter lipid profiles (i.e., decreased [HDL-C], increased [Triglycerides]). The hypertensive power athlete (e.g., heavy weight lifter or body builder) who has been prescribed a beta-blocker should understand the hemodynamic effects of static (isometric) exercise (i.e., increased total peripheral resistance and exacerbated arterial blood pressure response).

Legality. Beta-blockers are Prohibited by the IOC and the NCAA.

Ethanol

Ethanol (alcohol, C_2H_5OH) is a social drug that is consumed by many individuals. This section will provide a brief overview of the biochemistry and metabolism, evidence of ergogenicity, safety, and legality of ethanol as an ergogenic agent. For further information, the interested reader is referred to reviews by Reilly (1997) and M. H. Williams (1991, 1992).

Biochemistry. The glycolytic intermediate pyruvate has three major fates: (a) reduction to lactate, catalyzed by lactate dehydrogenase, (b) oxidative decarboxylation to acetyl CoEnzyme A, catalyzed by the pyruvate dehydrogenase complex, and (c) anaerobic decarboxylation/reduction, catalyzed by the enzymes pyruvate decarboxylase and alcohol dehydrogenase. The latter pathway, which occurs in fermentation of grain by yeast, produces ethanol, which has been known and consumed by individuals for thousands of years. Ethanol is water-soluble and quickly diffuses from the small intestine to the blood. Ethanol is catabolized primarily in the liver, where it is oxidized to acetaldehyde through the catalytic action of alcohol dehydrogenase. Acetaldehyde is subsequently oxidized by acetaldehyde dehydrogenase to acetate, which can either enter the tricarboxylic acid (Krebs) cycle for ATP production or serve as a building block for *de novo* synthesis of various biomolecules. Because catabolism of ethanol generates NADH H^+ for ATP synthesis by the mitochondrial electron transport chain, it is considered a food as well as a drug, with energy content of 7 kcal (~29 kJ)·gram^{-1}. The effects of acute and chronic ethanol consumption are most apparent in tissues with the greatest blood perfusion and the greatest uptake of ethanol, that is, brain, lungs, liver, kidney (Reilly, 1997).

Metabolic effects of ethanol. Ethanol is metabolized at a rate of ~100 mg·kg of body mass^{-1}·hr^{-1}. Although ethanol is an energy-containing substance, its role in energy metabolism is negligible. The most immediate acute effect of ethanol is as a central nervous system depressant. Ethanol depresses activity in the reticular activating system, which is responsible for physiologic arousal. Ethanol slows the velocity of neural action potentials and blocks the synthesis and release of acetylcholine, the neurotransmitter released at the neuromuscular synapse. Following ethanol consumption, there is a transient increase, followed by a decrease in central norepinephrine function. Because mood state is determined in part by brain catecholamines, the initial ethanol-related euphoria, followed by depression, is associated with this fluctuation. Ethanol also decreases the cerebral uptake of glucose, the main energy substrate of the brain, a decrease that is probably related to mental fatigue and loss of ability to concentrate following ethanol consumption (Reilly, 1997).

Evidence of ergogenicity. It has been suggested that the anti-inhibitory, antitremor, and anxiolytic action of ethanol may be potential ergogenic mechanisms. If so, competitors in target sports such as archery and shooting may benefit from ethanol consumption. Reilly and Halliday (1985) reported that improved holding time and loose (i.e., arrow release) were observed in archers with a blood alcohol content (BAC) of 0.02%, but noted that a BAC of 0.05% was deleterious to performance. Tasks requiring rapid reaction time, eye-hand coordination, complex information processing leading to a quick decision, and complex movement patterns are adversely affected by ethanol consumption (American College of Sports Medicine, 1982; Collins, Schroeder, Gilson, & Guedry, 1971; Moskowitz, Burns, & Williams, 1985; Reilly, 1997). Ethanol consumption on the day before competition may decrease muscle [glycogen] (Reilly). For this reason, the prudent course of action prior to competition is either abstinence or moderation, especially for endurance athletes who rely on glycogen stores for optimal performance (M. H. Williams, 1991). Reports of the effects of ethanol consumption immediately prior to submaximal exercise are inconsistent, but there are reports of higher VO_2 at a standard power output, due possibly to decreased mechanical efficiency. There is general agreement that moderate doses exert no effect on maximal cardiovascular response (i.e., VO_{2max}, V_{Emax}, Q_{max}, HR_{max}), but that high doses are clearly detrimental to performance. Ethanol is a diuretic and may compromise thermoregulatory function in a hot environment by inhibiting the release of arginine vasopressin (antidiuretic hormone) from the posterior pituitary gland. Ethanol consumption is also ill-advised in ambient cold because it increases cutaneous blood flow and exacerbates heat loss (Reilly, 1997; M. H. Williams, 1991).

Safety. Although moderate use (1–2 drinks·d^{-1}) has been associated with reduced mortality from cardiovascular disease and stroke (Klatsky, Armstron, & Friedman, 1989; Stampfer, Colditz, Willett, Speizer, & Hennekens, 1988), excessive use is associated with osteoporosis, various cancers, hypertension, cardiomyopathy, and fetal alcohol syndrome (Diamond, Satiel, Lunzer, Wilkinson, & Posen, 1989; Longnecker, Berlin, Orza, & Chambers, 1988).

Legality. Ethanol consumption is banned in sports such as archery where it may be ergogenic. The use of ethanol is not banned in endurance activity, but it is not ergogenic and may indeed be ergolytic to performance. For optimal health and performance, either moderation or abstinence is recommended. Athletes may want to consider abstaining from ethanol consumption on the day before competition.

Summary

Several contemporary ergogenic agents have been discussed in this chapter. Some agents have been shown in well-controlled studies to improve performance. Other purported ergogenic agents receive endorsement from anecdotal testimonials that have not been corroborated by controlled research. The association of adverse health-related outcomes with use of some ergogenic aids justifies a ban on use of these agents. The use of others is currently unregulated. Aside from the legality of a given substance, the athlete must also contend with the ethics of a decision to use ergogenic aids.

Throughout history, athletes have consumed many different substances in pursuit of enhanced performance. The list of agents discussed in this chapter is not exhaustive. Athletes of the future will be confronted with current and new substances that have real or purported ergogenic mechanisms. According to M. H. Williams (1989), appropriately conducted ergogenic research should include (a) a double-blind, placebo-control repeated-measures design, (b) investigation of differential doses to identify dose-response, (c) subjects who are representative of the parent athlete population, (d) dosages and ingestion schedules comparable to the ones actually used by the athletes, and (e) an appropriate performance measure for the group being studied. Responsibility ultimately belongs to the individual to be educated and aware of the efficacy, legality, health-related consequences, and ethics of use of a given ergogenic agent (United States Olympic Committee, 1996).

References

Abt, S. (1998). Top team expelled by Tour de France over drug charges. *The New York Times*. July 18, A1, C2.

Allen, J. D., McLung, J., Nelson, A. G., & Welsch, M. (1998). Ginseng supplementation does not enhance healthy young adults' peak aerobic exercise performance. *Journal of the American College of Nutrition, 17*, 462–466.

American College of Sports Medicine. (1982). Position statement on the use of alcohol in sports. *Medicine and Science in Sports and Exercise, 14*, ix–x.

Asano, K., Takahaski, T., Kugo, H., & Kuboyama, M. (1986). Effects of *Eleutherococcus sentocosus Maxim* on physical performance and resources in maximal and submaximal work. In *New Data on Eleutherococcus: Proceedings of the Second International Symposium on Eleutherococcus M. 1984* (pp. 229–239). Vladivostok: Far East Science Center, USSR Academy of Sciences.

Bahrke, M. S., & Morgan, W. P. (1994). Evaluation of the ergogenic properties of ginseng. *Sports Medicine, 18*, 229–248.

Balsom, P., Söderlund, K., & Ekblom, B. (1994). Creatine in humans with special reference to creatine supplementation. *Sports Medicine, 18*, 268–280.

Beltz, S. D., & Doering, P. L. (1993). Efficacy of nutritional supplements used by athletes. *Clinical Pharmacology, 12*, 900–908.

Bhasin, S., Storer, T. W., Berman, N., Callegari, C., Clevenger, B., Phillips, J., Brunnell, T. J., Tricker, R., Shirazi, A., & Caseburi, R. (1996). The effects of supraphysiologic doses of testosterone on muscle size and strength in normal men. *New England Journal of Medicine, 335*(1), 1–7.

Bradley, C. A., & Sodeman, T. M. (1990). Human growth hormone: Its use and abuse. *Clinical Laboratory Medicine, 10*, 473–477.

Brekhman, I. I., & Dardymov, I. V. (1969). New substances of plant origin which increase nonspecific resistance. *Annual Review of Pharmacology, 9*, 419–428.

Buckley, W. E., Yesalis, C. E., Friedl, K. E., Anderson, W. A., Streit, A. L., & Wright, J. E. (1988). Estimated prevalence of anabolic steroid use among male high school seniors. *Journal of the American Medical Association, 260*, 3441–3445.

Buick, F. J., Gledhill, N., Fronsoe, A. B., Spriet, L., & Meyers, E. C. (1980). Effect of induced erythrocythemia on aerobic work capacity. *Journal of Applied Physiology, 48*, 636–642.

Cable, N. T. (1997). Anabolic-androgenic steroids; ergogenic and cardiovascular effects. In T. Reilly & M. Orme (Eds.), *The clinical pharmacology of sport and exercise: Proceedings of the Esteve Foundation Symposium VII* (pp. 135–141). Amsterdam: Elsevier Science B. V.

Casey, A., Constantin-Teodosiu, D., Howell, S., Hultman, E., & Greenhaff, P. L. (1996). Creatine ingestion favorably affects performance and muscle metabolism during maximal exercise in humans. *American Journal of Physiology, 271*, E31–E37.

Chandler, J. V., & Blair, S. N. (1980). The effect of amphetamines on selected physiological components related to athletic success. *Medicine and Science in Sports and Exercise, 12*(1), 65–69.

Clemons, J. M., & Crosby, S. L. (1993). Cardiopulmonary and subjective effects of a 60 mg dose of pseudoephedrine on graded treadmill exercise. *Journal of Sports Medicine & Physical Fitness, 33*, 405–412.

Cohen, B. S., Nelson, A. G., Prevost, M. C., Thompson, G. D., Marx, B. D., & Morris, G. S. (1996). Effects of caffeine ingestion on endurance racing in heat and humidity. *European Journal of Applied Physiology, 73*(3–4), 358–363.

Collins, W. E., Schroeder, D. J., Gilson, R. D., & Guedry, F. E. (1971). Effects of alcohol ingestion on tracking performance during angular acceleration. *Journal of Applied Psychology, 6*, 559–563.

Conlee, R. K. (1991). Amphetamine, caffeine and cocaine. In D. R. Lamb & M. H. Williams (Eds.), *Perspectives in exercise science and sports medicine. Volume 4. Ergogenics: enhancement of performance in exercise and sport* (pp. 285–332). Dubuque, IA: WCM/Brown and Benchmark.

Cui, J., Garle, M., Eneroth, P., & Bjorkhem, I. (1994). What do commercial ginseng preparations contain? *Lancet, 344*, 134.

Diamond, T., Satiel, D., Lunzer, M., Wilkinson, M., & Posen, S. (1989). Ethanol reduced bone formation and may cause osteoporosis. *Annals of the Journal of Medicine, 86*, 282–287.

Dodd, S. L., Herb, R. A., & Powers, S. K. (1993). Caffeine and exercise performance: An update. *Sports Medicine, 15*(1), 14–23.

Dowling, E. A., Dedondo, D. R., Branch, J. D., Jones, S., McNabb, G., & Williams, M. H. (1996). The effect of *Eleutherococcus senticosus Maxim L* supplementation on physiological responses to submaximal and maximal exercise. *Medicine and Science in Sports and Exercise, 28*, 482–489.

DuRant, R. H., Escobedo, L. G., & Heath, G. W. (1995). Anabolic-steroid use, strength training and multiple drug use among adolescents in the United States, *Pediatrics, 96*, 23–28.

Elashoff, J. D., Jacknow, A. D., Shain, S. G., & Braunstein, G. D. (1991). Effects of anabolic-androgenic steroids on muscular strength. *Annals of Internal Medicine, 115*(5), 387–393.

Engels, H. J., & Wirth, J. C. (1997). No ergogenic effects of ginseng (*Panex ginseng C. A. Meyer*) during graded maximal aerobic exercise. *Journal of the American Dietetic Association, 97*, 1110–1115.

Evans, N. A. (1997). Gym and tonic: A profile of 100 male steroid users. *British Journal of Sports Medicine, 31*, 54–58.

Fogelholm, G. M., Naveri, H. K., Kiilavuori, K. T., & Harkonen, M. H. (1993). Low-dose amino acid supplementation: No effects on serum human growth hormone and insulin in male weightlifters. *International Journal of Sport Nutrition, 3*, 290–297.

Friedl, K. E., Dettori, J. R., Hannan, C. J., Patience, T. H., & Plymate, S. R. (1991). Comparison of the effects of a high dose of testosterone and 19-nortestosterone to a replacement dose of testosterone on strength and body composition in normal men. *Journal of Steroid Biochemistry and Molecular Biology, 40*, 607–612.

Gillies, H., Derman, W. E., Noakes, T. D., Smith, P., Evans, A., & Gabriels, G. (1996). Pseudoephedrine is without ergogenic effects during prolonged exercise. *Journal of Applied Physiology, 81*, 2611–2617.

Graham, T. E., & Spriet, L. L. (1995). Metabolic, catecholamine, and exercise performance responses to various doses of caffeine. *Journal of Applied Physiology, 78*(3), 867–874.

Green, A. L., Hultman, E., MacDonald, I. A., Sewell, D. A., & Greenhaff, P. L. (1996). Carbohydrate feeding augments skeletal muscle creatine accumulation during creatine supplementation in humans. *American Journal of Physiology, 271*, E821–E826.

Greenhaff, P. L. (1995). Creatine and its application as

an ergogenic aid. *International Journal of Sport Nutrition, 5*, S100–S110.

Hansen, P. A., Han, D. H., Nolte, L. A., Chen, M., & Holloszy, J. O. (1997). DHEA protects against visceral obesity and muscle insulin resistance in rats fed a high-fat diet. *American Journal of Physiology, 273*, R1704–R1708.

Haupt, H. A. (1993). Anabolic steroids and growth hormone. *American Journal of Sport Medicine, 21*, 468–474.

Hultman, E., & Sahlin, K. (1980). Acid-base during exercise. *Exercise and Sports Science Review, 8*, 41–128.

Hultman, E., Söderland, K., Timmons, J. A., Cederblad, G., & Greenhaff, P. L. (1996). Muscle creatine loading in men. *Journal of Applied Physiology, 81*, 232–237.

Jackman, M., Wendling, P., Friars, D., & Graham, T. E. (1996). Metabolic catecholamine and endurance responses to caffeine during intense exercise. *Journal of Applied Physiology, 81*(4), 1658–1663.

Jilka, S. M., Joyner, M. J., Nittolo, J. M., Kalis, J. K., Taylor, J. A., Lohman, T. G., & Wilmore, J. H. (1988). Maximal exercise response to acute and chronic beta-adrenergic blockade in healthy male subjects. *Medicine and Science in Sports and Exercise, 20*, 570–573.

Johnson, R. (1998). Demographics of creatine monohydrate users. Memorandum to Brett Hall, Experimental and Applied Sciences. July 30, 1998.

Karpovich, P. V. (1959). Effect of amphetamine sulfate on athletic performance. *Journal of the American Medical Association, 170*, 558–561.

Kelly, J. G. (1985). Choice of selective versus nonselective beta blockers: Implications for exercise training. *American Journal of Cardiology, 55*, 162D–166D.

Klatsky, A. L., Armstrong, M. A., & Friedman, G. (1989). Alcohol use and subsequent cerebrovascular disease hospitalization. *Stroke, 20*, 741–746.

Kockakian, C. D., & Murlin, J. R. (1935). Effect of male hormone on protein and energy metabolism of castrate dogs. *Journal of Nutrition, 10*, 437–459.

Lambert, M. I., Hefer, J. A., Millar, R. P., & Macfarlane, P. W. (1993). Failure of commercial oral amino acid supplements to increase serum growth hormone concentrations in male body-builders. *International Journal of Sport Nutrition, 3*, 298–305.

Linderman, J. K., & Gosselink, K. L. (1994). The effects of sodium bicarbonate ingestion on exercise performance. *Sports Medicine, 18*, 75–80.

Lombardo, J. A., Hickson, R. C., & Lamb, D. R. (1991). Anabolic/androgenic steroids and growth hormones. In D. R. Lamb & M. H. Williams (Eds.), *Perspectives in exercise science and sports medicine. Volume 4. Ergogenics: Enhancement of performance in exercise and sport* (pp. 249–284). Dubuque, IA: WCB/Brown and Benchmark.

Longnecker, M. P., Berlin, J. A., Orza, M. J., & Chambers, T. C. (1988). A meta-analysis of alcohol consumption in relation to risk of breast cancer. *Journal of the American Medical Association, 260*, 652–656.

Matson, L. G., & Tran, Z. V. (1993). Effects of sodium

bicarbonate on aerobic performance: A meta-analytic review. *International Journal of Sport Nutrition, 3*, 2–28.

McNaughton, L. R. (1992). Sodium bicarbonate ingestion and its effects on anaerobic exercise of various durations. *Journal of Sports Science, 10*, 425–435.

McNaughton, L., Dalton, B., & Palmer, G. (1999). Sodium bicarbonate can be used as an erogenic aid in high-intensity, competitive cycle ergonometry of 1 hr duration. *European Journal of Applied Physiology, 80*, 64–69.

Melchert, R. B., & Welder, A. A. (1995). Cardiovascular effects of anabolic-androgenic steroids. *Medicine and Science in Sports and Exercise, 27*(9), 1252–1262.

Melchert, R. B., Herron, T. J., & Welder, A. A. (1992). The effect of anabolic-androgenic steroids on primary myocardial cell cultures. *Medicine and Science in Sports Exercise, 24*(2), 206–212.

Middleman, A. B., Faulkner, A. H., Woods, E. R., Emans, S. J. & DuRant, R. H. (1995). High risk behaviors among high school students in Massachusetts who use anabolic steroids. *Pediatrics, 96*, 268–272.

Morris, A. C., Jacobs, I., McLellan, T. M., Klugerman, A., Wang, L. C., & Zamecnik, J. (1996). No ergogenic effect of ginseng ingestion. *International Journal of Sport Nutrition, 6*, 263–271.

Moskowitz, H., Burns, M. M., & Williams, A. F. (1985). Skills performance at low blood alcohol levels. *Journal of the Studies on Alcohol, 46*, 482–485.

Mujika, I., Chatard, J. C., Lacoste, L., Barale, F., & Geyssant, A. (1996). Creatine supplementation does not improve sprint performance in competitive swimmers. *Medicine and Science in Sports and Exercise, 28*, 1435–1441.

Nehlig, A., & Debry, G. (1994). Caffeine and sports activity: A review. *International Journal of Sports Medicine, 15*(5), 215–223.

Nestler, J. E., Barlascini, C. O., Clore, J. N., & Blackard, W. G. (1988). Dehydroepiandrosterone reduces serum low density lipoprotein levels and body fat but does not alter insulin sensitivity in normal men. *Journal of Endocrinology Metabolism, 66*, 57–61.

Ng, T. B., & Yeung, H. W. (1986). Scientific basis of the therapeutic effects of ginseng. In *Folk Medicine: The Art and the Science.* Washington, DC: American Chemical Society.

Nissen, S., Sharp, R., Ray, M., Rathmacher, J. A., Rice, D., Fuller, J. C., Connelly, A. S., & Abumrad, N. (1996). Effect of leucine metabolite beta-hydroxy-beta-methyl-butyrate on muscle metabolism during resistance-exercise training. *Journal of Applied Physiology, 81*, 2095–2104.

Papet, I., Ostaszewski, P., Glomot, F., Obled, C., Faure, M., Bayle, G., Nissen, S., Arnal, M., & Grizard, J. (1997) The effect of a high dose of 3-hydroxy-3-metylbutyrate on protein metabolism in growing lambs. *British Journal of Nutrition, 77*, 885–896.

Pasman, W. J., van Baak, M. A., Jeukendrup, A. E., & de Haan, A. (1995). The effect of different dosages of caffeine on endurance performance time. *International Journal of Sports Medicine, 16*(4), 225–230.

Reilly, T. (1997). Alcohol: Its influence in sport and exercise. In T. Reilly & M. Orme (Eds.), *The clinical pharmacology of sport and exercise: Proceedings of the Esteve Foundation Symposium VII* (pp. 281–292). Amsterdam: Elsevier Science B.V.

Reilly, T., & Halliday, F. (1985). Influence of alcohol ingestion on tasks related to archery. *Journal of Human Ergology, 14*, 99–104.

Rogol, A. (1989). Growth hormone: Physiology, therapeutic use and potential for abuse. *Exercise and Sports Science Review, 17*, 353–377.

Rudman, D., Feller, A. G., Nagraj, H. S., Gergáns, G. A., Lalitha, P. Y., Goldberg, A. F., Schlenker, R. A., Cohn, L., Rudman, I. W., & Mattson, D. E. (1990). Effects of human growth hormone in men over 60 years old. *New England Journal of Medicine, 323*, 1–6.

Sawka, M. N., Joyner, M. J., Miles, D. S., Robertson, R. J., Spriet, L. L., & Young, A. J. (1996). American College of Sports Medicine position stand: The use of blood doping as an ergogenic aid. *Medicine and Science in Sports and Exercise, 28*(6), i–viii.

SKW Trostburg. (1998). SKW Trostburg AG announces patent enforcement action, exposed inferior products and introduces Creapure™ brand creatine products. Memorandum, July 15.

Smith, D. A., & Perry, P. J. (1992). The efficacy of ergogenic aids in athletic competition. Part II. Other performance-enhancing agents. *Annals of Pharmacotherapy, 26*, 653–659.

Smith, G. M., & Beecher, H. K. (1959). Amphetamine sulfate and athletic performance. *Journal of the American Medical Association, 170*, 542–557.

Spence, J. C., & Gauvin, L. (1996). Drug and alcohol use by Canadian university athletes: A national survey. *Journal of Drug Education, 26*(3), 275–287.

Spriet, L. L. (1995). Caffeine and performance. *International Journal of Sport Nutrition, 5*, S84–S99.

Stampfer, M. J., Colditz, G. A., Willett, W. C., Speizer, F. E., & Hennekens, C. H. (1988). A prospective study of moderate alcohol consumption and the risk of coronary disease and stroke in women. *New England Journal of Medicine, 319*, 267–273.

Strauss, G. (1998, June 4). 1 in 3 pro sports teams say "no" to creatine. *USA Today*, 1A.

Tarnopolsky, M. A. (1994). Caffeine and endurance performance. *Sports Medicine, 18*(2), 109–125.

United States Olympic Committee. (1996). *United States Olympic Committee drug education handbook.* Colorado Springs, CO: Author.

Vandenberghe, K., Gillis, N., Vyan Leemputte, M., Van Hecke, P., Vanstapel, F., & Hespel, P. (1996). Caffeine counteracts the ergogenic action of muscle creatine loading. *Journal of Applied Physiology, 80*, 452–457.

Vandenberghe, K., Goris, M., Van Hecke, P., Van Leemputte, M., Van Gerven, L., & Hespel, P. (1997). Long-term creatine intake is beneficial to muscle performance during resistance training. *Journal of Applied Physiology, 83*, 2055–2063.

Welder, A. A., & Melchert, R. B. (1993). Cardiotoxic effects of cocaine and anabolic-androgenic steroids in the athlete. *Journal of Pharmacology and Toxicology Methods, 29*, 61–68.

Welder, A. A., Robertson, J. W., Fugate, R. D., & Melchert, R. B. (1995b). Anabolic-androgenic steroid-induced toxicity in primary neonatal rat myocardial cell cultures. *Toxicology and Applied Pharmacology, 133*(2), 328–342.

Welder, A. A., Robertson, J. W., & Melchert, R. B. (1995a). Toxic effects of anabolic androgenic steroids in primary rat hepatic cell cultures. *Journal of Pharmacology and Toxicology Methods, 33*(4), 187–195.

Williams, J. H. (1991). Caffeine, neuromuscular function and high-intensity exercise performance. *Journal of Sports Medicine and Physical Fitness, 31*, 481–489.

Williams, J. H., Wendling, P., Friars, D., & Graham, T. E. (1996). Metabolic, catecholamine, and endurance responses to caffeine during intense exercise. *Journal of Applied Physiology, 81*(4), 1658–1663.

Williams, M. H. (1989). Drugs and sports performance. In A. J. Ryan & F. L. Allman (Eds.), *Sports medicine* (pp. 183–210). San Diego, CA: Academic Press.

Williams, M. H. (1991). Alcohol, marijuana and beta blockers. In D. R. Lamb & M. H. Williams (Eds.), *Perspectives in exercise science and sports medicine. Volume 4. Ergogenics: Enhancement of performance in exercise and sport* (pp. 348–362). Dubuque, IA: WCM/Brown and Benchmark.

Williams, M. H. (1992). Alcohol and sport performance. *Sports Science Exchange, 4*, 1–4.

Williams, M. H. (1996). *Lifetime fitness and wellness* (4th ed.). Dubuque, IA: Brown and Benchmark Publishers.

Williams M. H. (1998). *The ergogenics edge: Pushing the limits of sports performance.* Champaign, IL: Human Kinetics.

Williams, M. H., Kreider, R. B., & Branch, J. D. (1999). *Creatine: The power supplement.* Champaign, Il: Human Kinetics.

Wilmore, J. H., Ewy, G. A., Freund, B. J., Hartzell, A. A., Jilka, S. M., Joyner, M. J., Todd, C. A., Kinser, S. M., & Pepin, E. B. (1985). Cardiorespiratory alterations consequent to endurance exercise training during chronic beta-adrenergic blockade with atenolol and propranolol. *American Journal of Cardiology, 55*, 142D–148D.

Wilmore, J. H., Freund, B. J., Joyner, M. J., Hetrick, G. A., Hartzell, A. A., Strother, R. T., Ewy, G. A., & Faris, W. E. (1985B). Acute response to submaximal and maximal exercise consequent to beta-adrenergic blockade: Implications for the prescription of exercise. *American Journal of Cardiology, 55*, 135D–141D.

Wyndham, C. H., Rogers, G. G., Benade, A. J. S., & Strydom, N. B. (1971). Physiological effects of the amphetamines during exercise. *South African Medical Journal, 45*, 247–252.

Yarasheski, K. E., Campbell, J. A., Smith, K., Rennie, M. J., Holloszy, J. O., & Bier, D. M. (1992). Effect of growth hormone and resistance exercise on muscle growth in young men. *American Journal of Physiology, 262*, E261–E267.

Yarasheski, K. E., Zachwieja, J. J., Angelopoulos, T. J., & Bier, D. M. (1993). Short-term growth hormone treatment does not increase muscle protein synthesis in experienced weight lifters. *Journal of Applied Physiology, 74*, 3073–3076.

Yen, S. S., Morales, A. J., & Khorram, O. (1995). Replacement of DHEA in aging men and women: Potential remedial effects. *Annals of the New York Academy of Science, 774*, 128–142.

Yesalis, C. E., & Bahrke, M. S. (1995). Anabolic-androgenic steroids. *Sports Medicine, 19*, 326–340.

Yesalis, C. E., Streit, A. L., Vicary, J. R., Friedl, K. E., Brannon, D., & Buckley, W. (1989). Anabolic steroid use: Indications of habituation among adolescents. *Journal of Drug Education, 19*(2), 103–116.

6
Exercise and Longevity

Daniel S. Rooks

Fred Kantrowitz

> All parts of the body which have a function, if used in moderation and exercised in labors to which each is accustomed, become thereby well-developed and age slowly; but if unused and left idle, they become liable to disease, defective in growth and age quickly.
>
> —Hippocrates, 460 B.C.

Living longer has been an obsession of many cultures throughout history. Alexander the Great searched for the pool of life, and Ponce de Leon pursued the fountain of youth. Today, scientists work to understand the genetic causes of aging and its consequences. Cultures with greater than average life spans continue to be studied in the attempt to identify health behaviors and other factors that could help extend life. The present desire to live longer has spawned the billion-dollar antiaging industry whose products, which are mostly untested, not validated, unregulated and usually expensive, promise ways to delay aging and prolong life.

A growing body of knowledge demonstrates that individuals who are physically active are healthier than individuals of similar or younger age who are sedentary. This enhanced physical and emotional health is present at all ages and can be quantified as improved cardiopulmonary efficiency (Blair, Kampert, et al., 1996; Hagan, Parrish, & Licciardone, 1991; Haskell et al., 1992; Warren et al., 1993), muscle strength (Frontera, Meredith, O'Reilly, Knuttgen, & Evans, 1988; Moritani, 1993; Rooks, Kiel, Parsons, & Hayes, 1997), neuromotor performance (Rikli & Edwards, 1991; Rooks et al. 1997; Spirduso, MacRae, MacRae, Prewitt, & Osborne, 1988), bone density (Kahn, 1992; Nelson et al., 1994), insulin resistance (Ivy, 1997; Mayer-Davis et al., 1998), mood (Cramer, Nieman, & Lee, 1991), and reduced incidence of depression (Camacho, Roberts, Lazarus, Kaplan, & Cohen, 1991). Based on the direct beneficial effect of exercise on body systems, it would be logical to propose that long-term exercise might have a protective effect against certain diseases and potentially may prolong life. The health-enhancing effect of exercise has led several investigators to examine the relationship of exercise participation to the incidence of certain chronic diseases and death due to any cause (i.e., all-cause mortality). Data from several longitudinal cohort studies supply evidence of an inverse association of physical activity or physical fitness to a lower risk for many chronic diseases and injuries, including several of the primary causes of death: cardiovascular disease (Blair, Kampert, et al., 1996; Blair, Kohl, Paffennbarger, et al., 1989; Sandvik et al., 1993), hypertension (Paffenbarger, Hyde, Wing, & Hsieh, 1986), cancer (Blair, Kohl, Paffenbarger, et al., 1989; Oliveria & Lee, 1997), and non-insulin-dependent diabetes (Helmrish, Ragland, Leung, & Paffenbarger, 1991; Ivy, 1997; Mayer-Davis et al., 1998).

Interestingly, the relationship between physical activity and longevity has existed for centuries. In the sixth century, a monk named Bodhidharma, the father of Zen Buddhism, walked over the mountains from India to China where he found monks who were in general ill health. Legend records that he instructed the monks in a form of physical exercise to improve their strength, endurance, and general health (Funakoshi, 1973). These exercises are reportedly the beginning of the martial arts, which are still practiced as a means of health enhancement. Earlier texts credit Hippocrates, the physician, with being a strong proponent of regular physical activity. Interestingly, he espoused the belief that *regular, moderate* exercise was essential to developing and maintaining good health. He is credited with observing the relationship between habitual physical activity and improved health and the delay in physical decline associated with aging (see quote at beginning of chapter). Although the concept of enhanced health developed through increased physical activity is not novel, epi-demiological data have been lacking to quantify the strength of the relationship between components of physical activity (volume, intensity, type) and the presence of health (e.g., lack of mortality). This chapter summarizes the available data that examine the relationship between physical activity and living longer in men and women.

The Relationship of Exercise to Longevity

Quantification of the relationship between physical activity and life span began with the comparison of disease and mortality rates among different occupations. Early studies reported less frequent disease and mortality in the more physically demanding jobs compared with those requiring sedentary activities (Morris, Heady, Raffle, Roberts, & Parks, 1953; Paffenbarger, Laughlin, Gima, & Black, 1970). This form of research was expanded to include quantifying leisure-time physical activity in cohorts of men and women of a wide range of ages in several countries.

The early seminal works by Morris and colleagues (Morris, Chave, et al., 1973; Morris, Everitt, Pollard, Chave, & Semmence, 1980; Morris, Heady, et al., 1953) in England and Paffenbarger and colleagues (Paffenbarger & Hale, 1975; Paffenbarger, Laughlin, et al., 1970; Paffenbarger, Wing, & Hyde, 1978) in the United States examined the relationship of occupational and leisure-time physical activity to health. Looking at coronary heart disease, Morris and his group (Morris & Crawford, 1958; Morris, Heady, et al., 1953) found a lower incidence of disease and associated death in bus conductors of the London transportation system whose jobs included repetitive climbing of stairs and constant movement, compared to the bus drivers who were relatively sedentary while performing their jobs. Findings showed that the conductors experienced approximately half the number of heart attacks as the drivers. Furthermore, of those who did experience heart attacks, drivers died at twice the rate of the conductors.

Morris and colleagues extended these observations to examine the relationship of leisure-time physical activity to chronic disease and mortality. The investigators categorized participants by whether they performed leisure-time physical activity of different intensities: sedentary, moderate, and vigorous. These data supported their previous finding of an inverse relationship between physical activity and the incidence of and associated death from coronary heart disease (Morris, Chave, et al., 1973; Morris, Everitt, et al., 1980).

The College Alumni Health Study is a longitudinal cohort study designed to elucidate the relationship between personal health habits and characteristics of adults and the incidence of chronic disease (Paffenbarger, Kampert, & Lee, 1997). The study began in 1960 and includes a sample of 57,500 men and women who were students at Harvard College (n=36,500) between 1916 and 1954 and at the University of Pennsylvania (n=21,000) between 1928 and 1944. The longitudinal design and comprehensiveness of the data collected allowed the investigators to report on associations of health habits (referred to as "lifeway patterns") as well as the effect of changes in health habits and their predisposition to chronic disease.

Examination of baseline data identified relationships between certain health behaviors and the incidence of chronic diseases. Findings showed the positive association of cigarette smoking, high body mass index (body weight/height^2), and elevated blood pressure to cardiovascular disease. Interestingly, a history of sports participation in college, a possible proxy for physical activity, was inversely related to coronary heart disease (CHD) incidence (Paffenbarger, Hyde,

Wing, & Steinmetz, 1984; Paffenbarger, Wing, et al., 1978).

In 1986, Paffenbarger and colleagues published key findings examining the theory that regular exercise participation contributes to longevity (Paffenbarger, Hyde, Wing, & Hsieh, 1986). Data were reported from 16,936 men aged 35 to 74 whose followup questionnaires assessed 12 to 16 years from baseline. Physical activity was measured as miles walked, number of stairs climbed, and hours of light and vigorous sports played. These variables were evaluated individually as categories and translated into calories expended, summed and reported as a "physical activity index." Classification from least active to most active showed gradient improvements in mortality risk within each variable. Individuals walking 3–8 miles per week had a 15% reduction in mortality, whereas those walking 9 or more miles a week showed a 21% lower mortality rate. Both light sports and vigorous sports participation showed graded reduction in all-cause mortality from no participation to 3 or more hours of play. Although it did not impact CHD incidence, participating an average of 1 to 2 hours per week in light sports activity resulted in a 24% reduction in other causes of death. This level was increased slightly to 30% with 3 or more hours. Vigorous sports activity also showed an inverse relationship to mortality—including CHD-related death.

The physical activity index, reported as caloric expenditure in blocks of 500 kilocalorie categories, further supported the finding of a progressively lower risk of death with increased physical activity. Dichotomizing the group into fewer than 2,000 kcals or 2,000 or more kcals expended per week revealed a 28% reduction in death from all causes in the more active group of middle-aged men. This relationship also was seen in older men. Those men aged 60 to 69 years who were most active had a mortality risk half (53%) that of their least active peers. Subjects aged 70 to 84 years had a similar risk (51%).

Habitual exercise was most important for longevity. The beneficial effect of exercise is related to current levels of exercise and not just a history. College athletes who did not continue to exercise after college were at greater risk for death than were those who maintained an exercise habit of moderate exercise (defined as 500–1,999 kcals/week of energy expenditure). Calculation of a lifestyle change from sedentary to physically active (> 2,000 kcals) predicted a 24% reduction in the risk of death. The "protective effect" of a physically active lifestyle was underscored by findings that showed participants with hypertension who exercised had a lower risk of death than did normotensive participants who were sedentary. This relationship also was seen in smokers.

The most provocative question around exercise and longevity is, "How many more years of life can a physically active lifestyle bring?" Analysis of 16-year followup data (Paffenbarger, Hyde, Wing, & Hsieh, 1986) compared the least active men (defined as weekly energy expenditures of < 500 kcals) with the most active (> 2,000 kcals/week). The authors reported a graded, progressive increase in life span in exercising men 35 to 80 years of age. In general, the group of more active men gained an average of 2.3 years of life (range 2.5–0.42 years). When data were dichotomized into groups of men who expended < 2,000 kcals per week and those who expended 2,000 or more kcals per week, the graded benefit was attenuated but still present (1.5 – 0.30 years). These values were consistent when considering the inclusion of vigorous sports participation. These findings support the theory of a dose-response relationship of exercise volume to health. Moreover, they support the thesis that caloric expenditure, regardless of the intensity of exercise—moderate or vigorous—is a key variable in determining the value of exercise to positive health benefit.

The inverse relationship of physical activity and longevity reported in men by Paffenbarger and colleagues has been substantiated in populations with other education and socioeconomic levels. In 1987, Pekkanen and colleagues (Pekkanen et al., 1987) examined the ability of habitual physical activity to predict CHD-related mortality in a group of 636 Finnish men ages 45–64. Unlike the participants in the alumni study, these men were from rural areas and mostly were involved in physically demanding occupations. Therefore, the categories of physical activity at work and during leisure time were relative to the sample and probably different from similar categories of the alumni study. Comparison between the most active and moderately/lightly active groups of middle-aged men resulted in an independent, inverse association between physical activity and mortality. Over the 20-year period, the most active group gained an average increase in life expectancy of 2.1 years. These additional years were due primarily to a reduction in deaths from CHD. Interestingly, although this was a different population, the calculated increase in years was similar to that seen in the larger alumni study.

Until recently, little data existed to draw conclusions on the relationship of physical activity and morbidity in women. Several studies have reported finding a positive relationship between physical activity and living longer in women. Reports from the Framingham Heart Study showed an inverse relationship between physical activity and mortality in women in their fifth decade of life and older (Kushi et al., 1997; Lissner, Bengtsson, Björkelund, & Wedel, 1996; Sherman, D'Agostino, Cobb, & Kannel, 1994a,b). In 1996, Lissner and colleagues (Lissner et al., 1996) reported data from 1,405 women who had been retested 6 years from baseline and followed for 20 years. Subjects who were moderately active during leisure-time activities had a 44% reduction in mortality risk compared with sedentary peers. Individuals who reduced their activity level during the 6 years were twice (RR=2.07) as likely to die from any cause than if they had maintained a more active lifestyle. These data underscore the risk of becoming more sedentary throughout life and provide further evidence that *moderate* levels of physical activity can reduce mortality risk in women.

Kushi and colleagues in the most definitive study on the relationship between physical activity and all-cause mortality in women, particularly older women, reported 7-year followup findings on 40,417 women ages 55–69 years (Kushi et al., 1997). Three levels of activity patterns (low, medium, and high) were identified based on frequency and intensity of moderate and vigorous activity. Findings showed a strong, graded, inverse relationship between physical activity and mortality, independent of the presence of baseline disease or the inclusion of vigorous physical activity. These data provide strong support of the efficacy of moderate-level physical activity, as little as once per week, to provide a protective effect against cardiovascular and respiratory disorders in women.

Exercise Type and Intensity

A variety of physical activities have been reported in the various studies documenting an association between exercise and mortality. Leisure-time physical activities have included walking city blocks, distance walking, jogging/running, climbing stairs, bicycling, cross-country skiing, swimming, playing racquet sports, and shoveling snow (Hakim et al., 1998; Paffenbarger, Hyde, Wing, & Hsieh, 1986; Paffenbarger, Hyde, Wing, Lee, et al., 1993; Pekkanen et al.,

1987). Most studies do not factor out occupational and leisure-time activities, but rather use the information to generate categories of total activity. Few studies have examined the relationship between a single form of exercise and mortality.

Paffenbarger and colleagues (Paffenbarger, Hyde, Wing, Lee, et al., 1993) examined the effect of walking on all-cause mortality rates in men ages 35 to 74 years over 9 years. Men who walked nine miles per week or more reduced their risk of death by 16% compared to men who walked fewer than nine miles per week. These findings of the benefits of walking were further clarified by a recent study by Hakim and colleagues (Hakim et al., 1998) that examined the relationship of walking on mortality in older men. Over a 12-year followup period, a group of retired, nonsmoking older men, 61 to 81 years old, who walked more than two miles daily, died at approximately half the rate (23.8% vs. 40.5%) as individuals who walked less than one mile.

Although recommendations exist on the intensity of exercise to bring about physiological and emotional benefits (Pate et al., 1995), data on the level of exercise intensity required to produce life extension are conflicting and inconclusive. Using prospective data from the Harvard Alumni Study, Lee and colleagues (Lee, Hsieh, & Paffenbarger, 1995) reported an inverse relationship between more intense exercise and all-cause mortality in middle-aged men. Activity was dichotomized in the alumni study to nonvigorous (< 6 METS) or vigorous (> 6 METS, e.g., brisk walking, running, jogging, swimming laps, playing tennis, and shoveling snow) levels. Total weekly energy expenditure was divided into quintiles of kilojoules per week (<630, 630<1,680, 1,680<3,150, 3,150<6,300, >6,300kj/wk). The investigators examined the contribution each level of exercise intensity made to the outcome of mortality. Findings suggested that individuals who expend more than 630 kJ/week of vigorous exercise have approximately 10% lower risk of death than their more sedentary peers do. The alumni data did not show a reduced mortality rate with nonvigorous activity alone. This may be due in part to the method of exercise-history collection—self-report at baseline—where subjects may have underestimated the level of exercise intensity.

The finding of efficacy associated with higher levels of physical activity and not with lower level activity in middle-aged men is supported by previous work, mostly in studies examining the effect of exercise on coronary heart disease (Morris, Everitt, et al., 1980; Siscovick et al., 1997). In one study looking at older adults, Siscovick and colleagues examined the relationship of exercise intensity to several cardiovascular disease risk-factor levels and subclinical disease in cross-sectional data. Using three categories (low, medium, and high) of exercise intensity to classify detailed self-report exercise histories resulted in a similar graded inverse relationship between exercise intensity and numerous coronary artery disease-related variables. These data lend support to a possible mechanism of action for the health benefits of intense exercise: physiological changes that improve the efficiency of the cardiorespiratory system.

Physical Fitness and Longevity

Until 1989, studies examining the association between mortality and physical activity used an estimated quantity of energy expenditure, with no objective marker of habitual activity. In 1989, Blair and colleagues reported the largest cohort study that examined the relationship between physical fitness, as measured by physiological performance on an exercise test, and mortality rate. The large study sample was composed of 10,244 men and 3,210 women, 20–60+ years of age, who had a maximum treadmill exercise test as part of a preventive medical exam at the Cooper Institute for Aerobics Research. Subjects were followed for an average of 8 years. Five fitness categories (quintiles) were created based on the length, in minutes, of the exercise test. Data were separated and analyzed by age and sex.

Findings showed a strong, graded, inverse relationship between fitness level and all-cause mortality in both men and women. Compared with the most fit within each gender group, the least fit men were 3.4 times and least fit women 4.7 times more at risk of death over the 8-year period from all causes. The biggest reduction in risk was seen between the least fit (Group 1) and the next quartile (Group 2) in both men (Relative Risk [RR] 3.4 vs. 1.4) and women (RR 4.7 vs. 2.4). These data support the theory that moderate exercise is sufficient to bring about a reduction in mortality risk in men and women. The protective effect of moderate fitness on mortality risk was further supported in more recent studies (Blair, Kampert, et al., 1996; Sandvik et al., 1993) that reported the independent risk of low fitness to cardiovascular-disease-related death.

In addition to all-cause mortality, fitness levels were strongly related to death by cardiovascular disease and cancer. When mortality from cardiovascular disease was examined, mortality rates in the least-fit groups were eight times that of the most-fit men and 9.25 times that of the most-fit women. Similarly, deaths from cancer were 4.3 times greater in the less fit men and 16 times greater in the less fit women (Blair, Kohl, Paffenbarger, et al., 1989). These findings offer further evidence that a sedentary lifestyle is a significant risk for premature death due to cardiovascular disease and cancer.

Changes in Physical Activity Patterns

If exercise participation is associated with measurable health benefit, such as a reduction in premature mortality, one would expect to see this effect in previously sedentary individuals who adopt a more physically active lifestyle. To date, two reports have examined this question. Paffenbarger and colleagues (Paffenbarger, Hyde, Wing, Lee, et al., 1993) examined the effect of changes in exercise habits on mortality from coronary heart disease and other causes. As in their 1986 reporting, physical activity patterns were categorized two ways—expending fewer than or more than 2,000 kilocalories per week and the intensity of physical activity (light vs. moderately vigorous). Total energy expended per week was based on questions relating to number of city blocks walked, flights of stairs climbed, and the type of sports activities participated in. Of the 20% who adopted a physically active lifestyle (moving from classifications of inactive to active), the risk of death was reduced by 15%. Although this inverse association of exercise adoption and mortality was not statistically significant due to a small number of deaths, it was consistent with changes in mortality risk seen with exercise intensity. Subjects who did not participate in moderately vigorous exercise at baseline and increased their activity intensity at followup had a 23% reduction of risk for death compared to those who continued to not participate in higher intensity activities. The relative risk of death from all causes in new exercisers was similar to that in individuals who continued to exercise at a moderately vigorous level (23% vs. 29%). Moreover, the individuals who adopted exercise showed a 41% reduction in cardiovascular-related mortality. These data support the theory that

adopting a more physically active lifestyle, at any age, reduces the incidence of death from any cause. In these data, the adoption or maintenance of a more active lifestyle translated into 4 additional months of life for those who included light activity alone, and to 9 months for those who included moderately vigorous activities. Comparatively, stopping smoking added an estimated 18 months of life.

The effect of changes in physical fitness level (physiological) on mortality risk was consistent with those of a change in physical activity (behavior) (Blair, Kohl, Barlow, et al., 1995). Using maximal treadmill exercise time as an objective measure of physical fitness, baseline data were compared to followup test performance taken an average of 4.9 years later in men 20–82 years of age. Men who remained unfit (unfit at both time points) had the highest death rate (122/10,000 man-years), whereas those who remained fit had the lowest (40/10,000 man-years). As anticipated, those individuals who improved from the unfit to the fit categories showed an encouraging, intermediate rate of death (67/10,000 man-years). This improvement in fitness translated to a calculated reduction in mortality risk of 44% for all-cause mortality and 52% for CHD-related mortality. Examination of improvements within individuals in the two lower fitness categories of the subjects classified as fit at baseline showed a decrease in mortality risk. Improvement among the fit categories showed a graded improvement in mortality risk with a change to a more fit category. Subjects who remained fit had a 28% reduction in risk from all-cause mortality and a 52% reduction in risk for CVD mortality. Every additional minute of treadmill time beyond baseline performance translated to a 7.9% reduction in mortality risk. This relationship between higher levels of fitness and reduced mortality risk was consistent even when the sample was dichotomized into those with clinical symptoms or history of disease ("unhealthy") and those without ("healthy").

The relationship of data collected at a single time point with events years beyond is potentially weakened by confounding factors such as the possibility of changes in physical activity habits between baseline measurement and followup and genetic predisposition. Using two time points and examining changes in physical activity or fitness reduce the potential impact of these confounding factors. Further support of the independent relationship of physical activity and mortality was seen in data from the Finnish twin cohort study (Kujala, Kaprio, Sarna, & Koskenvuo, 1998). Based on their self-reported physical activity habits, 7,925 healthy men and 7,977 healthy women in their third or fourth decade of life were classified in one of three groups (sedentary, occasional exercisers, conditioning exercisers). The cohort was followed for 17 years. Compared with a sedentary twin, exercisers showed a graded reduction in mortality risk of 21% in the occasional exercisers and 48% in the conditioning exercisers. These data provide further evidence of the independent relationship of physical activity and mortality.

Conclusion

A physically active lifestyle is inversely related to all-cause mortality in both men and women across the age spectrum. This graded, independent relationship has been demonstrated in groups using the total number of calories expended on physical activity, the intensity of activity, or the consequence of physical activity—physical fitness. These findings suggest that being physically active, and consequently more physically fit, may be the mechanism of action that prolongs life due to an effect on delaying or prevent-

ing the onset of several common chronic diseases. Although this inverse relationship may be one of cause and effect based on the consistency seen among study findings over the past 10 to 15 years; the data are not from randomized controlled trials and are not causal in nature. Therefore, data do not support the theory that physical activity directly extends life span.

Considering the estimated small number of added years of life calculated from exercise participation and the time taken to perform the necessary exercise, it appears that exercise is not an efficient method of life extension. However, with all of its consequent health benefits, regular physical activity is a keystone of "successful aging" (Rowe & Kahn, 1998). Therefore, it appears the greatest contribution exercise may make to extending life is its associated prevention of premature morbidity and prolongation of a higher level of body system function and positive attitude well into the later years.

References

Blair, S. N., Kampert, J. B., Kohl, H. W., Barlow, C. E., Macera, C. A., Paffenbarger, R. S., Jr., & Gibbons, L. W. (1996). Influences of cardiorespiratory fitness and other precursors on cardiovascular disease and all-cause mortality in men and women. *Journal of the American Medical Association, 276*(3), 205–210.

Blair, S. N., Kohl, H. W., Barlow, C. E., Paffenbarger, R. S., Gibbons, L. W., & Macera, C. A. (1995). Changes in physical fitness and all-cause mortality: A prospective study of healthy and unhealthy men. *Journal of the American Medical Association, 273*(14), 1093–1098.

Blair, S. N., Kohl, H. W., III, Paffenbarger, R. S., Clark, D. G., Cooper, K. H., & Gibbons, L. W. (1989). Physical fitness and all-cause mortality: A prospective study of healthy men and women. *Journal of the American Medical Association, 262*, 2395–2401.

Camacho, T. C., Roberts, R. E., Lazarus, N. B., Kaplan, G. A., & Cohen, R. D. (1991). Physical activity and depression: Evidence from the Alameda county study. *American Journal of Epidemiology, 134*, 220–231.

Cramer, S. R., Nieman, D. C., & Lee, J. W. (1991). The effects of moderate exercise training on psychological well-being and mood state in women. *Journal of Psychosomatic Research, 35*, 437–449.

Frontera, W. R., Meredith, C. N., O'Reilly, K. P., Knuttgen, H. G., & Evans, W. J. (1988). Strength conditioning in older men, skeletal muscle hypertrophy, and improved function. *Journal of Applied Physiology, 64*, 1038–1044.

Funakoshi, G. (1973). *Karate-Do kyohan: The master text*. Tokyo: Kodansha Int.

Hagan, R. D., Parrish, G., & Licciardone, J. C. (1991). Physical fitness is inversely related to heart disease risk: A factor analytic study. *American Journal of Preventive Medicine, 7(4)*, 237–243.

Hakim, A. A., Petrovitch, H., Burchfiel, C. M., Ross, G. W., Rodriguez, B. L., White, L. R., Yano, K., Curb, D., & Abbott, R. D. (1998). Effects of walking on mortality among nonsmoking retired men. *The New England Journal of Medicine, 338*(2), 94–99.

Haskell, W. L., Leon, A. S., Caspersen, C. J., Froelicher, V. F., Hagberg, J. M., Harlan, W., Holloszy, J. O., Regensteiner, J. G., Thompson, P. D., Washburn, R. A., & Wilson, P. W. F. (1992). Cardiovascular benefits and assessment of physical activity and physical fitness in adults. *Medicine and Science in Sports and Exercise, 24*, S201–S220.

Helmrish, S. P., Ragland, D. R., Leung, R. W., & Paffenbarger, R. S., Jr. (1991). Physical activity and reduced occurrence of non-insulin-dependent diabetes mellitus. *New England Journal of Medicine, 325*, 147–152.

Ivy, J. L. (1997). Role of exercise training in the prevention and treatment of insulin resistance and non-insulin-dependent diabetes mellitus. *Sports Medicine, 24*(5), 321–336.

Kahn, B. B. (1992). Facilitative glucose transporters: Regulatory mechanisms and dysregulation in diabetes. *Journal of Clinical Investments, 89*, 1367–1374.

Kujala, U. M., Kaprio, J., Sarna, S., & Koskenvuo, M. (1998). Relationship of leisure-time physical activity and mortality: The Finnish twin cohort. *Journal of the American Medical Association, 279*(6), 440–444.

Kushi, L. H., Fee, R. M., Folsom, A. R., Mink, P. J., Anderson, K. E., & Sellers, T. A. (1997). Physical activity and mortality in postmenopausal women. *Journal of the American Medical Association, 277*, 1287–1292.

Lee, I. M., Hsieh, C. C., & Paffenbarger, R. S., Jr. (1995). Exercise intensity and longevity in men: The Harvard alumni health study. *Journal of the American Medical Association, 273*(15), 1179–1184.

Lissner, L., Bengtsson, C., Björkelund, C., & Wedel, H. (1996). Physical activity levels and changes in relation to longevity: A prospective study of Swedish women. *American Journal of Epidemiology, 143*(1), 54–62.

Mayer-Davis, E. J., D'Agostino, R. Jr., Karter, A. J., Haffner, S. M., Rewers, M. J., Saad, M., & Bergman, R. N. (1998). Intensity and amount of physical activity in relation to insulin sensitivity: The insulin resistance atherosclerosis study. *New England Journal of Medicine, 279*(9), 669–674.

Moritani, T. (1993). Neuromuscular adaptations during the acquisition of muscle strength, power and motor tasks. *Journal of Biomechanics, 26*, S95–S107.

Morris, J. N., Chave, S. P. W., Adam, C., Sirey, C., Epstein, L., & Sheehan, D. J. (1973). Vigorous exercise in leisure-time and the incidence of coronary heart-disease. *Lancet, 1*(333), 339.

Morris, J. N., & Crawford, M. D. (1958). Coronary heart disease and physical activity of work: Evidence of a national necropsy survey. *British Medical Journal, 2*(1485), 1496.

Morris, J. N., Everitt, M. G., Pollard, R. A., Chave, S. P. W., & Semmence, A. M. (1980). Vigorous exercise in leisure time: Protection against coronary heart disease. *Lancet, 2*, 1207–1210.

Morris, J. N., Heady, J. A., Raffle, P. A. B., Roberts, C. G., & Parks, J. W. (1953). Coronary heart disease and physical activity of work: I. Coronary heart disease in different occupations. *Lancet, 2*, 1053–1057.

Nelson, M. E., Fiatarone, M. A., Morganti, C. M., Trice, I., Greenberg, R. A., & Evans, W. J. (1994). Effects of high-intensity strength training on multiple risk factors for osteoporotic fractures: A randomized controlled trial. *Journal of the American Medical Association, 272*(24), 1909–1914.

Oliveria, S. A., & Lee, I. M. (1997). Is exercise beneficial in the prevention of prostate cancer? *Sports Medicine, 23*(5), 271–278.

Paffenbarger, R. S., Jr., & Hale, W. E. (1975). Work activity and coronary heart mortality. *New England Journal of Medicine, 292*, 545–550.

Paffenbarger, R. S., Jr., Hyde, R. T., Wing, A. L., & Hsieh, C. C. (1986). Physical activity, all-cause mortality, and longevity of college alumni. *The New England Journal of Medicine, 314*(10), 605–401.

Paffenbarger, R. S., Jr., Hyde, R. T., Wing, A. L., Lee, I. M., Jung, D. L., & Kampert, J. B. (1993). The association of changes in physical-activity level and other lifestyle characteristics with mortality among men. *The New England Journal of Medicine, 328*(8), 538–545.

Paffenbarger, R. S., Jr., Hyde, R. T., Wing, A. L., & Steinmetz, C. H. (1984). A natural history of athleticism and cardiovascular health. *Journal of the American Medical Association, 252*(491), 495.

Paffenbarger, R. S., Jr., Kampert, J. B., & Lee, I. M. (1997). Physical activity and health of college men: Longitudinal observations. *International Journal of Sports Medicine, 18*(Suppl. 3), S200–S203.

Paffenbarger, R. S., Jr., Laughlin, M. E., Gima, A. S., & Black, R. A. (1970). Work activity of longshoremen as related to death from coronary heart disease and stroke. *New England Journal of Medicine, 282*, 1109–1114.

Paffenbarger, R. S., Jr., Wing, A. L., & Hyde, R. T. (1978). Physical activity as an index of heart attack risk in college alumni. *American Journal of Epidemiology, 108*, 161–175.

Pate, R. R., Pratt, M., Blair, S. N., Haskell, W. L., Macera, C. A., Bouchard, C., Buchner, D., Ettinger, W., Heath, G. W., King, A. C., Kriska, A., Leon, A. S., Marcus, B. H.,

Morris, J., Paffenbarger, R. S., Jr., Patrick, K., Pollock, M. L., Rippe, J. M., Sallis, J., & Wilmore, J. H. (1995). Physical activity and public health: A recommendation from the centers for disease control and prevention and the American College of Sports Medicine. *Journal of the American Medical Association, 273*(5), 402–407.

Pekkanen, J., Marti, B., Nissinen, A., Tuomilehto, J., Punsar, S., & Karvonen, M. J. (1987). Reduction of premature mortality by high physical activity: A 20-year followup of middle-aged Finnish men. *The Lancet,* (June 27, 1987), 1473–1477.

Rikli, R. A., & Edwards, D. J. (1991). Effects of a three-year exercise program on motor function and cognitive processing speed in older women. *Research Quarterly for Exercise and Sport, 62(1)*, 61–67.

Rooks, D. S., Kiel, D. P., Parsons, C., & Hayes, W. C. (1997). Self-paced resistance training and walking exercise in community dwelling older adults: Effects on neuromotor performance. *Journal of Gerontology, 52A*(3), M161–M168.

Rowe, J. W., & Kahn, R. L. (1998). *Successful aging.* New York: Pantheon Books.

Sandvik, L., Erikssen, J., Thaulow, E., Erikssen, G., Mundal, R., & Rodahl, K. (1993). Physical fitness as a predictor of mortality among healthy, middle-aged Norwegian men. *The New England Journal of Medicine, 328*(8), 533–537.

Sherman, S. E., D'Agostino, R. B., Cobb, J. L., & Kannel, W. B. (1994a). Does exercise reduce mortality rates in the elderly? Experience from the Framingham Heart Study. *American Heart Journal, 128*(5), 965–972.

Sherman, S. E., D'Agostino, R. B., Cobb, J. L., & Kannel, W. B. (1994b). Physical activity and mortality in women in the Framingham Heart Study. *American Heart Journal, 128*, 879–884.

Siscovick, D. S., Fried, L., Mittelmark, M., Rutan, G., Bild, D., & O'Leary, D. H. (1997). Exercise intensity and subclinical cardiovascular disease in the elderly: The cardiovascular health study. *American Journal of Epidemiology, 145*(11), 977–986.

Spirduso, W. W., MacRae, H. H., MacRae, P. G., Prewitt, J., & Osborne, L. (1988). Exercise effects on aged motor function. *Annals of New York Academy of Sciences, 515*, 363–375.

Warren, B. J., Nieman, D. C., Dotson, R. G., Adkins, C. H., O'Donnell, K. A., Haddock, B. L., & Butterworth, D. E. (1993). Cardiorespiratory responses to exercise training in septuagenarian women. *International Journal of Sports Medicine, 14*, 60–65.

7
Preparation for Labor and Delivery

Mara D. H. Smith

Giving birth is one of the most significant and challenging events in a woman's life. There are many facets to childbirth, with an almost infinite number of variables, making it a complex process in which to take part as well as to study. Childbirth is, in part, the physiological process in which the uterus contracts, the cervix opens, the fetus descends through the pelvis, and the mother helps push out the baby. The birth itself is a time-limited event. However, the birthing process has an effect long after the physical experience is over. The field of childbirth education has sought to give both women and their support person(s) a more active role in the birth experience while providing them with useful and usable information regarding childbirth.

The childbirth education movement grew out of two ideas: first, that childbirth was not intrinsically painful (Dick-Read, 1959) and, second, that with proper training, any woman could have a completely pain-free birth (Dick-Read, 1944; Lamaze, 1965). Over the years, research has shown that although encouraging in theory, painless childbirth is a rare exception (Beck, 1978; Cogan, 1976; Melzack, 1981). Even though we know that labor and delivery are painful for "prepared" women, this knowledge does not make childbirth education ineffectual. Women are

not necessarily looking for childbirth education to take away all the pain of birth, but to reduce anxiety and labor pain (Leiberman, 1990). No matter what type of labor a woman experiences, and each individual will be different, childbirth education should provide her with a framework to view the process as well as a repertoire of tools to use as labor progresses to delivery.

Much of the research on childbirth has a "problematic" focus—looking at outcomes such as pain or obstetrical complications. Suggested in the following is a focus on process and positive aspects of labor and delivery. Pregnancy is a unique physical state in which a healthy individual must come under the care of a physician. Pregnancy and childbirth are not "disabilities," but incredible abilities of the female body. There are questions regarding the prevailing norm among health care professionals that the critical element responsible for a "good birth experience" is solely the reduction of pain (Lieberman, 1990; Morgan, 1982). Some studies revealed that it was not the elimination of pain during labor, but feeling in control, which led to high birth satisfaction rates of new mothers (Leiberman, 1990). The issue arose as to whether a childbirth education program might be framed in a way to enhance the mother-to-be's control or feelings of mastery and accomplishment in labor. From personal experience and informal discussions with many new mothers, the need for a curriculum beyond different breathing patterns was clear. Coming from a background as an athlete, I conceived a sport framework for childbirth (no pun intended!). The analogy of sport, athletes, and the "hurts so good" aspect of training is the basis for the framework. The satisfaction an individual receives from training for or completing a physical challenge, or both, is undeniable, regardless of the type of activity. When an athlete is struggling, people do not offer drugs to help the athlete finish the chosen event; they offer encouragement and support. The sport framework is aimed at giving mothers-to-be and their support person(s) cognitive, affective, and psychomotor information and education on childbirth that is currently not utilized in standard childbirth education curriculum.

Clearly, every mother-to-be does not consider herself an athlete. However, giving birth is the most intense physical challenge a woman will probably encounter in her lifetime. Despite many efforts, research has failed to support correlations between a woman's physical condition and abilities to "manage" labor and delivery. A direct relationship is difficult because of confounding effects of exercise variables and other maternal, uterine, fetal, and obstetric factors known to influence labor (Clapp, 1990). Whether or not a woman prepares for childbirth, physiological mechanisms will take over and guide the process. Labor is unpredictable; even with the easiest of pregnancies, unforeseen situations or complications may arise. One of the best ways to prepare for childbirth is to be aware of possible situations, options available, and techniques to cope—in athletic terms, to formulate a "game plan." In childbirth as in an athletic event, there are many variables that cannot be controlled. Like

well-trained athletes and their ability to change with changing playing conditions, an expectant mother needs to be educated on the importance of the "flexibility" of that plan. In general, studies have repeatedly shown that patient preparation has been associated with favorable outcomes (Langer, 1980; Nichols, 1988; Williams, 1978). Obstetric outcome has also been shown to be favorably effected by education (Beck, 1979; Dick-Read, 1949; Hetherington, 1990; Lamaze, 1965; Nichols, 1988; Worthington, 1990). The comparison of childbirth to an athletic event seems a logical one; both present physical and psychological challenges. It would be highly unusual for an individual to attempt to participate in an athletic event without having trained for it; however, many pregnant women do not consider the possibility of "training" for their labor and delivery. It is interesting to note that we, as a society, are awed by (female) endurance athletes; however, a woman who chooses an unmedicated childbirth experience is often viewed as a "martyr" (Goer, 1999). As an athlete, an individual can set up a workout to strengthen herself physically and build endurance. Psychologically, one may employ mental "training" to improve focus and relaxation so the body can "perform" at optimal levels. It is this component that is missing from many childbirth education programs: positive psychological elements that can be used as specific techniques with which to approach labor and delivery. These include, but are not limited to, relaxation, imagery, positive self-talk, goal setting, and development of a game plan.

To use marathon running as a metaphor for the intense physical challenge of childbirth, there is a point when the runner (mother) becomes tired, discouraged, and ready to give up. Runners call it "the wall"; in childbirth it is known as "transition." Runners know this is a difficult and trying stage for which they need to prepare not only physically, but also mentally. During this time in childbirth, the cervix is dilating from 7 to 10 centimeters, contractions are at their strongest and longest, and there is very little time to rest between contractions. Most women find this the most tumultuous and difficult part of labor. As glycogen supplies to the muscles decrease, runners begin to feel dizzy, queasy, light-headed; they feel as though they cannot go on, much like the difficult period in labor known as transition. Just as an athlete needs to prepare for both the psychological and physical demands, so should a woman preparing for childbirth train for this exciting and challenging event.

An athlete needs to learn to control physiological responses to stress to enhance her performance. A woman in labor may also benefit from learning to both predict and handle these stressors. The gradual increase of pain and stress of labor serves an important function; it allows the laboring woman to acclimate slowly and steadily to the increasing demands that culminate in the birth. Stress hormones give the laboring mother stamina. Endorphins act as the body's built-in painkillers. Although endorphin levels of the mother rise throughout labor (Kofinas, 1985), the childbirth "high" that women describe is very similar to that described by runners (Morgan, 1981). It is possible to recognize the physiological changes that occur when an individual is under stress. Each person will have a different response. Childbirth education must encourage women to learn, as athletes do, not only to become aware of their individual responses to stress, but also to gain confidence in their bodies and abilities to handle this stress.

The environment affects the way a person perceives, is influenced by, and copes with life stress. It has been shown that individuals with good coping strategies and strong social support are better able to handle stressful events (Andrew, Tennant, Hewson, & Valliant, 1978). Research has also been conducted on the relationship between social support and health-related states, such as labor and delivery (Cogan, 1988, Kennell, 1991, Sosa, 1980). Studies show important perinatal benefits of constant human support during labor. These include fewer perinatal problems, fewer problematic labors; mothers with support were more alert following delivery and had more interactions with their newborns than did mothers who labored and delivered without a support person (Henneborn, 1978; Sosa, Kennell et al., 1984; Kennell, Klaus, & McGrath, 1991). There should be a trend toward engaging the labor companion to become more formally prepared to "coach" the mother through labor and delivery, taking an active role in the childbirth process. The purpose of an athletic coach is to come under the tutelage of an individual who knows as much, if not more about a particular sport. The concept of labor coaching reflects the importance of knowledge and understanding of the woman's need. The labor companion or coach is crucial to preparing for childbirth. The similarity of labor coaching to athletic coaching is strengthened in the area of support. The sports coaching literature emphasizes mutual trust and respect and the importance to viewing the athlete as an individual (Smith, 1983). Coaches need to be reminded of their importance. Even though fathers cannot experience childbirth, they must not become spectators. They should, by their interest and enthusiasm, be symbol, to the spirit of the "player," motivating the individual to want to participate at her optimal level. Labor coaches may understand their role more clearly, using the sport analogy; no coach just shows up for the "championship game." Coaches are there for practices, good and bad; they offer ideas and maintain enthusiasm and morale. The "coach" can have a great influence on the mother and provide invaluable assistance during labor and delivery. The coach must learn what helps the woman to relax and must help her to achieve a more relaxed and comfortable state and, most important, must provide a sense of reassurance and confidence. The focus of any childbirth education program should be the positive goal of the birth of a child (and not how the birth happens). Flow is a concept employed by Csikszentmihalyi (1990) to describe immersion and pleasurable involvement in a task that is in some way intrinsically rewarding. Everything the body can do is potentially enjoyable. However, many people disregard the body's incredible capacity and never use or explore their physical capabilities, never developing flow. It is important to note that the body does not produce or experience flow merely by its movements; the mind is always involved as well. It is the challenge to the activity that maintains the focus. The process of childbirth is very rhythmic, and women describe "getting into a groove." The pattern of counting a certain beat, or moving a limb back and forth in a rhythm is common. Being encouraged to feel a rhythm and allow it to happen can be helpful to the laboring woman.

Relaxation training has become an important component of therapy programs in several disciplines including medicine, rehabilitation, dentistry, and psychology. Relaxation is used to modify behavior as well as reduce an individual's symptoms to stress and anxiety (Gregg, 1979; Jacobson, 1938). When used as a primary treatment strategy, relaxation skills have been shown to be effective in reducing tension, anxiety, and pain perception (Benson, 1977; Paul, 1969; Richter, 1979). These results have been effective in the treatment of hypertension and insomnia as well as in the nonpathological condition of childbirth (Scott, 1979; Stevens, 1977; Wideman, 1984). Whether used as a main treatment or a component of stress reduction, relaxation training is aimed at lowering muscle activity and subsequently reducing autonomic activity. The hormonal chaos created by the body's natural response to stress can exhaust an athlete or a laboring woman at the very time when she needs the most energy. When balance between the sympathetic system and parasympathetic system exists, an individual is able to relax and rest, heart rate and breathing rates slow, and a sense of calm and focus ensues. Relaxation training is a self-regulating skill that can only be learned through individual effort and practice. As early in the pregnancy as possible, practice can begin. Because most women do not attend childbirth classes until the last trimester of pregnancy, unless they are familiar with the process, they have an average of 8 weeks to practice before the birth. Relaxation training should be approached from three facets: cognitive, affective, and psychomotor. Both mother and coach need a basic understanding of the nature of stress, the physiological changes it causes, their individual response to stress, and its detrimental effects during labor and delivery. If there is an understanding of the benefits of relaxation in reducing stress and decreasing pain perception, there may be more motivation to practice and acquire the necessary skills. Although the intensity of a uterine contraction cannot be replicated for practicing relaxation, other noxious stimuli may be introduced to demonstrate effectiveness. For example, after relaxation training, the coach may apply pressure above the knee or the trapezius muscle for a time period similar to that of a contraction ($1–1\frac{1}{2}$ minutes). When a woman uses a focal point, relaxation, and imagery, that pressure feels very different than it does when she is looking at the coach's hand pinching her knee. Cognitive restructuring may be used in the area of tension. During uterine contractions, the intensity a woman perceives in her uterus should be interpreted as the work of the uterus toward the positive goal of birth. Tension in muscles not involved in the specific process should be recognized and consciously released.

The affective element of relaxation includes the physical and emotional environment. The physical environment should positively affect the mother and coach in such a way that they can release tension. The mother must be physically comfortable with space and relative privacy. Labor is intense, yet surprisingly, many women are concerned with being loud or making sudden outbursts during labor. Where there is physical challenge, there may be noise; reassurance that grunting or moaning is normal is important. Having the coach assist in learning and practicing relaxation techniques can give the mother-to-be a greater sense of trust and confidence in her own abilities. The coach should assume a shared responsibility for practicing. This shared responsibility can increase the level of trust and develop a sense of teamwork so crucial to labor and delivery.

Physical comfort is the most important and basic component of all relaxation skills. Changing positions is invaluable in labor, and practicing relaxation skills in a variety of positions will give a mother and coach excellent preparations for different situations they will encounter during labor. Understanding neuromuscular reactivation, or the mind-body connection, is essential to relaxation skills. Mother and coach must be able to "tune in" to the mother's body and distinguish tense from relaxed. It is important to encourage each individual to predict (using past experiences) how she believes she will react to the stress of labor and delivery.

Not infrequently, the eyeballs begin to roll as soon as relaxation is mentioned. Inevitably, someone claims she does not need to practice relaxation because she is going to have an epidural. We live in times when women have many choices surrounding birth. Every physician should encourage a woman to see how far her body can take her on its own and then, if need be, get medicated. Again, the more tools a woman and her coach can enter into labor with, the better prepared they will both be to handle what may happen. Skills should be taught sequentially, mastering basic skills before progressing to skills of increasing difficulty. Mother and coach move from an awareness of breathing to an awareness of whole body, to major muscle groups, to individual areas, and to inner body. Verbal cues from the coach need to be clear and directed. Touch cues can also be used to encourage relaxation. A variety of techniques should be included in a practice regimen. Mother and coach should be aware of which techniques she prefers and will be most helpful during labor. Here are some examples.

Relaxation as Preparation for Childbirth

The fight-or-flight response is an incredible mechanism built into the human body. As cave people, confronting a saber-toothed tiger, we needed that mechanism to rally the resources in our body either to confront and slay the tiger or to get away from it. The stresses in our society are much more complex. Our bodies do not differentiate stressors according to whether they "make sense" or not. If an individual perceives something as a stressor, his or her body will react. We know we need to learn to relax. "I don't have the time" is a common response from those individuals who suffer from the effects of stress in their lives. Most people have to practice relaxation in order to master it, but everyone can learn to relax. Practicing regularly during the third trimester of pregnancy will teach the body the feeling of muscular release so that when labor begins, relaxation will be second nature.

Progressive Muscle Relaxation

Practice relaxation in any comfortable position. For a pregnant woman lying on one's back can impede circulation during late pregnancy. Semi-reclining with head and shoulders supported by coach or pillows and knees bent.

Take a deep cleansing breath by over oxygenating and filling the lungs completely and let it out with a sigh. Repeat.

1. Tense your feet. Press your heels forward and pull your toes toward your nose. Feel the muscular tension. (Hold for approximately 10 seconds.) Now relax your feet. Let your toes hang loosely from your feet and feel your feet hang from your ankles.
2. Tighten the muscles in your legs. Squeeze your inner thighs together and tighten the muscles on the tops of your thighs and around your knees. Try to breathe even though there is tension. Slowly relax your legs completely and feel the tightness melt away, allow your legs to fall open naturally (with your hips rotating out) and feel yourself being supported by the floor.
3. Contract your pelvic floor muscles. Squeeze tightly as if you have to urinate desperately, but someone is in the bathroom. (Feel the pelvic hammock lift between your legs.) Now, relax these muscles completely as if you can FINALLY go to the bathroom.
4. Squeeze your buttocks tightly together and tense your abdomen as well; you should rise a few inches. Feel the tension all the way around your body and the difficulty in breathing. Now tighten even a little bit more. Slowly release your buttocks and entire midsection, and take a deep cleansing breath to help you relax even more.
5. Tighten the muscles in your chest, try and pull your ribs together and give your baby a hug. Feel how this makes it difficult to breathe. Relax these muscles, and let the air escape. Allow your breathing to resume, and become aware of how your breastbone rises and your ribcage opens with each breath.
6. Shrug your shoulders up to your ears as if you are wearing your shoulders as earrings. Slowly let them fall back down to your collarbone, like wax melting. Let them feel heavy.
7. Stiffen your arms as if you had wet shirtsleeves outside on an icy day. Clench your fists tightly. In your mind, come in from the cold. Feel your arms soften with the warmth of the indoors. Unfurl your fingers.
8. Last, tighten all the muscles in your face and neck. Make your face as "small" as you possibly can. Allow all tension to drain from your face, and feel relief pass over as if you just got great news. Let the small muscles around your eyes relax, and let your jaw hang loosely. Smooth out the wrinkles in your forehead, and let your face grow smooth, calm, relaxed. Take a deep cleansing breath in and let it out with a sigh. Feel your whole body relaxed.

Touch Relaxation

Touch relaxation is another tool of relaxation. During pregnancy, as well as labor and delivery, the woman uses coach's touching, stroking, or massage as a nonverbal cue to relax. There are several types of touch relaxation; it is good to practice all of them because preferences could change during labor.

- Still touch. Coach holds hand(s) firmly in place until they feel a release of tension.
- Firm pressure. Coach applies pressure with fingertips or hand on tense area. Coach gradually releases pressure, and mother tries to replicate release of tension.
- Stroking. Coach strokes tense area, stroking away from center of mother's body.

- Massage. Coach firmly rubs and or kneads tense muscles.

Visualization and Imagery

Visualization and imagery are also important tools of relaxation that can help a mother-to-be cope with the intensity of labor and delivery. In sport, athletes may mentally rehearse a certain movement, a whole routine, or a relaxed response to a crisis. It is important to note that visualizations are not just daydreams about the perfect performance. They are usually carefully structured exercises that athletes practice every day. There are two different types of imagery: internal and external. Internal imagery is primarily kinesthetic; a person would imagine actually doing something within his or her own bodies. External imagery is visual; it would be as if a person were watching him- or herself doing something. Internal imagery is more effective as a relaxation tool as a mental picture can be filled in with sensory details. The more real the image, the more powerful the effect. (Make sure a tour of the labor and delivery unit or birthing center is done so those images may be integrated into practice.)

Encourage mothers-to-be and their partners to find images that will be helpful during labor and delivery. (Remember that everyone is different and what one person may find relaxing may be very uncomfortable or frightening to another.) Use internal imagery with as much sensory integration as possible. Here are some examples—encourage creativity!

1. The strength of a contraction is equal to the strength of a waterfall. (Could you crawl up a mighty waterfall?) Go with the waterfall and find yourself being carried from the torrent of the waterfall out into a peaceful lake.
2. Imagine a turtleneck being pulled over baby's head or a spring flower opening for the first time to imagine/encourage cervical dilation.
3. Contractions are like waves in the ocean: Once they begin (truly) there is no stopping them. Imagine riding those waves; feel the rhythm. Imagine how much fun it is to play in the waves when you are watching and expecting them. It is very different, however, when one slams you from behind as in not knowing or "getting psyched" for the most challenging phase of labor. It would seem that the importance of childbirth utilizing the least amount of pharmacologic agents to which mother and fetus are exposed is obvious. However, enduring labor without drugs is distinctly on childbearing's margins, at least among American women. Why is it that we are awed by female endurance athletes such as marathoners, triathletes, and even women who participate in the Ironman—2.4-mile swim, 112-mile bike, and 26.2-mile run? Family, friends and spectators offer encouragement and are inspired. Why is it, then, when a woman chooses to attempt the challenge of childbirth without medication she is "crazy" or a "martyr" (Goer, 1995, Chap. 13)? Some women want to embrace the challenge; some women are frightened and need encouragement. If someone told you she was going to run a marathon, would the first words out of your mouth be "just DRIVE the 26 miles"? An unmedicated childbirth within a framework of sport is not for everyone, but it should be used as the baseline for teaching. For some, childbirth can be the most profound physical challenge in a woman's life. Encouraging a woman to test her limits and do what she can with the tools she has is infinitely important. The implications are far-reaching and can be transforming. Give women a chance to challenge and use their bodies in this amazing "sport" we call childbirth.

References

Beck, N. C., E. A. Geden, et al. (1979). "Preparation for Labor: A Historical Perspective." *Psychosomatic Medicine* 41(3): 243–258.

Benson, H. (1977). *The Relaxation Response*. New York, Avon Books.

Clapp, J. F. (1990). "The Course of Labor After Endurance Exercise During Pregnancy." *American Journal of Obstetrics and Gynecology 163:* 1799.

Cogan, R. (1980). "Effects of Childbirth Preparation." *Clinical Obstetrics and Gynecology 21*(1).

Csikszentmihali, M. (1990). *Flow*. New York, NY, Harper & Row.

Dick-Read, G. (1959). *Childbirth Without Fear: The Principles and Practice of Natural Childbirth,* 2nd Edition. New York, Harper and Brothers.

Goer, H. (1995). *Obstetric Myths Versus Research Realities*. Westport, CT, Bergin & Garvey.

Gregg, R. H. (1979). Biofeedback and biophysical monitoring during pregnancy and labor. *Biofeedback Principles and Practice for Clinicians*. J. V. Basmajian. Baltimore, Williams and Wilkins Co.

Henneborn, W. J. a. C., R. (1975). "The Effect of Husband Participation on Reported Pain and Probability of Medication During Labor and Birth." *Journal of Psychosomatic Research 19:* 215–217.

Hetherington, S. E. (1990). "A Controlled Study of the Effect of Prepared Childbirth Classes on Obstetric Outcome." *Birth 17*(2): 86–91.

Jacobson, E. (1938). *Progressive Relaxation*. Chicago, IL, University of Chicago Press.

Kennell, J. K., Marshall (1991). "Continuous Emotional Support During Labor in a US Hospital." *JAMA 265:* 2197–2201.

Lamaze, F. (1965). *Painless Childbirth*. New York, Pocket Books.

Langer, E. J., Janis I. L. & Wolfer, J. A. (1975). "Reduction of Psychological Stress in Surgical Patients." *Journal of Personality and Social Psychology 11:* 155–165.

Lieberman, A. (1990). *Easing Labor Pain*. New York, Doubleday.

Melzack, R., P. Taenzer, et al. (1981). "Labour is Still Painful after Prepared Childbirth." *CMA Journal 125:* 357–363.

Morgan, W. P., M. L. (1977). "Psychologic Characterization of the Elite Distance Runner." *Annals of the New York Academy of Science 301:* 382–403.

Nichols, F. H. and S. S. Humenick, Eds. (1988). *Childbirth Education: Practice, Research and Theory*. Philadelphia, W.B. Saunders.

Richter, J. a. S. R. (1979). "A Relaxation Technique." *American Journal of Nursing 79:* 1960.

Scott, J. R. R. (1979). "Effect of Psychoprophylaxis on labor and delivery in primiparas." *New England Journal of Medicine 294:* 1295.

Smith, D. (1987). "Conditions that Facilitate the Development of Sport Imagery Training." *The Sport Psychologist 1:* 237–247.

Sosa, R., Kennell, J. H., Robertson, S. et al. (1980). "The Effect of a Supportive Companion on Perinatal Problems, Length of Labor and Mother-Infant Interaction." *New England Journal of Medicine 303:* 597–600.

Stevens, R. (1977). "Psychological Strategies for Management of Pain in Prepared Childbirth." *Birth 3:* 157–161.

Stevens, R. J. a. H., F (1977). "Analgesic characteristics of prepared childbirth techniques: Attention focusing and Systematic Relaxation." *Journal of Psychosomatic Research 21:* 429.

Wideman, M. a. S., J. (1984). "The role of psychological mechanisms in preparation for childbirth." *American Psychologist 39:* 1357.

Worthington, E., L. (1982). "Which Prepared Childbirth Coping Strategies are Effective." *Journal of Obstetric, Gynecologic and Neonatal Nursing 11*(Jan): 45.

8

Nutrition, Eating Disorders, & The Female Athlete Triad

Debra Wein

Lyle Micheli

The female athlete triad—disordered eating, amenorrhea, and osteoporosis—was first described at an American College of Sports Medicine (ACSM) conference in 1992 in Washington, DC, yet unfortunately has been silently observed and ignored since before 1992 (Yeager, Agostini, Nattiv, & Drinkwater, 1993). Each disorder within the triad can increase morbidity and mortality, but the three together can be extremely dangerous (Brandstater, 1995). At this time, there is still much to be learned about the causes, progression, and short- and long-term risks as well as effective treatments of the individual and combined disorders. In this chapter, we will discuss what is known regarding the prevalence, warning signs and symptoms, possible causes, consequences, and treatments of the three aspects of the female athlete triad.

Historically, athletes believed that their performance would increase in relation to their thinness, perhaps as a result of influences of other athletes, coaches, and/or parents. Today, restrictive or bulimic eating (taking in large amounts of food and then attempting to rid the body of the calories through vomiting, laxatives, diuretics, or ex-

cessive exercise) is estimated to occur in at least one half of the general population of young women and perhaps even up to 62% (Eichner, Loucks, Johnson, & Nelson Steen, 1997) in the athletic population. One large study of nearly 500 female elite swimmers, aged between 9 and 18, found that over 60% of those of "average weight" and nearly 18% of "underweight" girls were trying to lose weight; 62% of them were skipping meals whereas over 75% were eating smaller meals to lose weight. Nearly 13% were vomiting, 2.5% were using laxatives, and nearly 2% were ingesting diuretics (Dummer, 1987). In a very recent survey of almost 4,000 high school students across Massachusetts (Massachusetts Department of Education, 1998), nearly 3 in 10 (29%) described themselves as slightly or very overweight, yet 2 of every 5 students (43%) reported that they were trying to lose weight. Close to one third of the female students (30%), who did not even consider themselves overweight, were trying to lose weight! Between 6 and 7% of the girls reported having used vomiting, laxatives, or diet pills during the month preceding the survey. Although these statistics are truly alarming, most research is based on self-reports or other subjective information and unfortunately, these behaviors are most often denied and kept secret, and therefore, true prevalence statistics may be extremely difficult to obtain.

Eating Disorders

Description and Prevalence

Disordered eating can be viewed as if on a continuum. At one extreme are anorexia nervosa and bulimia nervosa, and at the other end are preoccupations with weight and restrictive eating. The development of the two other aspects of the triad, amenorrhea and subsequent osteoporosis, occur secondary to disordered eating (Eichner et al., 1997).

The diagnostic criteria to define anorexia nervosa, bulimia nervosa, and eating disorders not otherwise specified are found in the *Diagnostic and Statistical Manual of Mental Disorders, 4th Edition* (DSM-IV; American Psychiatric Association [APA], 1994). Eating disorders include anorexia nervosa where an individual demonstrates an intense fear of gaining weight even though she is underweight (at least 5% below normal weight for height and age) and thus skips meals or severely limits food consumption. Bulimia nervosa occurs when an individual binges on large amounts of food and then attempts to rid her body of the calories she has consumed through vomiting, laxatives, diuretics, or excessive exercise. Warning signs for anorexia include drastic weight loss, wearing of baggy or layered clothing, excessive exercise and avoidance of food-related social activities. Warning signs for bulimia nervosa include excessive concern about weight, bathroom visits after meals (sometimes for long periods with water running constantly), depressive moods, strict dieting followed by large binges, and increased criticism of one's body. See Table 8-1, which describes other warning signs for eating disorders.

To identify an athlete with an eating disorder, in addition to the criteria developed (APA, 1994), look for subtle physical signs such as a deceased pulse rate of 40 to 50 beats per minute, history of fainting, parotid swelling or "chipmunk cheeks," erosion of the tooth enamel or a large amount of dental work, Russell's sign (finger and nail changes on the first and second digits of the dominant hand; Brandstater, 1995), as well as medial signals such as abnormally low white blood cell counts, mild anemia, constipation, abdominal pain, high cholesterol, low mineral levels (especially magnesium, zinc, phosphates), and elevated amylase (APA, 1994).

Table 8-1. Warning Signs for Eating Disorders

• intense fears of gaining weight • repeated comments about feeling fat • preoccupation with food • complaints of feeling cold • excessive exercise outside of training • bulky clothing • emaciated appearance • food restriction • leaving table soon after finishing meal • tooth erosion	• dry skin • hair loss • brittle fingernails • lanugo (fine, downy hair on the body) • scarring on the back of the hand (bulimia) • mood swings, and irritability and depression • amenorrhea in women

These disorders may come at any time, but adolescents and young girls are the most vulnerable for developing eating disorders (Shisslak et al., 1998). Some recent and disturbing information reveals that body-image views and concerns develop well before puberty and that girls as young as 9 years old are following diets and restricting calories to lose weight (Sands, Tricker, Sherman, Armatas, & Maschette, 1997; author observations). Although eating disturbances increase as girls undergo puberty, it is the psychological perspective of the girl that actually determines whether the disordered eating becomes more intensified or subsides. Negative perceptions such as negative image, poor self-esteem, and psychopathology can enhance the disordered eating pattern (Sands et al.).

Girls may become less satisfied with their shape over time as a result of interrelated factors including familial knowledge and practices of nutrition, media images, self-efficacy, developmental integrity, actual height, current weight, and peer-group influences as well as other lifestyle influences (Sands et al.). Boys who identified themselves as gay or bisexual were also more likely to diet (35% vs. 13%), take diet pills (18% vs. 3%), and vomit or use laxatives (32% vs. 3%) This phenomenon is seen increasingly in adult males and is very prevalent in bodybuilders (Andersen, Barlett, Morgan, & Brownell, 1995). Almost half (46%) of the 49 all natural bodybuilders who participated in a questionnaire reported episodes of binge eating after competitions whereas more than three quarters (82%)

How Eating Disorders Differ From Disordered Eating
(Adapted from the National Eating Disorders Screening Program, 1996)

1. Essential distinction

Disordered Eating: A reaction to life situations; a habit

Eating Disorders: An illness

2. Psychological Symptoms

Disordered Eating: Infrequent thoughts and behaviors and thoughts about body, foods, and eating that do not lead to health, social, school, and work problems.

Eating Disorders: Frequent and persistent thoughts and behaviors about body, foods, and eating that do lead to health, social, school, and work problems.

3. Associated Medical Problems

Disordered Eating: May lead to transient weight changes or nutritional problems; rarely causes major medical complications.

Eating Disorders: Can result in major medical complications leading to the need for hospitalization or even death.

4. Treatment

Disordered Eating: Education and/or self-help group can assist; psychotherapy and nutritional counseling can be helpful but not always essential. Problem may go away without treatment.

Eating Disorders: Requires specific medical and mental health treatment. Problem does not go away without treatment.

reported being preoccupied with food sometimes, often, or always one week prior to competition (Andersen et al.).

Researchers are beginning to find a high incidence of subclinical eating disorders (Culnane & Deustsch, 1998; author observations) that do not exactly match the standard criteria set by the DSM-IV (APA, 1994), yet can still be harmful for athletes and young girls (Yeager et al., 1993). It, therefore, becomes important to seek out not only those individuals whose patterns match the set criteria but also those who regularly calorie restrict, are slightly preoccupied with food, have a less than ideal body image, and possess poor attitudes about food.

Possible Causes

Psychological issues including poor coping skills, low self-esteem, and lack of identity as well as physical or sexual abuse can lead an individual to an eating disorder (Eichner et al., 1997). Girls, aged 13–16 years old, were more likely to diet if they perceived pressures from their parents to diet or fit a certain mold whereas those girls who were taught self-confidence and autonomy were less likely to diet (Paxton, 1998). The stress leading to disordered eating could stem from an intense determination to succeed at sports, in academics, or even in social situations, but

Table 8-2. Factors Placing Athlete at Greater Risk of Eating Disorder

- poor coping skills
- lack of self-esteem
- poor identity
- necessity to meet inappropriate weight goals
- pressure to succeed
- perceived societal expectations
- trying to fit into established norms
- inability to deal with stress properly

a closer look at certain requirements of sport reveals that athletes especially may be at even greater risk. Although exercise provides numerous benefits to the individual who partakes in sensible and balanced activities, extreme intense physical activity can cause delayed puberty, menstrual disorders, stress fractures, and early onset of non-age-related osteoporosis (Myszkewycz & Koutedakis, 1998). Athletes involved in at-risk sports include those in which revealing clothing is the uniform, such as in ballet and other dance, figure skating, diving, and swimming; those in which performance is based on subjectivity, such as with dancers, gymnasts, divers, and synchronized swimmers; those in which weight can be a hindrance to performance, such as with distance runners, ballet dancers, figure skaters, cross-country skiers; or those in which weight classifications are built in such as with rowing, bodybuilding, and the martial arts.

Although research reveals that those who participate in activity are more likely to have high self-esteem and feel more positive about their bodies than are those who do not (Biddle, 1993; Sands et al., 1997;), research also describes athletes as having a higher prevalence of eating disorders than the general population (Shangold, 1990). It seems that even though a woman's conditioning level may be very high, she may also be very dissatisfied with her body (Finkenberg, 1993). See Table 8-2 for factors placing athletes at greater risk of developing an eating disorder.

Consequences and Treatment

The athlete's body requires peak nutrition in order to meet the needs of intense training and exercise. Disordered eating and inadequate caloric intake can impair athletic performance by decreasing endurance, strength reaction time, speed, and ability to concentrate. Lightheadedness, very low blood pressure and pulse, dehydration (Mitchell, Seim,

Colon, & Pomeroy, 1987), electrolyte imbalances, and fatigue—all detrimental to performance—could also occur. Although a decrease in athletic ability may not result immediately after an athlete restricts intake or employs other unhealthy techniques of weight management, over time, more severe consequences will surface (Van De Loo & Johnson, 1995). These consequences can include menstrual dysfunction, potentially irreversible bone loss, psychological complications such as depression, gastrointestinal, and thermoregulatory changes, and a risk of death. In nonathletes treated for eating disorders, the death rate is reported at 18% (Van De Loo & Johnson) and according to the National Institutes of Mental Health (1993), about 1 in 10 cases of eating disorders leads to death from cardiac arrest, starvation, or suicide.

As implied by the title "eating disorder," some well-meaning individuals may wrongly try to "treat" the disorder by suggesting the athlete resume normal eating practices, eat more, or merely stop participating in these risky behaviors, as if the suggestion could actually make it so. Clinically, however, eating disorders are considered to be a mental disorder and are often an expression of underlying emotional distress, thereby ensuring that the treatment must address issues such as concerns related to food-intake patterns, food- and weight-related behaviors, body image, and weight reduction (ADA, 1994).

Outpatient treatment is adequate for most individuals working through their eating disorder; however, for some, the comprehensive support and treatment available through hospitalization become necessary. The decision, made on a case-by-case basis, should be made by members of the treatment team, which could include the doctors, registered dietitians, mental health professionals, coaches, and parents. Typically, those with bulimia nervosa do not require hospitalization whereas those with anorexia nervosa are more likely candidates. Issues used by the medical team to decide whether to admit a patient include amount of lost weight, body mass index, rapidity of progressive weight loss (1–2 lb. weight loss despite concomitant psychotherapy), weight less than 20% below average weight for height, severe metabolic disturbances, certain cardiac dysfunctions, syncope, psychomotor retardation, severe depression or suicide risk, severe bingeing and purging (with risk of aspiration), psychosis, family crisis, inability to perform normal daily functions, or lack of response to outpatient programs (ADA, 1994).

Amenorrhea

Definition and Prevalence

Amenhorrea, a potential consequence of and sometimes a warning sign for eating disorders, is defined as the absence of menstrual bleeding. Many athletes, not realizing the potential dangers associated with this condition, often welcome this as one less hassle to deal with and find it a desirable effect of intense training. Menarche should occur approximately 2 years after a young girl begins to develop breasts (Van De Loo & Johnson, 1995). When menstruation does not occur by the age of 16 years old, the individual is diagnosed with primary amenorrhea. Secondary amenorrhea, on the other hand, is the absence of at least three to six consecutive menstrual cycles in females who have already begun to menstruate (Van De Loo & Johnson). The prevalence of secondary amenorrhea is between 2 and 5% in the general population as compared to a staggering 3 and 66% of the athletic population (Shangold, Rebar, Wentz, & Schiff, 1990). Oligomenorrhea, another type of menstrual irregularity often seen in athletes with eating disorders, is menstrual cycles lasting longer than 36 days.

Some causes of menstrual dysfunction, unrelated to exercise and poor nutritional habits, include pregnancy, pituitary tumors, thyroid dysfunction, polycystic ovary disease, and premature ovarian failure. The causes must be ruled out before a diagnosis of amenorrhea secondary to an eating disorder is made (Shangold et al., 1990).

Possible Causes

Women who fail to meet their energy needs due to inadequate calorie intake develop amenorrhea (Van De Loo & Johnson, 1995). However, amenorrhea has also been linked to poor nutrition, low body weight, low caloric intake, hormonal status, and psychological and physiological stress (Myszkewycz & Koutedakis, 1998). Whether a threshold of caloric balance exists for a female athlete to maintain menses and, thus, reproductive health is still questionable. However, balancing calories consumed with those expended is of utmost importance in helping athletes to restore regular menses and thus preventing the triad from continuing and leading to osteoporosis (Eichner et al., 1997). Athletes who underconsume calories and then begin to take in extra calories to meet energy requirements have not shown weight gain (author observations).

Amenorrhea is an overt sign of decreased estrogen production (Yeager et al., 1993) and causes estrogen levels to drop to levels similar to those of postmenopausal women. Bone density tests show that the spinal density of some young athletes may be similar to those of women in their 80s (Shangold et al., 1990). Estrogen plays a significant role in maintaining skeletal integrity and strength (Myszkewycz & Koutedakis, 1998). Thus, a long-term decrease in estrogen levels often leads to a reduction in bone mineral density and possibly osteoporosis (Myszkewycz & Koutedakis). For the best health of the athlete and in order to avoid further progression

of the triad to osteoporosis, treatment must be immediate and aggressive.

Consequences and Treatment

It is believed that by increasing energy intake approximately 10–20% (or by decreasing training), the female can restore normal menses (Eichner et al., 1997), but not necessarily replace all decreases in bone density (Shangold, 1990). Because of the link of estrogen and bone integrity, many clinicians are prescribing oral contraceptives to treat amenorrhea and prevent osteoporosis (Eichner et al., 1997).

Long-term consequences of the estrogen-depleted body are still not clearly defined. Although a potentially irreversible bone loss could occur, estrogen depletion could also be linked to problems of the cardiovascular system and reproductive organs (Van De Loo & Johnson, 1995).

Osteoporosis

Description and Prevalence

Osteoporosis is characterized by a decreased bone mass and an increased susceptibility to fractures (National Institutes of Health [NIH], 1984). A fall, a blow, or a lifting action that would not cause strain in an individual with normal bone density would cause one or more bones to break in an individual with osteoporosis (NIH, 1984).

In addition to water, fat protein (70%), calcium (10%), phosphorous, potassium, zinc, and magnesium (combined 20%) all contribute to the development of bone (Myszkewycz & Koutedakis, 1998). Therefore, restricted eating can severely affect the natural formation of bone. The strongest predictor of peak bone density is believed to be genetics (Seeman, Hopper, & Bach, 1989), although menstrual history is also important (Van De Loo & Johnson, 1995). Bone mass acquisition (development) is gradual in early childhood, and accelerates during adolescence until sexual maturity is reached. Nearly 50% of all adult skeletal mass is formed during the second decade of life (Van De Loo & Johnson). Peak accumulation is thought to occur during the first three decades of life with 95% of the maximum density reached by age 18 (Brandstater 1995). With recent trends towards increasing reliance on fast foods to meet busy schedules as well as increased television viewing and decreased sport participation and physical activity in schools, our adolescents have become more susceptible to poor bone mass acquisition.

Possible Causes

Osteoporosis in the young female athlete may occur as a result of amenorrhea or oligomenorrhea (Van De Loo & Johnson, 1995) and may be explained by the failure of the female body to attain a sufficiently high bone mineral content during growth or through an excessive bone loss in early adulthood (Myszkewycz & Koutedakis, 1998). A decrease in estrogen, as seen in amenorrhea, results from the bone's increased release of calcium ions, which are essential to proper growth (Myburgh, Bachrach, Lewis, Kent, & Marcus, 1993).

Consequences and Treatment

Fracture frequency increases as bone density decreases (Myszkewycz & Koutedakis, 1998). In one study, athletes who suffered from oligomenorrhea were six times more likely to sustain a stress fracture and the likelihood of stress fractures increased to eight times if the athlete also had a restrictive diet (Van De Loo & Johnson). Inactivity, caused by the fracture, could further lead to problems, such as depression and further restriction of intake, potentially furthering the severity of the triad.

Prevention is key because osteoporosis, as a result of amenorrhea or oligomenorrhea,

cannot be reversed even if menstruation is resumed, estrogen is present, or calcium is supplemented (Van De Loo & Johnson, 1995). The best method to prevent osteoporosis is to develop a healthy skeleton during growth and maturation (Myszkewycz & Koutedakis, 1998), yet in those who already suffer from osteoporosis, reducing exercise, improving nutrient intake, and increasing body weight can help to improve bone mineral density although these levels may never return to normal (Eichner et al., 1997; Shangold et al., 1990).

Not all amenorrheic athletes have low bone mass (Otis et al., 1997), and it is known that high-intensity exercise can increase the bone mass density of an athlete in specific sites despite amenorrhea. This was seen in a group of skaters who had higher bone mass density than controls despite their menstrual function (Van De Loo & Johnson, 1995). It is still important to try to restore regular menses because longer-term information is not available. Therefore, health professionals must not rely solely on the argument that amenorrhea causes low bone density because although the bone density may be normal, other risks may still be prevalent.

Female Athlete Triad: Treatment Issues

In order to truly prevent the female athlete triad, a multidisciplinary team approach is not optional but necessary. For recognition of the disorder(s), more than a survey or questionnaire may be necessary, and research may take the shape of an open-ended discussion between a skilled health professional and each athlete who joins a new team or athletic community.

The team members, at a minimum, should include a physician, a registered dietitian, and a mental health professional. A physician should be available to coordinate treatment and monitor overall progress; a mental health professional can aid the athlete in uncovering the underlying issues causing the disorder; and a registered dietitian can aid the athlete in learning to fuel her body for health, well-being, and performance. For treatment purposes, a physician can serve as a case manager to monitor the medical progress of the interrelated issues and ensure compliance of the individual with treatment.

A registered dietitian/nutritionist is imperative to the team to provide the athlete with an adequate understanding of the body's needs during exercise as well as information on how to optimally fuel the body for the sport in which the athlete is participating. In their position statement on intervention in the treatment of anorexia nervosa, bulimia nervosa, and binge eating, the American Dietetic Association (ADA, 1992) outlines specific objectives that should be addressed by the nutritional counselor working with the eating-disordered athlete. The nutritionist should perform a comprehensive history in order to collect relevant information regarding history of weight changes and eating and exercise patterns as well as purging behaviors. Developing a therapeutic alliance with the patient is important to successfully resolve food fears and develop goals for weight and behavior changes. Correct concepts and principles of food, nutrition, and weight control must be taught, and myths should be dispelled.

Over the course of nutritional treatment, the athlete needs to understand the symptoms of, and the body's response, to starvation, metabolism, abnormal and normal hunger, day-to-day weight fluctuations, a healthy weight range, the minimum food intake needed to stabilize weight and metabolic rate, optimal food intake for health, etc. Examples of individuals who have successfully recovered from an eating disorder should be presented to the athlete including what this individual's hunger patterns, typical food intake patterns, and total caloric intakes might resemble. Educating the family is another objective important to the successful recovery of the individual. The nutritionist could offer suggestions on meal planning, nutrient needs, and strategies for dealing with inappropriate food- and weight-related behaviors, which should be addressed with both the athlete and her family.

The psychologist/mental health professional is necessary to deal with and help the athlete come to terms with the root of the problems bringing on the disorder in the first place. Decreasing stress at meal times and helping the family work towards a supportive rather than confrontational environment are important goals. A patient's ability to make changes in food intake, weight, and behaviors may decrease in the event that disturbing emotions surface; therefore, supportive and understanding professionals allow the athlete to feel more comfortable about stopping and resuming therapy (ADA, 1994).

Coaches, parents, athletic training staff, teachers, administrators, physical therapists, choreographers, and dance instructors all need to be involved in the team in identifying, addressing, and helping to monitor recovery from the triad. They must all be aware of the components of the triad as well as the symptoms, the risks, the consequences, and the severity as well as proper approaches to take with athletes including resources available locally. Members of the team must also do their best to separate their biases and needs when determining the appropriate treatment for the athlete.

To increase weight gradually and aid in the recovery of the triad, the following should be encouraged: a decrease in training and activity by 10 to 20%, a gradual increase in calorie intake, a weight increase of about 2 to 3% of current weight, calcium intake of 1,500 mg/day through food or supplementation, and a moderate strength-training regimen to aid in bone mineralization (Eichner et al., 1997).

Female Athlete Triad: Prevention Issues

Team prevention strategies (ADA, 1994)

The following techniques and strategies should be considered when working with each new athlete:

- Separate food- and weight-related behaviors from feelings and psychological issues. Having the athlete appreciate the difference can help her to learn to separate facts and move toward a better understanding of how to get better.
- Teach the connection between food intake and health and the requirement of nutrients in food for the optimal functioning of our bodies.
- Incorporate education with behavior change. For example, teach the need for nutrients and energy before suggesting an increase in caloric intake.
- Work on small changes rather than making gross alterations in the athlete's lifestyle. Discourage an athlete from wanting to change everything at once. Small changes are more likely to be adapted and maintained.
- Explain that setbacks are normal and can be used as learning tools to resculpt responses to cues.
- Teach self-monitoring techniques such as a food diary and behavior records so that the individual can feel a sense of control over her treatment and choices. You can include food, exercise, and behaviors such as frequency of bingeing and/or purging as well as weight gain/fluctuation.
- Use weight and eating contracts, but avoid using these techniques if the individual becomes too overinvolved and you feel that it may be counterproductive.
- Slowly increase or decrease weight to prevent the individual from feeling a loss

of control and potentially cause her to withdraw from therapy.
- Teach athletes how to maintain a weight that is healthful. Encourage regular meal times, variety and moderation of intake, and gradual reintroduction of foods (typically those most recently excluded from the diet are best received).
- Evaluate and change your approach as necessary throughout treatment and with each individual.
- Strive, ultimately, for the individual to be comfortable in social eating situations where she does not have total control.

Some important messages you can share with your athletes:

- Sports participation includes physical and mental health.
- Winning at all costs is not an ideal philosophy.
- Successful performance relates to optimal nutrient intakes of all of the macro- and micronutrients.
- Strength, stamina, and body composition are more important than body weight.
- Sexual maturation is normal.
- Changes in eating, activity levels, menstrual patterns, or performance should be addressed with an appropriate professional as soon as possible.

In approaching an individual you suspect has an eating disorder, keep in mind the following (Wein, 1996):

- An individual with a solid and positive relationship with the athlete will be the ideal individual to approach her.
- Approach her in a relaxed manner and in private. Go by yourself rather than in an intimidating group.
- Always approach her from your point of view. For example, say, "I am concerned about your well-being" or "I feel that . . . ". This approach is much less

confrontational than "You have done this. . . ." The athlete will find it harder to argue with your feelings. How can she say you are wrong? You are simply expressing your feelings.

• Explain that you are there for her, not against her. Assure her that no matter what she says. you will not criticize her or make her feel bad or embarrassed.

• Use terms like "well-being" rather than "disorder" or "sickness." Approach her rather than accuse her.

• Don't use terms such as "bingeing," "fasting," or "purging" as they make her defensive.

• If you are not in the position of making a

Table 8-3. National Resources on the Female Athlete Triad

American Anorexia/Bulimia Association
www.members.aol.com/amanbu
Provides national referrals to therapists, hospitals, and treatment centers. Offers a quarterly newsletter, support groups, and community outreach nationwide.

American College of Sports Medicine
317-637-9200   www.acsm.org
Position statement on the Female Athlete Triad, slides for presentations, and other resources.

American Dietetic Association
800-877-1600   www.eatright.org
Position statement on the treatment of eating disorders, referrals to local dietitians, and other resources. A separate practice group covering eating disorders and related issues, SCAN: Sports Cardiovascular and Wellness Nutritionists.

Anorexia Nervosa and Related Eating Disorders Inc.
541-344-1144   www.anred.com
An information clearinghouse; offers a free booklet.

Eating Disorders Awareness and Prevention
206-382-3587   www.members.aol.com/EDAPinc
Sponsors Eating-Disorders Awareness Week every February and provides screening materials for distribution.

International Association of Eating Disorders Professionals
800-800-8126 or 561-338-6494
Provides national and international referrals.

National Association of Anorexia Nervosa and Associated Disorders
847-831-3438   www.healthtouch.com
Has a hotline, free phone counseling for you and the patient/client, informational brochures, referrals to local professionals and support groups, and prevention programs.

National Collegiate Athletic Association
913-339-1906   www.ncaa.org
Videos, handouts, and other printed materials available.

National Eating Disorders Organization
918-481-4044   www.laureate.com
Will find support, education, treatment, and/or referrals for people with eating disorders.

specific diagnosis, then don't. Simply ask if she needs help rather than tell her she has a problem or try to diagnose her.

- Do not try to gather evidence by catching her in the act of bingeing or purging. Sometimes even mentioning these activities may cause her to feel more pressure and to become more defensive.
- No matter the outcome, give her the phone number of a qualified psychologist, eating-disorder specialist, or resource organization in your area that she can use in the future should she decide she wants to contact someone. See Table 8-3 for organizations providing resources and referrals for eating disorders.
- Most important, let her know that you are there if and when she is ready to talk.

As sports medicine professionals, we have the opportunity to help athletes maximize their nutritional intake and fitness regimen by focusing them on healthy habits and lifestyles. We can teach our athletes to adopt enjoyable eating and exercise behaviors to reduce disease risk and improve well-being in the long run. We can help them to think of every action as permanent lifestyle habits rather than a temporary behavior. We can be sensitive to an athlete's changes in mood and energy level—a sign that she may be pushing herself a bit too aggressively. We can learn to reward our athletes for even small successes and to deal with lapses in healthy eating by problem solving not sabotaging. We can teach our athletes to use social support systems—friends, relatives, team members, and support groups—to help them stay on track, maintain new habits, and get out feelings, appreciating that it is OK to seek a professional to sort through ill feelings.

Referring to another health professional allows us to work together to pool knowledge and share responsibility as well as provide a model of team collaboration for our athlete(s). A cohesive treatment plan must include individuals who share philosophies similar to our own about intervention, treatment, and recovery. In working together, the recognition, treatment, and prevention of the female athlete triad are more likely. With our help, athletes can learn to plan a well-balanced life filled with proper amounts of food and exercise as a means of optimizing sports performance, which can also provide much pleasure as well.

References

American Psychiatric Association. (1994). *Diagnostic and statistical manual of mental disorders* (4th ed.). Washington, DC: Author.

American Dietetic Association. *Position Statement on Intervention in the Treatment of Anorexia Nervosa, Bulimia, and Binge Eating.* October 18, 1987, and reaffirmed on September 12, 1992.

Andersen, R. E., Barlett, S. J., Morgan, G. D. & Brownell, K. D. (1995) Weight loss, psychological, and nutritional patterns in competitive male body builders. *International Journal of Eating Disorders, 18*(1), 49–57.

Biddle, S. (1993). Children, exercise and health. *International Journal of Sport Psychology, 24*, 200–216.

Brandstater, M. E. (1995). Female athlete triad. *Western Journal of Medicine, 162*(2), 149–150.

Culnane, C. & Deutsch, D. (1998). Dancer disordered eating. *Journal of Dance Medicine and Science, 2*(3), 95–100.

Dummer, G. M., Rosen, L. W., Huesner, W. W., Roberts, P. J., & Counsilman, J. E. (1987). Pathogenic weight control behaviors of young competitive swimmers. *The Physician and Sports Medicine, 15*(50), 75–86.

Eichner, E. R., Loucks, A. B., Johnson, M., & Nelson Steen, S. (1997). The female athlete triad. *Sports Science Exchange Roundtable, 8*(1), 27–31.

Finkenberg, M., DiNucci, J., McCune, S., & McCune, D. (1993). Body esteem and enrollment in classes with different levels of physical activity. *Perceptual and Motor Skills, 76*, 783–792.

Massachusetts Department of Education. (1998). *1997 Massachusetts youth risk behavior survey results.* Boston: U.S. Centers for Disease Control & Prevention Division of Adolescent & School Health [U87/CCU 109035-02].

Mitchell, J., Seim, H., Colon, E., & Pomeroy, C. (1987). Medical complications and medical management of bulimia. *Annals of Internal Medicine, 107*, 71–77.

Myburgh, K. H., Bachrach, L. K., Lewis, B., Kent, K., & Marcus, R. (1993). Low bone mineral density at axial and appendicular sites in amenorrheic athletes. *Medicine and Science in Sports and Exercise, 25*(1), 1197–1202.

Myszkewycz, L., & Koutedakis, Y. (1998). Injuries, amenorrhea and osteoporosis in active athletes: An overview. *Journal of Dance Medicine and Science, 2*(3), 88–94.

National Eating Disorders Screening Program. (1996, Feb. 1–8). *Eating disorders newsletter* and slide presentation. National Mental Illness Screening Project.

National Institutes of Health. (1984). Osteoporosis consensus conference. *Journal of the American Medical Association, 252*(6), 799–802.

National Institutes of Mental Health. (1993). *Eating disorders* [DHHS Publication No. (NIH) 93–3477]. Washington, DC: U.S. Department of Health & Human Services.

Otis, C. L., Drinkwater, B., Johnson, M., Loucks, A., & Wilmore, J. (1997). The American College of Sports Medicine position stand: The female athlete triad. *Medicine and Science in Sports and Exercise, 29,* i–ix.

Paxton, S. J. (1998). Current issues in eating disorders research. *Journal of Psychsomatic Research, 44,* 297–299.

Sands, R., Tricker, J., Sherman, C., Armatas, C., & Maschette, W. (1997). Disordered eating patterns, body image, self-esteem, and physical activity in preadolescent school children. *International Journal of Eating Disorders, 21*(2), 159–166.

Seeman, E., Hopper, J. L., & Bach, L. A. (1989). Reduced bone mass in daughters of women with osteoporosis. *New England Journal of Medicine, 320,* 554–558.

Shangold, M., Rebar, R. W., Wentz, A. C., & Schiff, I. (1990). Evaluation and management of menstrual dysfunction in athletes. *Journal of the American Medical Association, 263,* 1665–1669.

Shisslak, C. M., Crago, M., McKnight, K. M., Estes, L. S., Gray, N., & Parnaby, O. G. (1998). Potential risk factors associated weight control behaviors in elementary and middle school girls. *Journal of the Psychosomatic Research, 44*(3/4), 301–313.

Van De Loo, D. A., & Johnson, M. D. (1995). The young female athlete. *Clinics in Sports Medicine, 14*(3), 687–707.

Wein, D. (1996, April). Clients with eating disorders. *IDEA Today, 13*(4), 22–23.

Yeager, K., Agostini, R., Nattiv, A., & Drinkwater, B. (1993). The female athlete triad: Disordered eating, amenorrhea and osteoporosis. *Medicine and Science in Sports and Exercise, 25* (7), 775–777.

9

Orthopedic Considerations in Sport Performance

William K. Thierfelder

Michael Gaudette

Imagine driving a golf ball 360 yards or throwing a baseball over 100 miles per hour. Aside from having the right parents, there are innumerable variables that make this level of performance possible. This chapter will help define these variables and explain how their interaction can either lead to extraordinary performance or increase the probability of injury.

Typically, we think of the term *orthopedic* as dealing with injury of the bones and joints. However, this rather narrow perspective tends to reduce our view to a specific body part rather than see the body as a dynamic unbroken chain, commonly referred to as the kinetic chain. Low back pain and the 360-yard drive would normally be considered mutually exclusive events when, in fact, they should be more accurately described as two extremes on the same sport-performance continuum. This will be described in greater detail as the chapter unfolds, tying together the structural, functional, and cognitive factors influencing sport performance and orthopedic injury.

Generating maximum power, whether for driving a golf ball or throwing a baseball, requires coiling and uncoiling specific body parts in a precise sequence and with exact timing. Understanding this process necessitates an integration and working knowledge of the components controlling the kinetic chain, namely, anatomy, biomechanics, physiology, neurology, and psychology. People working in the fields of orthopedics and physical rehabilitation tend to utilize the disciplines listed above in dealing with the disease state. Health and fitness experts use the same information to improve general wellness, whereas sport performance specialists use it to improve athletic performance. Understanding the kinetic chain's multitude of reactions is the first step toward realizing high-level sport performance and minimizing the risk of injury. The term *kinetic chain* refers to the linking of body segments, just like links in a chain. Movement of one link effectuates a movement in the links that are attached to it. The kinetic chain can be either open or closed. In an open kinetic chain, muscles are contracting, bones are moving, and the distal end is free to move. Throwing a baseball is an example of an open-chain activity because the hand is the last link and it is free to move. In contrast, the distal segment is not free to move in the closed kinetic chain, such as during a push-up. The hand is firmly planted on the floor, and the body moves about the fixed hand, placing different demands on the muscular system. However, the key to maximizing performance depends upon the application of scientific knowledge to the athlete's kinetic chain to control and optimize a series of specific reactions. The difference between what the athlete did (actual performance) and what the athlete wanted to do (ideal performance) is the problem. Bridging that gap is the solution. Determining the athlete's actual performance involves an accurate assessment from a multidisciplinary perspective. This might include the initial evaluation, athlete's self-report, kinesthetic awareness, observer's feedback, video, and more. Due to the interaction of many confounding variables, ideal performance is more accurately described as an approximation that is based on the athlete's initial evaluation and established scientific knowledge in the various disciplines mentioned above. The difference between actual and ideal performances helps to accurately identify the causes for less than "ideal" performance and provides a tangible structure for effective intervention.

This text is not meant as a comprehensive list of conditions that affect the performance of athletes. Rather, it is presented in a manner to conceptually educate and stimulate the readers' thought process, utilizing their own sound understanding of the body's systems. Although the tendency is to focus on the physical sciences, a rudimentary knowledge of psychology is important to fully understand how orthopedic factors influence sport performance. One tenet of sport performance is that movement, in its simplest or most complex form, is based on and affected by the kinetic chain system. Therefore, injuries, particularly the chronic or overuse type, are the result of kinetic chain dysfunction.

Working with athletes in the sport perfor-

mance arena can be both frustrating and rewarding. Athletes and clinicians are often unsure of where to find the most reliable information and delivery of sport performance services. Many programs are "packaged" well but lack substance and comprehensiveness. In today's world, sport medicine and science have the knowledge and tools to do far more than prescribe generic exercise programs. Skilled sport-performance specialists recognize problems or barriers to ideal performance and, therefore, customize the athlete's program, based on specific evaluation findings, to help make significant improvements and maximize performance.

For elite athletes, improvements usually come in smaller increments that have a greater overall impact relative to the performance of their competitors. Although achieving small performance gains can be quite significant, such achievement requires excellent planning and much hard work. The saying "great athletes are born and not made" is misleading because it assumes that the science of sport performance has been readily accessible to all athletes. There is clear evidence from the old Soviet and Eastern Bloc countries that many athletes had been "made" through the use, and sometimes abuse, of sport medicine and science. Surprisingly, elite American athletes appear to have risen through the sport ranks by attrition rather than design. Even at this elite level, a systematic evaluation can help to identify glaring problems within the many components that constitute performance.

Observing the athlete during a training session or competition, prior to completing an in-depth evaluation, will reveal most of the obvious problems involving flexibility, strength, speed, agility, biomechanics, and motor control. These problems should be closely assessed during the evaluation to further define the discrepancy between actual and ideal performances. This will make it possible to design and implement a plan that will create positive changes in performance. The goal in working with athletes of all abilities is to maximally improve their present level of performance and longevity. In the context of an athlete's long-term participation and enjoyment, realizing short-term gains at the expense of future improvements is usually not a wise decision.

The purpose of the evaluation and assessment is to assist the clinician in finding the causative factors of the sub par performance and address them systematically. A comprehensive and integrated evaluation should start with a complete medical history that elicits pertinent information through direct questioning:

- Are previous injuries causing the athlete to perform or compensate in an undesirable way?
- Are there any medical problems that specifically affect the athlete's performance, such as diabetes?
- Is the athlete currently in pain? What is the pattern of that pain? What makes it better or worse?
- Is the athlete taking any medications?
- Are there any problems with vision or hearing that may impact performance?
- Determine the athlete's training patterns based on types of exercises or drills, intensity, volume, duration, and recovery.
- Can the athlete's training patterns be traced to overuse problems?
- Does the athlete have an understanding of periodization?
- Has the athlete noticed a plateau or reduction in performance levels?

The answers to these and other training questions will help establish a clearer picture of the factors that have contributed to current performance levels and provide a direction for future improvements.

The physical assessment portion of the evaluation establishes a baseline. A postural assessment done in relaxed stance should show potential problem areas that will require a more in-depth exam. Problems such as scoliosis, forward head posture, rounded shoulders, excessive kyphosis or lordosis, anterior pelvic tilt, femoral anteversion or retroversion, genu recurvatum or varum/valgum, or excessive pronation can have a major impact on performance. These postural problems often result in poor mechanics by causing the athlete to compensate. Range of motion and flexibility measurements are important to assure that there is an adequate amount of movement needed at all applicable areas of the athlete's body. Joint or muscle tightness will often cause the surrounding areas to compensate, sometimes resulting in a hypermobility of those tissues. This creates an imbalance with some areas being hypermobile and some being hypomobile. A strength assessment of the major muscle groups will determine their ability to develop the force needed for a given sport. This assessment should also include assessing the smaller muscles responsible for controlling motion, assisting in maintaining joint integrity, fine-tuning the segmental movements, and reducing strain on the larger muscles and tendons. Maintaining joint congruency and integrity is important for developing and transferring force to subsequent segments. If the smaller muscles effectively do their job, they will prevent injuries, primarily the overuse type. Aerobic capacity and muscular endurance can significantly affect performance and should, therefore, be measured and considered in the development of the program.

A neuromuscular control and learning assessment can provide information about muscular function that is not ascertained from an isolated strength assessment. Athletes should perform specific skills that imitate the physical and mental demands of their sport. Skill acquisition can be assessed by observing the athlete's speed and accuracy while performing one of these sport-specific tasks. For example, a tennis player may perform a high-intensity footwork drill whereas a basketball player works on a one-on-three ball handling drill. A less skill-specific, but valuable, test might include a comparison of single-leg balancing with eyes open and then closed. This type of skill assessment provides information about the integrity of the neuro-muscular feedback mechanisms and how the athlete compensates for any deficits.

Functional training should be included in the plan as it incorporates strengthening components at multiple joints, in multiple planes of motion, and is done in a way that mimics the normal movements of a specific sport. Functional training improves strength and allows the athlete to practice the transfer of force. The result is a complete training benefit for developing, transferring, and imparting force. This force can be used in a variety of sport-specific ways such as striking a ball or pushing and pulling water through the swim stroke.

Proper flexibility is an important aspect of individual muscle function that also plays a significant role in synergistic movement patterns that sequentially move body segments toward the desired goal. Flexibility allows each segment of the body to go through an adequate range of motion and achieve the "windup" that is required for preloading the muscles. It will also prevent tearing when the muscles are quickly stretched and contracted. Optimal performance requires that a muscle be trained in a manner similar to the way it will be used during an activity. This includes aspects such as speed, duration, resistance, and range. For example, high-resistance, low-speed biceps exercise in the 30° to 90° of flexion range has little carryover to pitching a baseball where the ideal performance criterion is low-resistance, high-speed

deceleration of the elbow from 30° to 0° of extension. Specificity of training has been well documented, suggesting the need to look at a multitude of factors when designing exercise programs, especially for elite athletes. Neglecting to correct specific deficits creates an unstable base and prevents the successful training of movement patterns beneficial to ideal performance. After eliminating these deficits, progress can be made toward integrating all of the body segments into a synergistic whole.

Knowing the movements involved in the particular sport will help determine the power demands. Is lower body power as important as upper body power? Is flexibility very important? Observing athletes in their natural training and competition environment frequently reveals great mechanical and psychological insights that may otherwise be missed. Recognizing the psychological barriers to optimal performance can be a major part of achieving success as a sport performance specialist. For most athletes, sport becomes their identity. Consequently, fear of an injury or other psychological issues can commonly underlie physical problems. Note the mechanical and physiological demands including power, agility, speed, fine motor control, flexibility, endurance, and their combined interaction. This practical experience also enables the clinician to learn the "culture and language" of the sport and cultivate a deeper, more trusting relationship with those athletes.

The comprehensive evaluation process provides the critical information needed to design a challenging, yet achievable, individualized training program. This approach will often allow the clinician to effectively address the athlete's deficits in a way that no one else has tried in the past. Although two clinicians have the same qualifications, they may have very different approaches to dealing with the same problem. Athletes need to be aware that a skilled clinician can sometimes miss the cause of their problem. They may need to seek a second or third opinion in order to gain a different perspective and solution for the same problem. For example, if a car breaks down, it is usually brought to a mechanic for repair, but if the problem is not adequately fixed, would the car be abandoned or brought to another mechanic? Although athletes may become skeptical or frustrated during this process, a skilled clinician can quickly re-engage them by teaching a practical exercise or drill that results in some immediate improvement.

To make significant long-term gains in sport performance, athletes must develop an acute, kinesthetic awareness of their bodies in order to know what they did during the actual performance. Kinesthetic awareness is the athlete's ability to precisely "feel" the performance as accurately as the evaluator can see the performance. Focus and attention play a vital role by filtering out extraneous information and highlighting the essential aspects of the performance. Through learning and incorporating various physical and mental skills into the training program, the athlete can dramatically improve this skill. Initially, training to process information faster and more accurately requires an undesirable level of conscious thought. Through accurate repetition, this skill gradually becomes unconscious, enabling the athlete to enter a "flow" state and move closer to the ideal performance. Although it is beyond the scope of this chapter, selecting mental skills that employ visual, auditory, and tactile cues will help the athlete to master movement and more efficiently use the kinetic chain to optimize sport-specific biomechanics.

Lack of proper instruction during the earliest stages of biomechanical development can have enduring negative effects on performance and may necessitate intervention. Making major changes in the natural mechanics of the elite athlete is usually not a good idea. Current compensatory mechanics are often long-term adaptations to the athlete's body structure and physiology. Even though the athlete may require major changes because the present performance level is predicated on bad habits, the decision to intervene must be weighed carefully. However, making some minor changes may prevent future injury and improve the athlete's overall performance. The decision to intervene will usually depend on the athlete's age, present level of performance, or injury status.

It is best to take the "big picture" approach when working with the athlete rather than focus on the painful or problem area. Problems may exist due to poor or compensatory mechanics above or below the injured body part in the kinetic chain.

Looking at the whole body as a kinetic chain will greatly increase the clinician's success rate in working with athletes. For instance, a problem in the upper body can lead to a problem in the lower body due to the reciprocal nature of gait. A limitation in one shoulder or arm may decrease its natural swing during walking or running. This will reduce the excursion of movement in the contra-lateral lower extremity and alter the entire gait cycle. Finally, abnormal strain will be placed on the area compensating for the upper extremity limitation. To observe this phenomenon, have an athlete run with both arms crossed over the chest. Notice the significant decrease in performance and compensatory overuse of the lower extremities.

Physiological factors including energy stores, energy release, body fluids, muscular contractions, neuromuscular control, cardiorespiratory function, training effects, environmental factors, nutritional status, and ergogenic aids all control and greatly influence the development of muscular force. Applying that force to an intact biomechanical system results in functional movement.

Appropriate force production first requires that a muscle be stretched to a relatively lengthened position. In a perfect world, the force produced at each segment builds on the peak force produced at the more proximal segment, or perhaps in the lower body, creating a cumulative effect. This precise timing will allow the athlete to reach a much higher level of force or velocity, expressed in a more global sense as the combined development of force being maximized at the moment of impact.

Many athletic events require that significant power be developed in the lower body and then transferred to each segment in the kinetic chain, often to the upper extremity. Most sports-specific movements begin with a combined "winding" of the segments of the body away from the end result to place the muscles on stretch. From that position, forces are produced within each segment that move the body in the direction of the desired movement. A crucial link in the transfer of force from the lower extremities to the upper body is the area between the pelvis and upper torso controlled by the abdominal musculature. This area is often referred to as the *core* of the body. The core is vital to both high-level sport performance and injury prevention. Building strength and neuromuscular control will help prevent injury. As with every link in the kinetic chain, it is necessary for the core to receive and control momentum from the previous segment. The new segment contributes to the total force and then passes it on to the next segment in the kinetic chain. Inefficiency can cause a dissipation of force tangential to the optimal line of force transfer or the absorption of this energy by the discs, ligaments, and joints, resulting in injury.

Analysis of the sport event is essential to the design and content of the training program. In golf, the object of the swing is to hit a stationary ball. There is an opportunity to take time aligning the body, club, and ball. There is a coiling, an uncoiling, and finally an imparting of the cumulative force through the club head to the ball. Accurately striking a golf ball with a club at high speed requires proper alignment of the hips to the feet, the shoulders to the hips, the arms to the shoulders, the club to the arms, and, last, the club to the ball. If there is poor alignment at any of these areas during the transfer of force or at the moment of impact, energy will be lost or misdirected through the object, resulting in a poor outcome. Compensations in the swing can minimize some problems with setup and delivery, but the loss of power and accuracy will result in a performance that is below average.

In tennis, the object of the swing is to hit a moving ball. The right body position, relative to the ball, is critical for setting up the swing and avoiding compensatory mechanics. Good foot speed enables the athlete to achieve that appropriate body position to meet the demands of variable ball movement and velocity. Although contact with the ball is important, greater emphasis and skill are placed on the setup and ball placement in the opponent's court.

All sports have unique requirements for applying force; however, there is a common process for developing a maximal total force that involves the entire body. There is a coiling and centralizing of the body mass used to preload the muscles. The initiation of motion toward the desired goal begins the uncoiling phase, designed to develop, transfer, and build force development. The force developed through the lower body opens the hip and pelvis toward the final target while the upper body and throwing arm lag behind, undergoing a further stretch and preload. When the lead foot is planted, the lower body momentum is abruptly stopped, accelerating the forward rotation of the upper torso. The abdominals contract to flex and rotate the upper torso toward the target as the chest and anterior shoulder muscles accelerate the lead arm through in a whip-like fashion.

Anatomically, having an intact musculotendinous unit and proper osseous alignment is essential for this efficient application of force and accurate movement. Misalignments causing problems should be corrected, or the athlete will compensate, possibly leading to poor performance and injury. One common lower extremity problem that affects sport performance is excessive pronation. Pronation, or *pes planus*, is a slight flattening of the medial longitudinal arch of the foot that helps the body to absorb force and adapt to the surface it is walking or running over. In a closed-chain environment, when the calcaneus everts, the talus adducts, and the plantar flexes, the medial longitudinal arch falls; and the tibia internally rotates. Some of this motion is normal and, in fact, necessary. However, when it becomes excessive or poorly timed, it presents a problem. The foot becomes too mobile and inefficient in transmitting force to the ground. A customized biomechanical foot orthotic can be effectively utilized to support the foot and control this excessive amount and speed of pronation. Soft tissue in the foot will break down if overloaded by an excessively high amount or rate of force. Most athletic events require that force production in the lower extremity be transmitted through the foot to the ground to initiate movement of the body. During excessive pronation, the potential energy that is established with preload of the lower extremities is lost as it changes to kinetic energy during the initiation of movement. Whether the ground gives way or the shoe slips on the surface, the energy is lost. Slipping on a wet floor is a good example of energy loss through improper force transfer.

To illustrate the chain reaction that occurs in the lower extremity, picture a batter preparing to hit a baseball. Weight is shifted to the back leg, which externally rotates with supination of the foot. The gastrocnemius and soleus produce a force that is applied through the Achilles tendon to the calcaneus, causing slight plantar flexing. Ultimately, the foot intrinsic musculature and plantar fascia keep the foot supinated to provide a rigid lever for transferring force to the ground, initiating the swing. At the same time, the slightly flexed stance leg will extend, adding to the power that has already been developed. The center of mass is displaced laterally by a strong contraction of the supporting leg's gluteus medius and an abductory thrust of the front leg toward the pitcher's mound. As the center of mass is moved toward the pitcher's mound, the weight shifts from the lateral to the medial border of the foot. The peroneus longus contracts to hold the first ray rigidly against the ground. This process is vital to preventing excessive pronation and allowing appropriate force transfer. Excessive pronation due to an alignment problem or muscular insufficiency will "unlock" the bones in the foot and allow the force to be dissipated rather than transferred up the kinetic chain. This demonstrates Newton's third law of motion: For every action, there is an equal and opposite reaction. Running on the beach is a good example of inefficient energy transfer because substantial energy is lost when the sand underneath the foot gives way.

Structural varus deformities in the tibia, calcaneus (rearfoot), or metatarsals (forefoot) can result in excessive pronation of the foot with obligatory lower extremity internal rotation. Abnormal alignments farther up the kinetic chain can also add to the loss of energy or momentum transfer. Genu valgum or varum may affect lateral movement by shifting the center of gravity relative to the plant foot, or it may affect the extension moment of the knee by altering patellofemoral tracking. Likewise, excessive pronation of the foot with accompanied lower extremity internal rotation will move the trochlear groove medially, out from underneath the patella. Weakness in the hip abductors and external rotators will result in poor eccentric control of the lower extremity's internal rotation, resulting in the same mechanical problems and pain in the anterior knee. Moving up the kinetic chain, abdominal weakness and poor neuromuscular control of the trunk will result in an abnormal position and length relationship of the hip muscles attaching from the pelvis to the femur. This will cause a lack of lower extremity control and increase the probability of injury to the back, hip, knee, ankle, or foot. In some sports where the goal of the movement is to transmit force to the upper extremity, problems in the lower extremities can cause compensatory movements resulting in upper extremity overload.

An upper extremity problem equivalent to pronation is scapulo-thoracic dysfunction. The scapula is the proximal base of the upper extremity and, as such, must provide the stability for proper distal function of the arm. The complex nature of upper extremity function, however, dictates that it also work dynamically. This is a difficult balance to achieve, albeit a critical one. The muscles must be trained to maintain a stable scapula that can dynamically move to keep an optimal congruence of the glenohumeral joint. This maximizes bony stability and keeps the muscles in a proper alignment to do their job, exerting the force they have developed. The muscles that move and stabilize the scapula are important because they have the potential to improve the position and function of the glenohumeral joint and rotator cuff.

Dysfunction along the body's kinetic chain, and its effect on performance or injury, are not limited to the above examples of scapulo-thoracic instability in the upper quarter or excessive pronation of the foot in the lower extremity. The main concept to remember is to avoid focusing on a singular body part.

Every segment is interdependent on the segments proximal and distal to that segment. No segment of the kinetic chain works in isolation. Dysfunction of one link may cause breakdown of another. Conversely, reestablishing the stability of one link may improve function in other links.

The expression "a chain is only as strong as its weakest link" certainly holds true for both ideal performance and injury prevention. Treating the athlete's symptoms may offer short-term relief, but to avoid compensatory changes and reoccurrence of injury, the underlying cause for dysfunction must be identified and corrected. The successful sport performance specialist considers all the variables until the ideal performance is realized.

References

Bandy, W. D., Lovelace-Chandler, V., & McKitrick-Bandy, B. (1990). Adaptation of skeletal muscle to resistance training. *Journal of Orthopedic and Sports Physical Therapy, 12*(6), 248–255.

Bobbert, M. F., & van Ingen Schenau, B. A. (1988). Coordination in vertical jumping. *Journal of Biomechanics, 21*(3), 249–262.

Bompa, T. O. (1993). *Periodization of strength.* Toronto, Ontario: Veritas Publishing.

Duncan, P. W., Chandler, J. M., Cavanaugh, D. K., Johnson, K. R., & Buehler, A.. G. (1989). Mode and speed specificity of eccentric and concentric exercise training. *Journal of Orthopedic and Sport Physical Therapy, 11*(2), 70–75.

Gould, J. A. (1990). (1990). *Orthopaedic and sports physical therapy* (2nd ed.) Philadelphia: C. V. Mosby Company.

Gray, G. W. (1992, October). Chain reaction course.

Hoppenfeld, S. (1976). *Physical examination of the spine and extremities.* New York: Appleton-Century-Crofts.

Komi, P., Ed. (1992). *Strength and power in sport.* Blackwell Scientific Publications.

Kraemer, W. J., Duncan, M. D., & Volek, J. S. (1998). Resistance training and elite athletes: Adaptations and program considerations. *Journal of Orthopedic and Sport Physical Therapy, 28*(2), 110–119.

Mair, S. D., Seaber, A. V., Glisson, R. F., & Garrett, W. E. (1996). The role of fatigue in susceptibility to acute muscle strain injury. *American Journal of Sports Medicine, 24*(2), 137–143.

Moffroid, M. T., & Whipple B. A. (1970). Specificity of speed of exercise. *Physical Therapy, 50*, 1692–1700.

Morrissey, M. C., Harman, E. A., & Johnson, M. J. (1995). Resistance training modes: Specificity and effectiveness. *Medicine and Science in Sports and Exercise, 27*(5), 648–660.

Rooney, K. J., Herbert, R. D., & Belnave, R. J. (1994). Fatigue contributes to the strength training stimulus. *Medicine and Science in Sports and Exercise, 26*(9), 1160–1164.

Schmidt, R. (1982). *Motor control and learning: A behavioral emphasis* (2nd ed.). Champaign, IL: Human Kinetics Publisher.

Tippett, S. R., & Voight, M. L. (1995). *Functional progression for sport rehabilitation.* Champaign, IL: Human Kinetics.

Wilson, G. J., Newton, R. U., Murphy, A. J., & Humphries, B. J. (1993). The optimal training load for the development of dynamic athletic performance. *Medicine and Science in Sports and Exercise, 25*(11), 1279–1286.

Wojtys, E. M., Huston, L. J., Taylor, P. D., & Bastian, S. D. (1996). Neuromuscular adaptations in isokinetic, isotonic, and agility training programs. *American Journal of Sports Medicine, 24*(2), 187–192.

Zatsiorsky, V. (1995). *Science and practice of strength training.* Champaign, IL: Human Kinetics Publisher.

10
Youth Strength Training

Avery D. Faigenbaum

The development of muscular strength in children has received increasing public and medical attention in recent years. Despite the previously held beliefs that children would not benefit from strength training or that the risk of injury was too great, research conducted over the past decade clearly demonstrates that strength training can be a safe and effective method of conditioning for children, provided that appropriate guidelines are followed (Blimkie, 1992, 1993; Faigenbaum & Bradley, 1998; Kraemer & Fleck, 1993; Webb, 1990). The American College of Sports Medicine (2000), the American Academy of Pediatrics (1990), the American Orthopedic Society for Sports Medicine (1988), and the National Strength and Conditioning Association (Faigenbaum, Kraemer, et al., 1996) support children's participation in appropriately designed and competently supervised youth strength-training programs. Further, current public health objectives discussed in the Surgeon General's report entitled *Physical Activity and Health* aim to increase the number of children age 6 and older who regularly participate in physical activities that enhance and maintain muscular strength and muscular endurance (U.S. Department of Health and Human Services, 1996).

For the purpose of this chapter, strength training (also known as resistance training) is defined as a specialized method of physical conditioning that involves the progressive use of resistance to increase one's ability to exert or resist force. This term encompasses a wide range of resistive loads (from light manual resistance to depth jumping) and a variety of training modalities (free weights, weight machines, hydraulics, pneumatics, elastic tubing, body weight, and plyometrics). The term *strength training* should be distinguished from the sports of weight lifting and power lifting in which individuals routinely train at high intensities and attempt to lift maximal amounts of weight in competition. The term *preadolescence* refers to a period of life prior to the development of secondary sex characteristics (roughly up to the age of 11 in girls and 13 in boys) and the term *adolescence* refers to the period between childhood to adulthood. For ease of discussion, the terms *children* and *youth* are broadly defined in this chapter to include both the preadolescent and adolescent years.

Although a growing number of boys and girls are participating in strength-training programs to improve their health and fitness, lingering concerns related to the efficacy, benefits, and risks associated with youth strength training persist. In this chapter, issues related to the trainability of children, the mechanisms underlying training-induced strength gains, and the potential benefits and risks of youth strength training will be addressed. Misperceptions will be dispelled, and age-specific strength-training guidelines will be outlined. This chapter will solely address the topic of youth strength training and will not address other important youth fitness issues related to the development of aerobic power and flexibility. Selected aspects of these issues have been reviewed by Rooks and Micheli (1988) and Rowland (1990).

Effectiveness of Youth Strength Training

For many years, the prevailing dogma among the medical community was that strength training was inappropriate for preadolescent boys and girls due to their physical immaturity. Although the value of strength training for adolescents was recognized (Gallagher & DeLorme, 1949), it was presumed that training-induced strength gains before puberty were not possible due to insufficient levels of circulating androgens (American Academy of Pediatrics, 1983). In 1978, Vrijens wrote, "It seems that strength development is closely related to sexual maturation. Therefore, specific strength training can only be effective in the post-pubescent age" (p. 152). The results from several studies supported this claim, despite the fact that methodological limitations such as poor experimental design (e.g., short study duration) or inadequate training program (e.g., low training volume [sets × repetitions × load]) may have influenced the results (Docherty, Wenger, Collis, & Quinney, 1987; Hetherington, 1976). In light of the fact that muscular strength normally increases as muscle mass increases with age (Malina & Bouchard, 1991), it seems that a more appropriate conclusion from the aforementioned reports may be that training–induced strength gains from a short-duration, low-volume strength-training program may not be distinguishable from gains attributable to growth and maturation. Muscular strength typically peaks by age 20 in females and between the ages of 20 and 30 in males (Servedio, 1997).

More recent scientific investigations using longer study durations and higher training volumes have quite conclusively proven that apparently healthy preadolescent boys and girls can, in fact, improve their muscular strength above and beyond growth and maturation, provided that the strength-training stimulus is sufficient (see Table 1).

Furthermore, strength training appears to be an effective therapeutic modality for children with surgically corrected congenital heart disease (Koch, Galioto, Vaccaro, Vaccaro, & Buckenmeyer, 1988) or cerebral palsy (Darrah, Fan, Chen, Nunweiler, & Watkins, 1997). In general, scientific investigations and clinical impressions from physicians and therapists support the premise that training-induced strength gains are possible in young weight trainers. Two meta-analyses on youth strength training (Falk & Tenenbaum, 1996; Payne, Morrow, Johnson, & Dalton, 1997) and several qualitative reviews of literature (Blimkie, 1992, 1993; Faigenbaum & Bradley, 1998; Kraemer, Fry, Frykman, Conroy, & Hoffman, 1989; Sale, 1989; Webb, 1990) have indicated that well-designed strength-training programs can enhance the muscular strength of preadolescents beyond what is normally due to growth and maturation.

Children as young as age 6 have benefited from strength training (Falk & Mor, 1996; Weltman et al., 1986), and studies have lasted up to 10 months (Morris, Naughton, Gibbs, Carlson, & Wark, 1997). Different combinations of sets and repetitions from one set of 10 repetitions (Westcott, 1992) to five sets of 15 repetitions (Isaacs, Pohlman, & Craig, 1994) and a variety of training modalities including adult-size weight machines (McGovern, 1984; Pfeiffer & Francis, 1986; Ramsay, Blimkie, Smith, Garner, & MacDougall, 1990; Sewall & Micheli, 1986; Williams, 1991), child-size weight machines (Faigenbaum, Westcott, Micheli, et al., 1996; Faigen-

Table 1. Studies That Demonstrated Strength Improvements in Healthy Preadolescents Following Strength Training

Reference	Age	Sex	Training Mode	Duration
Westcott (1979)	8–13	F	weights	3 wk
Nielson et al. (1980)	7–19	F	isometric	5 wk
Baumgartner & Wood (1984)	grades 3–6	M,F	calisthenics	12 wk
Clarke et al. (1984)	7–9	M	wrestling	12 wk
McGovern (1984)*	grades 4–6	M,F	weights	12 wk
Servedio et al. (1985)*	11.9	M	weights	8 wk
Pfeiffer & Francis (1986)	8–11	M	weights	8 wk
Sewall & Micheli (1986)	10-11	M,F	weights, pneumatic	9 wk
Weltman et al. (1986)	6–11	M	hydraulic	14 wk
Funato et al. (1987)	6–11	M,F	isometric	12 wk
Sailors & Berg (1987)	12.6	M	weights	8 wk
Siegal et al. (1988)	8.4	M,F	weights, calisthenics	12 wk
Ramsay et al. (1990)	9–11	M	weights	20 wk
Williams (1991)*	10.5	M	weights	8 wk
Westcott (1992)	9–13	M,F	weights	7 wk
Queary & Laubach (1992)	7–11	F	weights	4 wk
Faigenbaum et al. (1993)	8–12	M,F	weights	8 wk
Ozmun et al. (1994)	9–12	M,F	weights	8 wk
Stahle et al. (1995) *	7–9/10-12	M	weights	9 mo
Falk & Mor (1996)	6–8	M	calisthenics	12 wk
Faigenbaum et al. (1996)	7–12	M, F	weights	8 wk.
Morris et al. (1997)	9–10	F	weights, calisthenics	10 mo
Lillegard et al. (1997)	9–11	M, F	weights	12 wk
Treuth et al. (1998)	7–10	F	weights	5 mo

Age range is reported when available; * abstract.
Abbreviations: F = females, M = males, wk = weeks, mo = months

baum, Zaichkowsky, Westcott, Micheli, & Fehlandt, 1993; Westcott, 1992), free weights (barbells and dumbbells; Brown et al., 1992; DeRenne, Hetzler, Buxton, & Ho, 1996; Ramsay et al., 1990; Sailors & Berg, 1987; Servedio et al., 1985), hydraulic machines (Weltman et al., 1986), pneumatic machines (Sewall & Micheli, 1986), isometric contractions (Funato, Fukunaga, Asami, & Ikeda, 1987; Hetherington, 1976; Nielsen, Nielsen, Behrendt-Hansen, & Asmussen, 1980); wrestling drills (Clarke, Vaccaro, & Andresen,

1984), modified pull-ups and push-ups (Baumgartner & Wood, 1984; Falk & Mor, 1996), and calisthenics (Siegal, Camaione, & Manfredi, 1989) have proven to be effective. In terms of gender differences, there is no clear evidence of any difference in muscle fiber size (Servedio, 1997) or strength (Blimkie, 1989; Sale, 1989) between preadolescent boys and girls.

Strength gains of roughly 30 to 40% have been typically observed in preadolescent children following short-term (8 to 20 weeks) strength-training programs, although gains up to 74% have been reported (Faigenbaum, Zaichkowsky, Westcott, Micheli, et al., 1993). The variability in degree of training-induced strength gain may be due to several factors including the program design, quality of instruction, study duration, specificity of testing and training, background level of physical activity, and whether or not the researchers accounted for the learning effect. Overall, it appears that the relative (percent improvement) strength gains in preadolescent children are quantitatively similar to if not greater than gains made by older populations (Nielsen et al., 1980; Pfeiffer & Francis, 1986; Westcott, 1979). Conversely, when compared on an absolute basis, it appears that adolescents and adults make greater gains than preadolescents do (Sailors & Berg, 1987; Sale, 1989; Vrijens, 1978). Although the issue of whether training-induced strength gains should be compared on a relative or absolute basis is debatable, it seems unrealistic to expect a child to make the same absolute increases in strength as those of a larger adult who probably has at least twice the absolute strength of a child.

The evaluation of strength changes in children following the temporary or permanent reduction or withdrawal of the training stimulus (known as detraining) is complicated by the concomitant growth-related increases in strength during the same time period. At this time, limited data suggest that training-induced strength gains in children are impermanent and tend to regress to untrained control-group values during the detraining period (Blimkie, Martin, Ramsay, Sale, & MacDougall, 1995; Faigenbaum, Westcott, Micheli, et al., 1996; Isaacs et al., 1994; Sewall & Micheli, 1986). In one report, researchers noted rapid and significant decreases in upper and lower body strength of preadolescent boys and girls after discontinuation of an 8-week strength-training program (Faigenbaum, Westcott, Micheli, et al., 1996). Even though children in this study participated in physical education classes and organized sports during the 8-week detraining period, the magnitude of strength loss averaged 3% per week. Although the precise mechanisms responsible for this detraining response remain unclear, it seems likely that changes in neuromuscular functioning would be at least partly responsible. These findings underscore the importance of a strength maintenance program for children who want to persevere with training-induced strength gains.

In terms of program evaluation and testing, there has been concern that maximal strength testing in children could be potentially injurious to the immature skeletons of young weight trainers. Even though physical educators and rehabilitation therapists routinely perform strength tests on children to assess physical fitness or evaluate the degree of muscle disability, the concept of maximal strength testing in children needs to be explored. Most concerns regarding strength testing in children stem from earlier case-study reports in which children were injured while they attempted to lift maximal or near-maximal amounts of weight (Jenkins & Mintowt-Czyz, 1986; Rowe, 1979; Ryan & Salciccioli, 1976). However, no injuries have occurred while children performed competently supervised maximal strength tests (i.e., 1 repetition maximum [RM] tests, maximal isometric tests, and maximal isokinetic tests) in any prospective youth strength-training studies (DeRenne et al., 1996; Faigenbaum, Westcott, Long, et al., 1998; Morris et al., 1997; Ozmun, Mikesky & Surburg, 1994; Ramsay et al., 1990; Treuth, Hunter, Pichon, Figueroa-Colon, & Goran, 1998). Instead of heeding the emotional reaction to accidents that may have been prevented if appropriate guidelines were followed (e.g., adequate warm-up, gradual progression of loads, and close supervision), a review of the related scientific literature and anecdotal reports from teachers and therapists reveals that appropriately performed maximal strength tests can be used to evaluate changes in muscular strength consequent to training. Conversely, unsupervised and poorly performed maximal strength tests should not be performed under any circumstances because of the potential for serious injury (Risser, 1991).

Mechanisms Underlying Strength Gains

Because it is generally accepted that preadolescent boys and girls will become stronger if they participate in a strength-training program of adequate intensity and duration, recent efforts have attempted to determine the precise underlying mechanisms of training-induced strength gains in young weight trainers. Although muscle hypertrophy can explain, in part, training-induced strength gains in adolescents and adults (Sale, 1989), it is unlikely that muscle hypertrophy is primarily responsible for training-induced strength gains (at least up to 20 weeks) in younger populations. Without adequate levels of circulating testosterone to stimulate increases in muscle size, preadolescents experience more difficulty increasing their muscle mass consequent to a strength-training program as compared to older populations

(Ozmun, et al., 1994; Ramsay et al., 1990; Vrijens, 1978).

In the most comprehensive study on this topic, Ramsay et al. (1990) have suggested that neural adaptations and possibly intrinsic muscle adaptations (i.e., changes in excitation or contraction coupling, myofibrillar packing density, and muscle fiber composition) are primarily responsible for training-induced strength gains in preadolescents. After 20 weeks of strength training, it was reported that a trend towards increased motor unit activation and changes in motor unit co-ordination, recruitment, and firing were primarily responsible for the observed strength gains in prepubescent boys (Ramsay et al.). It was also noted that improvements in motor skill performance and the coordination of the involved muscle groups could be partly responsible for the observed strength gains. In another study, significant strength gains in preadolescent children were associated with increases in the electromyographic (EMG) amplitude of the trained muscle group (Ozmun et al., 1994). In support of these findings, several reports have indicated significant strength improvements in pre-adolescents without concomitant increases in limb circumference, as compared to age-matched controls (Faigenbaum, Zaichkowsky, Westcott, Micheli, et al., 1993; McGovern, 1984; Ozmun et al.; Ramsay et al.; Sailors & Berg, 1987; Weltman et al., 1986). These data suggest that the maturation of neural influences (e.g., motor nerve myelination) is an important factor in the development of muscular strength in children. In an excellent review of this topic, Sale (1989) suggested that preadolescents may have more of a potential for an increase in strength owing to neural rather than hypertrophic factors because pre-adolescents have more difficulty activating their muscles as well as adults do.

Although a majority of the evidence suggests that neuromuscular mechanisms, in contrast to hypertrophic factors, are primarily responsible for strength gains in preadolescent children (at least during the first 20 weeks of training), some findings are at variance with this suggestion (Fukunga, Funato, & Ikegawa, 1992; Mersch & Stoboy, 1989). Thus, it cannot be stated a priori that strength training will not result in muscle hypertrophy in preadolescent children. It is possible that longer study durations, more intensive training programs, and advanced measuring techniques (e.g., computerized imaging) may be needed to uncover the potential for training-induced hypertrophy in preadolescent children. However, during and after puberty, training-induced strength gains in males are typically associated with an increase in fat-free mass because hormonal influences on muscle mass are operant (Kraemer et al., 1989). In females, the magnitude of training-induced muscle hypertrophy is limited by lower levels of androgens (Sale, 1989).

Potential Benefits

The potential benefits of youth strength training extend beyond an increase in muscular strength and include the potential to influence positively many other health- and fitness-related measures. Limited data suggest that participation in a youth strength-training program may improve motor skills and sports performance; may reduce injuries in sports and recreational activities; and may favorably alter cardiorespiratory fitness, body composition, bone mineral density, blood lipids, and other selected parameters (see reviews by Blimkie, 1992, 1993; Faigenbaum & Bradley, 1998; Kraemer et al., 1989).

Motor skills and sports performance. The potential for strength training to enhance the motor skills and sports performance of children is of growing interest to clinicians and youth sport coaches. Because most sports have a significant strength or power component, it is intuitively attractive to assume that

a stronger child will perform better in selected sports and recreational activities. Several reports have indicated significant improvements in selected motor performance skills such as the long jump or vertical jump following a youth strength-training program (Falk & Mor, 1996; Hetzler et al., 1997; Lillegard, Brown, Wilson, Henderson, & Louis, 1997; Nielsen et al., 1980; Weltman et al., 1986; Williams, 1991) and others noted improvements in sprint speed (e.g., the 30-m dash) and agility run time (Lillegard et al.; Williams). Improvements in flexibility have also been reported in strength-training studies that included stretching exercises (Lillegard et al.; Stahle, Roberts, Davis, & Rybicki, 1995; Weltman et al., 1986). In contrast, two studies involving prepubescent children reported significant increases in muscular strength without concomitant improvements in motor performance skills (Brown et al., 1992; Faigenbaum, Zaichkowsky, Westcott, Micheli, et al., 1993).

These inconsistent findings may be explained, in part, by the design of the strength-training program. Because factors such as the choice of exercise, speed of movement, and volume of training can influence the outcome of a youth strength-training program, the question of training specificity must be addressed when evaluating the potential for strength training to enhance motor performance skills and sports performance. As noted in adults (Sale & MacDougall, 1981), it seems that training adaptations in children may be specific not only to the movement pattern, but also to the velocity of movement, contraction type, and contraction force. The specific nature of the training effect in children was observed by Nielsen et al. (1980), who studied young girls who trained for a specific test (i.e., isometric strength, vertical jump, or sprint acceleration) by running, jumping, or performing isometrics. Following 5 weeks of training, the greatest improvements were made in the activity for which the subjects trained. Although not well documented, youth strength-training programs that incorporate relatively fast speed movements (i.e., plyometrics and medicine ball exercises) that are specific to the test may be more likely to improve selected motor performance skills (e.g., sprint speed and vertical jump) as compared to a strength-training program characterized by slow speed movements and less specific exercises.

If strength training can improve selected motor performance skills of children, it seems reasonable to assume that a contemporary corollary of youth strength training would be an improvement in sports performance. Although comments from children and parents suggest that strength training enhances athletic ability, scientific reports of this observation are limited because athletic performance is a such a multivariate gestalt. To date, only a few studies have evaluated the effects of strength training on sports performance in children (Ainsworth, 1970; Blanksby & Gregor, 1981; Bulgakova, Vorontsov, & Fomichenko, 1990; Ford & Puckett, 1983; Queary & Laubach, 1992). Two studies have reported favorable changes in swim performance in age-group swimmers (Blanksby & Gregor; Bulgakova et al.), and one study noted improvements in selected gymnastics events (Queary & Laubach). Conversely, other studies failed to show any significant improvement in sports performance following participation in a youth strength-training program (Ainsworth; Ford & Puckett).

Although conclusions regarding the effects of youth strength training on sports performance are equivocal, limited direct and indirect evidence suggests that a sports-specific youth strength-training program will not have a negative effect on sports performance and, in all likelihood, will result in some degree of improvement. Participation in a youth strength-training program may enhance sports performance by increasing muscular strength (Falk & Tenenbaum, 1996; Payne et al., 1997), increasing cardiorespiratory endurance (Docherty et al., 1987; Weltman et al., 1986), improving motor performance skills (Falk & Mor, 1996; Nielsen et al., 1980; Weltman et al., 1986; Williams, 1991), improving body composition (Faigenbaum, Zaichowsky, Westcott, Micheli, et al., 1993; Siegal et al., 1989), increasing resistance to injury (Cahill & Griffith, 1978; Dominguez, 1978; Hejna, Rosenberg, Buturusis, & Krieger, 1982) decreasing time for rehabilitation (Hejna et al.), and enhancing mental health and wellbeing (Faigenbaum, 1995; Holloway, Beuter, & Duda, 1988). Further, strength training during the preadolescent years (and the associated neuromuscular adaptations) may provide the foundation for dramatic strength gains during the adolescent years.

If appropriate youth strength-training guidelines are followed, children may be better prepared (both physically and mentally) to handle the sport-specific demands of their chosen activity, and therefore, they may be more likely to have a positive sports experience. It is intuitively attractive to assume that children who are better prepared to experience the enjoyment of physical activity are more likely to continue participating in sports and less likely to drop out due to frustration, embarrassment, failure, and possible injury. Unfortunately, however, the focus of many youth programs in the United States is on the development of sport-specific skills rather than on the development of fundamental fitness abilities (speed, strength, and power). For over two generations, many parents and coaches have argued that early sports specialization is the key to later success in sport. Interestingly, however, research has shown that involvement in a variety of skills and activities was more related to later sports success than was early sports specialization (Magill & Anderson, 1995).

Emphasizing sport skills instead of fundamental skills not only discriminates against children whose motor skills are not as well developed, but it may also lead to acute and overuse injuries. The American College of Sports Medicine (1993) has estimated that over 50% of overuse injuries sustained by children could be prevented if more emphasis were placed on fundamental fitness as opposed to sport-specific training. Although the concept of preseason conditioning for children may seem a bit bizarre, in many cases children who enroll in organized sports are generally unfit and ill-prepared to handle the demands of their chosen sport. Although participation in youth sports has the potential to offer many social, psychological, and health benefits (Baxter-Jones & Helms, 1996), sports and recreation injuries are the second most frequent cause of emergency room visits among children in the United States (Guyer & Ellers, 1990).

With caring and competent instruction, children can have fun, develop fundamental skills, and acquire the abilities they need for successful and enjoyable participation in recreational activities and organized sports that demand moderate to high levels of physical conditioning. This recommendation may be particularly important for aspiring young female athletes, who appear to be at greater risk for major sports-related injuries, most of which involve the knee (DeHaven & Lintner, 1986). A comprehensive review of the theory and practice of physical and motor skill development in children can be found in a recent paper by Zaichkowsky and Larson (1995).

Prevention of injuries. Every year approximately 3 million injuries occur during sports participation among preadolescents in the United States (Hergenroeder, 1998). Although there are many mechanisms to potentially reduce sports injuries (e.g., preseason medical examination, coaching education, and proper equipment), the establishment of general physical fitness (including preparatory muscle conditioning) as a preventive health measure should not be overlooked. Progressive resistance exercise (PRE) has been used traditionally by physicians and therapists to restore and improve musculoskeletal function after an injury, and limited data suggest that participation in a youth strength-training program may increase a healthy child's resistance to injury (Cahill & Griffith, 1978; Dominguez, 1978; Hejna et al., 1982). In one report involving 13- to 19-year-old males and females (Henja et al.), it was observed that athletes who strength trained had a lower injury rate and required less time for rehabilitation when compared to their teammates who did not strength train. Others noted that strength training decreased the number and severity of knee injuries in high school football players (Cahill & Griffith) and the incidence of shoulder pain in 13- to 18-year-old swimmers (Dominguez). Even though these reports involved adolescents, it seems that similar protective effects could be seen in preadolescents provided that appropriate training guidelines are followed. The likelihood that conditioning may prevent more serious sports-related injuries has not yet been explored.

Although factors such as training errors, improper footwear, and hard playing surfaces are recognized risk factors for overuse injuries in youth sport (Micheli, 1983), the fitness level of young sports participants must also be considered. The upper body strength of American children is reportedly decreasing (Rupnow, 1985), and only about one half of young people in the United States (ages 12–21) regularly participate in vigorous physical activity (Heath, Pratt, Warren, & Kann, 1994). Further, the incidence of childhood obesity is increasing (Troiano,

1995), and sedentary pursuits such as television viewing and "surfing the net" continue to occupy a growing amount of time during childhood (Dietz, 1990). Although the elimination of youth sports injuries is an unrealistic goal, the addition of strength training to a child's fitness program may better prepare the young athlete to handle the duration and magnitude of forces that develop during practice and game situations, but because of interindividual differences in stress tolerance and the fact that the threshold intensity of exercise that might cause an injury is not known, the frequency, volume, intensity, and progression of the strength-training program needs to be carefully prescribed because strength training adds to the chronic repetitive stress placed on the young musculoskeletal system. Strength training should not simply be added onto a child's exercise regimen, but rather incorporated into a preventive program that varies in volume and intensity throughout the year. Additional clinical trials are needed to determine the optimal way to reduce the incidence of sports-related injuries in children.

Health-related benefits. Youth strength training, along with many other forms of exercise, has been shown to influence positively several measurable indices of health including cardiorespiratory fitness (Weltman et al., 1986), body composition (Faigenbaum, Zaichkowsky, Westcott, Micheli, et al., 1993, Siegal et al., 1989), bone mineral density (Morris et al., 1997), blood lipids, (Fripp & Hodgson, 1987; Weltman, Janney, Rians, Strand, & Katch, 1987), and selected psychosocial measures (Holloway et al., 1988; Westcott, 1992). Intuitively, the development of muscular strength should enable children to perform life's daily physical activities with more energy and vigor. Although the health-related benefits of youth strength training have not been unequivocally established, a growing body of evidence supports the con-

tention that the overall health of a child is more likely to improve than be adversely affected by strength training provided that appropriate guidelines are followed.

Common misperceptions related to strength training are the concerns that it could result in chronic hypertension or stunt the statural growth of children. Although blackouts and chronic hypertension have been reported in adult competitive weightlifters (Compton, Hill, & Sinclair, 1973), reports indicate that strength training has no adverse effect on the resting blood pressure of children (Faigenbaum, Zaichkowsky, Westcott, Micheli, et al., 1993; Rians et al., 1987; Servedio et al., 1985). Hagberg et al. (1984) reported a decrease in the resting blood pressure of hypertensive adolescents who participated in a strength-training program, and others have recommended low-intensity, high-repetition strength-training programs for hypertensive adolescents who want to strength train (Zahka, 1987). Overall, it seems that the resting blood pressure of children will remain unchanged or will decrease following several weeks of strength training.

Perhaps the most common misperception related to youth strength training is the belief that it could stunt the statural growth of children. This myth seems to have come from an earlier report that indicated that children who performed heavy labor in remote areas of Japan experienced damage to their epiphyseal plates, which resulted in significant decreases in stature (Kato & Ishiko, 1964). However, etiologic factors such as nutrition were not controlled for in this study. Current observations indicate no evidence of a decrease in stature in children who performed repetitive lifting in controlled environments (American Orthopaedic Society for Sports Medicine, 1998; Blimkie, 1993; Faigenbaum, Kraemer, et al., 1996). In all likelihood, participation in physical activity programs (including strength training) will have a favorable influence on growth at any stage of development but will not affect the genotypic maximum (Bailey & Martin, 1994; Ekblom, 1969).

Although the effects of intense physical training in children remain unknown, it is clear that physical stress is required for normal bone development in young populations. Sports and activities characterized by high-impact loading on the skeleton seem to result in greater bone mineral density than sports producing low loads (Grimstone, Willows, & Hanley, 1993). Even gymnasts as young as age seven have been found to have a higher bone mineral density than that of age-matched controls (Cassell, Benedict, & Specker, 1996). Strength training has been shown to enhance the bone mineral density of adults (Gutin & Kasper, 1992; Snow-Harter & Marcus, 1991), and some data, although not all (Blimkie et al., 1995), suggest that this type of exercise may have a positive influence on the bone mineral density of children and adolescents (Conroy et al., 1993; Loucks, 1988; Morris et al., 1997; Virvidakis, Georgiu, Korkotsidis, Ntalles, & Proukakis, 1990).

In one of the few reports providing direct evidence that exercise enhances bone accrual in children, participation in a 10-month, high-impact, strength-building exercise program resulted in significant improvements in strength and bone mineral density in preadolescent girls as compared to that of an age-matched control group (Morris et al., 1997). The authors of this report suggested that preadolescence may be an opportune time for the bone modeling and remodeling process to respond to the mechanical loading of high-impact physical activities. In support of this contention, Bass et al. (1998) noted that participation in gymnastics before puberty may confer residual benefits in bone density during adulthood, and others have observed that

the skeletal benefits of tennis and squash training were twice as great if training began before menarche rather than after (Kannus, Haapasalo, & Sankelo, 1995). Although peak bone mass is strongly influenced by genetics (Snow-Harter & Marcus, 1991), it seems that regular participation in a high-impact exercise program (e.g., aerobic dance and strength training) during preadolescence has the potential to be a potent osteogenic stimulus. Although more data are needed, these findings are especially important for young women who are at increased risk of developing osteoporosis (Gutin & Kasper, 1992).

Another potential health benefit of strength training is its influence on body composition. As the prevalence of childhood obesity in the United States continues to increase (Troiano, 1995), the effects of strength training on body fat have received increased attention. Several strength-training studies—but not all (Ramsay et al., 1990; Vrijens, 1978; Weltman et al., 1986)—have noted significant decreases in body fatness as measured by skinfold thicknesses in preadolescent children (Faigenbaum, Zaichkowsky, Westcott, Micheli, et al, 1993; Lillegard et al., 1997; Sailors & Berg, 1987; Siegal et al., 1989).

In adult populations, strength training has been shown to increase the resting metabolic rate (Pratley et al., 1994), but only limited data are available regarding the effects of strength training on metabolic parameters in children. In one report, a low-volume strength-training exercise intervention increased the muscular strength of obese preadolescent girls but did not significantly improve energy expenditure that was measured by 24-hour calorimetry and doubly labeled water (Treuth et al., 1998). Because this finding may be explained in part by a low training volume, it is possible that higher volumes of training would have a more favorable influence on energy expenditure. Although the type of training that increases daily energy expenditure in obese children remains undefined, unpublished data from our laboratory suggest that overweight children enjoy strength training because it is not aerobically taxing and it provides an opportunity for all children to experience success and feel good about their performance (Faigenbaum, unpublished observations).

Perhaps the most overlooked benefit of youth strength training is its potential impact on psychosocial health. Data from studies involving adults indicate that strength training can result in favorable changes in selected psychometric measures (e.g., self-concept, self-esteem, and body cathexis; Melnick & Mookerjee, 1991; Stein & Motta, 1992; Tucker, 1983), and it seems possible that similar benefits could occur in children. In one study involving untrained adolescent girls, significant improvements in self-efficacy and general self-esteem were observed following 12 weeks of strength training (Holloway et al., 1988), and other reports suggest that the socialization and mental discipline exhibited by children who strength trained were similar to the experiences of children who participated in team sports (Rians et al., 1987). Further, observations from parents of preadolescents who strength trained suggest that their sons and daughters were more willing to do their homework and household chores on the days that they strength trained (Faigenbaum, 1995; Weltman et al., 1986). Whereas some evidence (Holloway et al, 1988; Westcott, 1992), although not all (Faigenbaum, Zaichkowsky, Westcott, Long, et al., 1997), suggests that participation in a youth strength-training program will favorably influence selected psychosocial measures, scientific data supporting this contention are wanting.

It is possible that the potential psychosocial effects of youth strength training may depend on the intensity, frequency, and duration of the training program as well as the initial levels of muscular strength and psychosocial well-being. As previously observed in adult populations (Tucker, 1983, 1987), strength training may have its greatest influence on children who begin with relatively low levels of muscular strength and poor body attitudes. Although there is not enough information to state unequivocally that strength training will have a positive influence on the psychosocial well-being of children, if the program is well designed and competently supervised, strength training may offer psychosocial benefits comparable to those gained from other sports and activities. Conversely, unethical coaching practices and excessive pressure to perform at a level beyond one's capabilities may lead to the abuse of performance-enhancing drugs (Faigenbaum, Zaichkowsky, Gardner, & Micheli, 1998; Melia, Pipe, & Greenberg, 1996), burnout (Gould, 1993), and other untoward consequences (Tofler, Stryer, Micheli, & Herman, 1996).

Risks and Concerns

For many years, strength training was deemed inappropriate if not unsafe for children because of the fear that this type of activity would be injurious. Case study reports (George, Stakiw, & Wright, 1989; Jenkins & Mintowt-Czyz, 1986; Rowe, 1979; Ryan & Salciccioli, 1976) of injured young weight trainers and injury surveillance surveys from the U.S. Consumer Product Safety Commission fueled the belief that all strength-training activities—regardless of supervision or program design—were dangerous for children. However, a careful review of these reports suggests that most of the reported injuries were due to improper lifting techniques, maximal lifts, or lack of qualified adult supervision. Further, data from injury surveillance surveys did not distinguish between injuries associated with strength training and those associated with the competitive sports of power lifting and weight lifting. Although data from these reports suggest that the unsupervised use of heavy weights may be injurious, it is misleading to generalize these findings to appropriately designed and supervised youth strength-training programs.

Current findings indicate that youth strength training is relatively safe when compared with many other sports and activities in which children regularly participate (Hamill, 1994; Zaricznyj, Shattuck, Mast, Robertson, & D'Elia, 1980). A retrospective evaluation of strength-training injuries incurred by primarily 13- to 16-year-olds revealed that strength training was remarkably safer than many other sports, including soccer, basketball, and football (Hamill). Paradoxically, it seems that the forces placed upon the joints of children during sports participation may be far greater than those generated from moderate-intensity strength-training programs. Thus it seems unjustifiable to deter children from supervised strength-training activities for fear of injury when sport-specific forces may be potentially more stressful to their immature musculoskeletal system. At a time when many children seem to be ill prepared for sports participation, the belief that strength training is unsafe is not consistent with the needs of young athletes and the documented risks associated with this type of training.

A traditional concern associated with youth strength training involves the potential for injury to the epiphyseal plate or growth cartilage. Because this area of bone is less strong than the surrounding tissue, these growth centers are prone to injury. Damage to this area of the bone could disrupt the bone's blood and nutrient supply and could cause the epiphysis to fuse, resulting in limb defor-

mity and/or the cessation of limb growth (Singer, 1984). Although the number of epiphyseal plate fractures as result of strength training is small compared to the number that occur in sports such as football, hockey, and basketball (Benton, 1982), retrospective case-study reports noting epiphyseal plate fractures in adolescent weight trainers are of concern. In general, injuries to young weight trainers were typically caused by improper lifting techniques and/or the performance of heavy overhead lifts in unsupervised settings (Brady, Cahill, & Bodnar, 1982; Gumbs, Segal, Halligan, & Lower, 1982; Jenkins & Mintowt-Czyz, 1986; Rowe, 1979; Ryan & Salciccioli, 1976). An epiphyseal plate fracture has not been reported in any prospective youth strength-training study characterized by an appropriate progression of training loads and close supervision. Although all children are susceptible to epiphyseal plate fractures, Micheli (1988) noted that this type of injury is less likely to occur during preadolescence than during adolescence because the growth plates of younger children may actually be stronger and more resistant to shearing-type forces that have been implicated as the causal factor of many injuries involving the growth cartilage (Mueller & Blyth, 1981). If children are taught how to strength train properly under the watchful eye of a qualified adult, it appears that the risk of an epiphyseal plate injury is low.

The greatest concern for young weight trainers may be the risk for repetitive-use soft-tissue injuries (Brady et al., 1982; Brown, & Kimball, 1983; Jackson, Wiltse, Dingeman, & Hayes, 1981; Mason, 1977; Risser, 1991). Because this type of injury does not always result in physician visits, the incidence of repetitive-use soft-tissue injuries is difficult to determine. Nevertheless, retrospective data suggest that the risk of developing a lower back soft-tissue injury while strength training is noteworthy (Brady et al.; Risser). In one report involving adolescent power lifters who presumably trained with maximal or near-maximal weights, 50% (49 of 98) of the reported injuries were to the lower back region, 18% to the upper extremity, 17% to the lower extremity, and 14% to the trunk (Brown & Kimball). In another study, 67% (29 of 43) of high school athletes developed lumbosacral pain as a result of their conditioning program; however, the improper use of a device designed to improve jumping ability may have placed undue stress on the extended lumber spine (Brady et al.). Although these studies involved adolescents, who are typically bigger and often attempt more challenging skills than do preadolescents, similar injuries could occur in preadolescents if appropriate training guidelines are not followed.

Prospective studies involving children suggest that strength training has a relatively low risk of injury. In most of the studies, no serious clinical injuries occurred even through various training modalities and exercise regimens were used during the strength-training programs. However, all of the programs were closely supervised, and the training loads were individually prescribed. In one report, the safety of youth strength training was evaluated via biphasic musculoskeletal scintigraphy and the measurement of creatine phosphokinase (CPK), which is a muscle enzyme that is released during muscle necrosis (Rians et al., 1987). Following 14 weeks of strength training, there was no evidence of damage

to bones, epiphyses, or muscles; and CPK levels were not elevated. To date, only two published prospective studies have noted strength-training injuries in children (see Table 2). Overall, it seems that the risk of injury consequent to strength training is low, provided that children adhere to established guidelines.

On the other hand, unsupervised training programs and poorly designed training equipment can result in catastrophic injuries. Physicians, therapists, and coaches who recommend home strength-training programs should ensure that the child is supervised by a competent adult and that appropriate training loads are used. During a 1-year period, 11 adults died of asphyxia caused by barbell compression of their neck or chest as they performed heavy bench presses at home without a spotter (Lombardi, 1995), and an unsupervised nine-year-old boy died when a barbell rolled off a bench press support and fell on his chest (George et al., 1989). Although any exercise for children carries some degree of risk, accidents such as this underscore the importance of close supervision and safe training equipment.

General Youth Strength-training Guidelines

A variety of strength-training programs have been developed and recommended for children (Faigenbaum & Bradley, 1998; Kraemer & Fleck, 1993; Rooks & Micheli, 1988).

Table 2. Injuries to Youth in Prospective Strength-Training Studies

Reference	Injury	Exercise
Rians et al. (1987)	Shoulder strain that resolved within 7 days	Shoulder press
Lillegard et al. (1998)	Shoulder strain that resolved within 5 days	Barbell curl

Different types of equipment and various combinations of the acute program variables (e.g., choice of exercise, order of exercise, number of sets, load, and rest period between sets) have proven to be safe and effective when age-specific guidelines are followed. Although there is no minimal age requirement for participation in a youth strength-training program, all participants should have the emotional maturity to follow directions and undergo the stress of a training program. In general, if a child is ready for participation in sports (e.g., ballet class or Little League baseball), then he or she is ready for some type of strength training. A pretraining medical examination is not mandatory for apparently healthy children, but is recommended for children with known or suspected health problems (Faigenbaum, Kraemer, et al., 1996).

Youth strength-training programs should be specific to each child's individual needs. No matter how big or strong a child is, adult training guidelines and training philosophies (e.g., "No pain, no gain") should not be imposed on young weight trainers. Too often, the volume and intensity of training exceed a child's abilities, and the recovery periods are inadequate for a child's fitness level. It is always better to underestimate the physical abilities of children and gradually increase the volume and intensity of training than to overestimate their abilities and risk an injury. The focus of youth strength-training programs should be on learning proper form and technique rather than on the amount of weight lifted. During each session, instructors should teach children about their bodies, promote lifetime fitness, and provide a stimulating program that gives children a more positive attitude toward strength training and exercise in general. Instead of competing against each other, children should learn to embrace self-improvement and feel good about their performances. Ideally, strength training should be incorporated into a well-rounded fitness program that includes aerobic, flexibility, and agility exercises.

Three important areas of concern related to the development of a youth strength-training program are the quality of instruction, mode of training, and rate of progression. Instructors must have a thorough understanding of youth strength-training guidelines and safety procedures. They must speak to children at a level the children understand and should keep the program fun and challenging. Exercises must be clearly explained and properly demonstrated. Children should be encouraged to ask questions, and all of their concerns should be addressed. During the first few weeks of a youth strength-training class, an instructor-to-child ratio of 1 to 10 has been recommended (Faigenbaum, Kraemer, et al., 1996); however, additional instruction may be needed if all the children in class are learning the exercises for the first time.

A variety of strength-training modalities, including body weight exercises, elastic tubing, free weights, and modified adult-size machines, are available for children. In addition, child-size youth strength-training equipment is now available from several manufacturers. Although child-size equipment may not necessarily be safer than other modes of training, researchers who have used child-size equipment have reported relatively large gains in strength in 7 to 8 weeks (Faigenbaum, Zaichkowsky, Westcott, Micheli, et al., 1993; Westcott, 1992). Youth strength-training equipment may be biomechanically superior for preadolescents and, therefore, may afford the opportunity for greater gains in strength. Whatever type of equipment is used, instructors should be cognizant of the exploratory nature of children and should remove or disassemble any potential hazards or broken equipment from the exercise area. Above all else, sound teaching methodologies, enforcement of rules, and competent supervision appear to be more important for the safety and effectiveness of youth strength training than does the actual mode of training.

Another area of concern relates to the concept of progressive overload. A fundamental principle of strength training is that as the muscle adapts to the strength-training stimulus, the demands placed on the muscle need to become more challenging in order to maintain the same relative training intensity. Increasing the resistance, the number of repetitions, or the number of sets is necessary to make continual gains. This does not mean that every exercise session needs to be more intense or voluminous than the previous session, however. Although it is important to keep the program fresh and challenging, children should be given the opportunity to develop proper form and coordination with minimal muscle soreness. A summary of youth strength-training guidelines is presented in table 3.

Only limited data are available regarding the relationship between repetitions and selected percentages of the 1 repetition maximum (RM) in children. In adults, it appears that the number of repetitions that can be performed at a given percentage of the 1 RM are specific for a given exercise (Hoeger, Barette, Hale, & Hopkins, 1987), and similar observations have been noted in children (Faigenbaum, Westcott, Long, et al., 1998). In one study, preadolescent boys and girls performed a significantly greater number of repetitions at 50% 1 RM on the leg-press exercise as compared to the chest-press exercise (87.2 vs. 39.2), yet at 75% of the 1 RM there was no significant difference in the number of repetitions performed on the leg-press and chest-press exercises (18.2 vs. 13.4) (Faigenbaum, Westcott, Long, et al., 1998). These findings suggest that a given number of repetitions may not always be associated with the same percentage of the 1 RM in

Table 3. Summary of Strength-Training Guidelines for Children

- Children should understand the benefits and concerns associated with strength training.
- Children should have realistic expectations and should be reminded that it takes time to learn a new skill.
- Children should be encouraged to provide feedback about the training program.
- Competent and caring adult supervision should be present at all times.
- Children should focus on learning the technique of each exercise, not on the amount of weight lifted.
- All sessions should begin with 5 to 10 minutes of general warm-up exercises and stretching.
- Because children learn best by doing, have them demonstrate each exercise under observation.
- Start with one set of several upper and lower body exercises that focus on the major muscle groups.
- Begin with light loads (e.g., 12 to 15 repetitions) to allow for appropriate adjustments to be made.
- Increase the resistance gradually (e.g., 5 to 10%) as strength improves.
- Depending on individual needs and goals, one to three sets of 6 to 15 repetitions on a variety of single- and multijoint exercises can be performed.
- Two to three nonconsecutive training sessions per week are recommended.
- Exercises should be performed throughout the full range of motion (or pain-free range of motion).
- Repetitions should not be continued if the exercise technique is compromised.
- When necessary, adult spotters should be nearby to actively assist the young weight trainer in the event of a failed repetition.
- Vary the strength-training program by periodically changing the choice of exercises, order of exercises, or number of sets and repetitions.

children (at least at intensities below 75% 1 RM). Thus, it is possible that the minimal strength threshold—when expressed as a percentage of the 1 RM—may vary between muscle groups, possibly due to the amount of muscle mass involved with each exercise. In terms of prescribing a strength-training program for children, the best approach may be to first establish the repetition training range (e.g., 10 to 12) and then, by trial and error, determine the maximal load that can be handled for the prescribed range.

Because of the incidence of shoulder and lower back injuries, prehabilitation exercises for the shoulder and torso should be included in the strength-training program. In other words, exercises that would be prescribed for the rehabilitation of shoulder injuries (e.g., lateral raise, internal rotation, and external rotation) and back injuries (e.g., pelvic tilt and abdominal curl) should be performed beforehand as part of a preventive health measure. Once a child has mastered the basic exercises, multijoint structural exercises (e.g., squat) can be introduced into the program. However, when performing new exercises, children should start with an unloaded bar or a broomstick in order to develop the neuromuscular coordination and skill technique required to safely and correctly perform these exercises. Advanced multijoint lifts (e.g., Olympic-style cleans, pulls, and presses) may be incorporated into the program provided that qualified coaching is available, appropriate loads are used, and the child is mature enough to learn advanced exercises. Further, coaches should be aware of the time required to safely and effectively teach advanced multijoint lifts to children. The details of comprehensive youth strength-training programs are beyond the scope of this chapter but are available elsewhere (Faigenbaum & Westcott, 2000; Kraemer & Fleck, 1993).

Conclusion

Youth strength training is a safe and worthwhile activity for preadolescents and adolescents, provided that appropriate training guidelines are followed and qualified adult supervision is present. Despite traditional concerns that strength training would be ineffective or unsafe for children, a growing body of evidence suggests that this type of exercise offers significant health and fitness benefits for boys and girls. Although a variety of training methods and modalities have proven to be effective, the importance of competent and caring adult supervision should not be overlooked. Youth strength training is a specialized method of conditioning that should be recommended as part of a total fitness program that includes aerobic, flexibility, and agility exercises.

References

Ainsworth, J. (1970). *The effects of isometric resistive exercise with the Exer-Genie on strength and speed in swimming.* Unpublished doctoral dissertation, University of Arkansas.

American Academy of Pediatrics. (1983). Weight training and weight lifting: Information for the pediatrician. *The Physician and Sports Medicine, 11,* 157–161.

American Academy of Pediatrics. (1990). Strength training, weight and power lifting, and bodybuilding by children and adolescents. *Pediatrics, 86,* 801–803.

American College of Sports Medicine. (1993). The prevention of sports injuries of children and adolescents. *Medicine and Science in Sports and Exercise, 25* (Suppl. 8), 1–7.

American College of Sports Medicine. (2000). *ACSM's guidelines for exercise testing and prescription* (6th ed.). Baltimore: Lippincott, Williams & Wilkins.

American Orthopaedic Society for Sports Medicine. (1988). *Proceedings of the conference on strength training and the prepubescent.* Chicago: Author.

Bailey, D., & Martin, A. (1994). Physical activity and skeletal health in adolescents. *Pediatric Exercise Science, 6,* 330–347.

Bass, S., Pearce, G., Bradney, M., Hendrich, E., Delmas, P., Harding, A., & Seeman, E. (1998). Exercise before puberty may confer residual benefits in bone density in adulthood: Studies in active prepubertal and retired female gymnasts. *Journal of Bone and Mineral Research, 13*(3), 500–507.

Baumgartner, T., & Wood, S. (1984). Development of shoulder-girdle strength-endurance in elementary children. *Research Quarterly for Exercise and Sport, 55,* 169–171.

Baxter-Jones, A., & Helms, P. (1996). Effects of training at a young age: A review of the training of young athletes study (TOYA) study. *Pediatric Exercise Science, 8,* 310–327.

Benton, J. (1982). Epiphyseal plate fracture in sports. *Physician and Sports Medicine, 10,* 63–67.

Blanksby, B., & Gregor, J. (1981). Anthropometric, strength, and physiological changes in male and female swimmers with progressive resistance training. *Australian Journal of Sport Science, 1,* 3–6.

Blimkie, C. (1989). Age- and sex-associated variation in strength during childhood: Anthropometric, morphologic, neurologic, biomechanical, endocrinologic, genetic, and physical activity correlates. In C. Gisolfi & D. Lamb (Eds.), *Perspectives in exercise science and sports medicine* (Vol. 2, pp. 99–163). Indianapolis: Benchmark.

Blimkie, C. (1992). Resistance training during pre- and early puberty: Efficacy, trainability, mechanisms and persistence. *Canadian Journal of Sport Sciences, 17,* 264–279.

Blimkie, C. (1993). Benefits and risks of resistance training in youth. In B. Cahill & A. Pearl (Eds.), *Intensive participation in children's sports* (pp. 133–167). Champaign: Human Kinetics.

Blimkie, C., Martin, J., Ramsay, D., Sale, D., & MacDougall, D. (1995). The effects of detraining and maintenance weight training on strength development in prepubertal boys. *Canadian Journal of Sport Sciences, 14,* 104P.

Blimke, C., Rice, S., Webber, C., Martin, J., Levy, D., Gorgon, C. (1993). Effects of resistance training on bone mass and density in adolescent females. *Medicine and Science in Sports and Exercise, 25,* S48.

Brady, T., Cahill, B., & Bodnar, L. (1982). Weight training related injuries in the high school athlete. *The American Journal of Sports Medicine, 10,* 1–5.

Brown, E., Lillegard, W., Henderson, R., Wilson, D., Lewis, E., Hough, D., & Stringer, K. (1992). Efficacy and safety of strength training with free weights in prepubescents to early post pubescents. *Medicine and Science in Sports and Exercise, 24,* S82.

Brown, E., & Kimball, R. (1983). Medical history associated with adolescent power lifting. *Pediatrics, 72(5),* 636–644.

Bulgakova, N., Vorontsov, A., & Fomichenko, T. (1990). Improving the technical preparedness of young swimmers by using strength training. *Soviet Sports Review, 25,* 102–104.

Cahill, B., & Griffith, E. (1978). Effect of preseason conditioning on the incidence and severity of high school football knee injuries. *The American Journal of Sports Medicine, 6,* 180–184.

Cassell, C., Benedict, M., & Specker, B. (1996). Bone mineral density in elite 7- to 9-yr-old female gymnasts and swimmers. *Medicine and Science in Sports and Exercise, 28,* 1243–1246.

Clarke, D., Vaccaro, P., & Andresen, N. (1984). Physiologic alterations in 7- to 9-year old boys following a season of competitive wrestling. *Research Quarterly for Exercise and Sport, 55,* 318–322.

Compton, D., Hill, P., & Sinclair, J. (1973). Weightlifters' blackout. *Lancet, 2,* 1234–1237.

Conroy, B., Kraemer, W. Maresh, C., Fleck, S., Stone, M., Fry, A., Miller, P., & Dalsky, G. (1993). Bone mineral density in elite junior Olympic weightlifters. *Medicine and Science in Sports and Exercise, 25,* 1103–1109.

Darrah, J., Fan, J., Chen, L., Nunweiler, J., & Watkins, B. (1997). Review of the effects of progressive resisted muscle strengthening in children with cerebral palsy: A clinical consensus exercise. *Pediatric Physical Therapy, 9(1),* 12–17.

DeHaven, K., & Linter, D. (1986). Athletic injuries: Comparison by age, sport and gender. *American Journal of Sports Medicine, 14,* 218–224.

DeRenne, C. Hetzler, R., Buxton, B., & Ho, K. (1996). Effects of training frequency on strength maintenance in pubescent baseball players. *Journal of Strength and Conditioning Research, 10,* 8–14.

Dietz, W. (1990). Children and television. In M.Green & R. Hagerty (Eds.), *Ambulatory pediatrics IV* (pp. 39–41). Philadelphia: W. B. Saunders.

Docherty, D., Wenger, H., Collis, M., & Quinney, H. (1987). The effects of variable speed resistance training on strength development in prepubertal boys. *Journal of Human Movement Studies, 13,* 377–382.

Dominguez, R. (1978). Shoulder pain in age group swimmers. In B. Erikkson & B. Furberg (Eds.), *Swimming medicine IV* (pp. 105–109). Baltimore: University Park Press.

Ekblom, B. (1969). Effects of physical training in adolescent boys. *Journal of Applied Physiology, 27,* 350–355.

Faigenbaum, A. (1995). Psychosocial benefits of prepubescent strength training. *Strength and Conditioning, 17,* 28–32.

Faigenbaum, A., & Bradley, D. (1998). Strength training for the young athlete. *Orthopedic Physical Therapy Clinics of North America, 7(1),* 67–89.

Faigenbaum, A., Kraemer, W. Cahill, B., Chandler, J., Dziados, J., Elfrink, L., Forman, E., Gaudiose, M., Micheli, L., Nitka, M., & Roberts, S. (1996). Youth resistance training: Position statement paper and literature review. *Strength and Conditioning, 18,* 62–75.

Faigenbaum, A., & Westcott, W. (2000) *Strength and power for young athletes.* Champaign, IL: Human Kinetics.

Faigenbaum, A., Westcott, W., Long, C., Loud, R., Delmonico, M., & Micheli, L. (1998). Relationship between repetitions and selected percentages of the one repetition maximum in healthy children. *Pediatric Physical Therapy, 10,* 110–113.

Faigenbaum, A., Westcott, W., Micheli, L., Outerbridge, A., Long, C., LaRosa-Loud, R., & Zaichkowsky, L. (1996). The effects of strength training and detraining on children. *Journal of Strength Conditioning Research, 10,* 109–114.

Faigenbaum, A., Zaichkowsky, L., Gardner, D., & Micheli, L. (1998). The use of anabolic steroids by middle school students. *Pediatrics*, *101*, e6.

Faigenbaum, A., Zaichkowsky, L.,Westcott, W., Long, C., LaRosa-Loud, R., Micheli, L., & Outerbridge, A. (1997). Psychological effects of strength training on children. *Journal of Sport Behavior, 70,* 164–175.

Faigenbaum, A., Zaichkowsky, L.,Westcott, W., Micheli, L., & Fehlandt, A. (1993). The effects of a twice per week strength training program on children. *Pediatric Exercise Science, 5*, 339–346.

Falk, B., & Mor, G. (1996). The effects of resistance and martial arts training in 6 to 8 year old boys. *Pediatric Exercise Science, 8*, 48–56.

Falk, B., & Tenenbaum, G. (1996). The effectiveness of resistance training in children. A meta-analysis. *Sports Medicine, 22*, 176–186.

Ford, H., & Puckett, J. (1983). Comparative effects of prescribed weight training and basketball programs on basketball skill test scores of ninth grade boys. *Perceptual and Motor Skills, 56*, 23–26.

Fripp, R., & Hodgson, J. (1987). Effect of resistive training on plasma lipid and lipoprotein levels in male adolescents. *The Journal of Pediatrics, 111,* 926–931.

Fukunga, T., Funato, K., & Ikegawa, S. (1992). The effects of resistance training on muscle area and strength in prepubescent age. *Annals of Physiological Anthropology, 11*, 357–364.

Funato, K., Fukunaga, T., Asami, T., & Ikeda, S. (1987). Strength training for prepubescent boys and girls. *Proceedings of the Department of Sports Science* (pp. 9–19). Tokyo, Japan: University of Tokyo.

Gallagher, J., & DeLorme, T. (1949). The use of progressive resistance exercise in adolescence. *The Journal of Bone and Joint Surgery, 31-A*(4), 847–858.

George, D., Stakiw, K., & Wright, C. (1989). Fatal accident with weight-lifting equipment: Implications for safety standards. *Canadian Medical Association Journal, 140*, 925–926.

Gould, D. (1993). Intensive sport participation and the prepubescent athlete: Competitive stress and burnout. In B. Cahill & A. Pearl (Eds.), *Intensive participation in children's sports* (pp. 19–38). Champaign: Human Kinetics.

Grimstone, S., Willows, N., & Hanley, D. (1993). Mechanical loading regime and its relationship to bone mineral density in children. *Medicine and Science in Sports and Exercise, 25*, 1203–1210.

Gumbs, V., Segal, D., Halligan, J., & Lower, G. (1982). Bilateral distal radius and ulnar fractures in adolescent weight lifters. *American Journal of Sports Medicine, 10*, 375–379.

Gutin, B., & Kasper, M. (1992). Can vigorous exercise play a role in osteoporosis prevention? A review. *Osteoporosis International, 2*(2), 55–69.

Guyer, B., & Ellers, B. (1990). Childhood injuries in the United States: Morbidity, mortality, and cost. *American Journal of Diseases in Children, 144*, 649–652.

Hagberg, J., Ehsani, A., Goldring, D., Hernandez, A., Sinacore, D., & Holloszy, J. (1984). Effect of weight training on blood pressure and hemodynamics in hypertensive adolescents. *The Journal of Pediatrics, 104*, 147–151.

Hamill, B. (1994). Relative safety of weight lifting and weight training. *Journal of Strength and Conditioning Research, 8*, 53–57.

Heath, G., Pratt, M., Warren, C., & Kann, L. (1994). Physical activity patterns in American high school students. *Archives of Pediatric and Adolescent Medicine, 148*, 1131–1136.

Hejna, W., Rosenberg, A., Buturusis, D., & Krieger, A. (1982). The prevention of sports injuries in high school students through strength training. *National Strength and Conditioning Journal, 4*, 28–31.

Hergenroeder, A. (1998). Prevention of sports injuries. *Pediatrics, 101*(6), 1057–1063.

Hetherington, M. (1976). Effect of isometric training on the elbow flexion force torque of grade five boys. *Research Quarterly, 47*, 41–47.

Hetzler, R., DeRenne, C., Buxton, B., Ho, K., Chai, D., & Seichi, G. (1997). Effects of 12 weeks of strength training on anaerobic power in prepubescent male athletes. *Journal of Strength and Conditioning Research, 11*(3), 174–181.

Hoeger, W., Barette, S., Hale, D., & Hopkins, D. (1987). Relationship between repetitions and selected percentages of the one repetition maximum. *Journal of Applied Sport Science Research, 1*, 11–13.

Holloway, J., Beuter, A., & Duda, J. (1988). Self-efficacy and training in adolescent girls. *Journal of Applied Social Psychology, 18*, 699–719.

Isaacs, L., Pohlman, R., & Craig, B. (1994). Effects of resistance training on strength development in prepubescent females. *Medicine and Science in Sports and Exercise, 26*, S210.

Jackson, D., Wiltse, L., Dingeman, R., & Hayes, M. (1981). Stress reactions involving the pars interarticularis in young athletes. *The American Journal of Sports Medicine, 9*, 304–312.

Jenkins, N., & Mintowt-Czyz, W. (1986). Bilateral fracture separations of the distal radial epiphyses during weight-lifting. *British Journal of Sports Medicine, 20*, 72–73.

Kannus, P., Haapasalo, H., & Sankelo, M. (1995). Effect of starting age of physical activity on bone mass in the dominant arm of tennis and squash players. *Annals of Internal Medicine, 123*, 27–31.

Kato, S., & Ishiko, T. (1964). Obstructed growth of children's bones due to excessive labor in remote corners. In S. Kato (Ed.), *Proceedings of the International Congress of Sports Sciences*. Tokyo: Japanese Union of Sports Sciences.

Koch, B., Galioto, F., Vaccaro, P., Vaccaro, J., & Buckenmeyer, P. (1988). Flexibility and strength measures in children participating in a cardiac rehabilitation program. *The Physician and Sports Medicine, 16*(2), 139–147.

Kraemer, W., Fry, A., Frykman, P., Conroy, B., & Hoffman, J. (1989). Resistance training and youth. *Pediatric Exercise Science, 1*, 336–350.

Lillegard, W., Brown, E., Wilson, D., Henderson, R., & Lewis, E. (1997). Efficacy of strength training in prepubescent to early postpubescent males and females: Effects of gender and maturity. *Pediatric Rehabilitation, 1*(3), 147–157.

Lombardi, V. (1995). Recreational weight training injuries and deaths: Trends over the most recent decade in the U.S. *Medicine and Science in Sports and Exercise, 27*, S98.

Loucks, A. (1988). Osteoporosis prevention begins in childhood. In E. Brown & C. Brown (Eds.), *Competitive sports for children and youth* (pp. 213–223). Champaign: Human Kinetics.

Magill, R., & Anderson, D. (1995). Critical periods as optimal readiness for learning sports skills. In F. Smoll & R. Smith (Eds.), *Children and youth in sport: A biopsychosocial perspective* (pp. 57–72). Madison, WI: Brown & Benchmark.

Malina, R., & Bouchard, C. (1991). *Growth, maturation and physical activity.* Champaign: Human Kinetics.

Mason, T. (1977). Is weight lifting deleterious to the spines of young people? *British Journal of Sports Medicine, 5*(61), 54–56.

McGovern, M. (1984). Effects of circuit weight training on the physical fitness of prepubescent children. *Dissertation Abstracts International, 45*, 452A–453A.

Melia, P., Pipe, A., & Greenberg, G. (1996). The use of anabolic androgenic steroids by Canadian students. *Clinical Journal of Sports Medicine, 6*, 9–14.

Melnick, M., & Mookerjee, S. (1991). Effects of advanced weight training on body cathexis and self-esteem. *Perceptual and Motor Skills, 72*, 1335–1345.

Mersch, F., & Stoboy, H. (1989). Strength training and muscle hypertrophy in children. In S. Oseid & K. Carlsen (Eds.), *Children and exercise XIII* (pp. 165–182). Champaign: Human Kinetics.

Micheli, L. (1983). Overuse injuries in children's sports: The growth factor. *Orthopedic Clinics of North America, 14*, 337–360.

Micheli, L. (1988). Strength training in the young athlete. In E. Brown & C. Branta (Eds.), *Competitive sports for children and youth* (pp. 99–105). Champaign: Human Kinetics.

Morris, F., Naughton, G., Gibbs, J., Carlson, J., & Wark, J. (1997). Prospective ten-month exercise intervention in premenarcheal girls: Positive effects on bone and lean mass. *Journal of Bone and Mineral Research, 12*(9), 1453–1462.

Mueller, F., & Blyth, C. (1981). Epidemiology of sports injuries in children. *Clinical Sports Medicine, 15*, 229–233.

Nielsen, B., Nielsen, K., Behrendt-Hansen, M., & Asmussen, E. (1980). Training of "functional muscular strength" in girls 7–19 years old. In K. Berg & B. Eriksson (Eds.), *Children and exercise IX* (pp. 69–77). Baltimore: University Park Press.

Ozmun, J., Mikesky, A., & Surburg, P. (1994). Neuromuscular adaptations following prepubescent strength training. *Medicine and Science in Sports and Exercise, 26*, 510–514.

Payne, V., Morrow, J., Johnson, L., & Dalton, S. (1997). Resistance training in children and youth: A meta-analysis. *Research Quarterly for Exercise and Sport, 68*(1), 80–89.

Pfeiffer, R., & Francis, R. (1986). Effects of strength training on muscle development in prepubescent, pubescent and postpubescent males. *The Physician and Sports Medicine, 14*, 134–143.

Pratley, R., Nicklas, M., Rubin, J., Miller, A., Smith, M., Smith, B., & Hurley, B. (1994). Strength training increases resting metabolic rate and norepinephrine levels in healthy 50- to 60-yr-old men. *Journal of Applied Physiology, 76*, 133–137.

Queary, J., & Laubach, L. (1992). The effects of muscular strength/endurance training. *Technique, 12*, 9–11.

Ramsay, J., Blimkie, C., Smith, K., Garner, S., & MacDougall, J. (1990). Strength training effects in prepubescent boys. *Medicine and Science in Sports and Exercise, 22*, 605–614.

Rians, C., Weltman, A., Cahill, B., Janney, C., Tippet, S., & Katch, F. (1987). Strength training for prepubescent males: Is it safe? *The American Journal of Sports Medicine, 15*, 483–489.

Risser, W. (1991). Weight training injuries in children and adolescents. *American Family Physician, 44*, 2104–2110.

Rooks, D., & Micheli, L. (1988). Musculoskeletal assessment and training: The young athlete. *Clinics in Sports Medicine, 7*, 641–677.

Rowe, P. (1979). Cartilage fracture due to weight lifting. *British Journal of Sports Medicine, 13*, 130–131.

Rowland, T. (1990). *Exercise and children's health.* Champaign: Human Kinetics.

Rupnow, A. (1985). Upper body strength: Helping kids win the battle. *Journal of Physical Education, Recreation and Dance, 56*, 60–63.

Ryan, J., & Salciccioli, G. (1976). Fractures of the distal radial epiphysis in adolescent weight lifters. *American Journal of Sports Medicine, 4*, 26–27.

Sailors, M., & Berg, K. (1987). Comparison of responses to weight training in pubescent boys and men. *Journal of Sports Medicine, 27*, 30–37.

Sale, D. (1989). Strength training in children. In G. Gisolfi & D. Lamb (Eds.), *Perspectives in exercise science and sports medicine* (pp. 165–216). Indianapolis: Benchmark Press.

Sale, D., & MacDougall, D. (1981). Specificity in strength training: A review for the coach and athlete. *Canadian Journal of Applied Sport Sciences, 6*, 87–92.

Servedio, F. (1997). Normal growth and development. *Orthopedic Physical Therapy Clinics of North America, 6*(4), 417–435.

Servedio, F., Bartels, R., Hamlin, R., Teske, D., Shaffer, T., & Servedio, A. (1985). The effects of weight training, using Olympic style lifts, on various physiological variables in pre-pubescent boys. *Medicine and Science in Sports and Exercise, 17*, 288.

Sewall, L., & Micheli, L. (1986). Strength training for children. *Journal of Pediatric Orthopedics, 6*, 143–146.

Siegal, J., Camaione, D., & Manfredi, T. (1989). The effects of upper body resistance training in prepubescent children. *Pediatric Exercise Science, 1*, 145–154.

Singer, K. (1984). Injuries and disorders of the epiphyses in young athletes. In M. Weiss and D. Gould (Eds.), *Sport for children and youths* (pp. 141–150). Champaign, IL: Human Kinetics.

Snow-Harter, C., & Marcus, R. (1991). Exercise, bone mineral density and osteoporosis. In J. Hollowszy (Ed.), *Exercise and sports science reviews* (Vol. 19, pp. 351–388). Philadelphia: Williams & Wilkins.

Stahle, S., Roberts, S., Davis, B., & Rybicki, L. (1995). Effect of 2 versus 3 times per week weight training program in boys aged 7 to 16. *Medicine and Science in Sports and Exercise, 27*, S114.

Stein, P., & Motta, R. (1992). Effects of aerobic and non-aerobic exercise on depression and self-concept. *Perceptual and Motor Skills, 74*, 79–89.

Tofler, I., Stryer, B., Micheli, L., & Herman, L. (1996). Physical and emotional problems of elite female gymnasts. *New England Journal of Medicine, 335*, 281–283.

Treuth, M., Hunter, G., Pichon, C., Figueroa-Colon, R., & Goran, M. (1998). Fitness and energy expenditure after strength training in obese prepubertal girls. *Medicine and Science in Sports and Exercise, 30*(7), 1130–1136.

Troiano, R. (1995). Overweight prevalence and trends for children and adolescents. *Archives of Pediatric and Adolescent Medicine, 149*, 1085–1091.

Tucker, L. (1983). Effect of weight training on self-concept: A profile of those influenced most. *Research Quarterly for Exercise and Sport, 54*, 389–397.

Tucker, L. (1987). Effect of weight training on body attitudes: Who benefits most? *Journal of Sport Medicine, 27*, 70–78.

U.S. Department of Health and Human Services. (1996). *Physical activity and health: A report from the Surgeon General.* Atlanta: U.S. Department of Helath and Human Services, Centers for Disease Control and Prevention, National Center for Chronic Disease Prevention and Health Promotion.

Virvidakis, K., Georgiu, E., Korkotsidis, A., Ntalles, K., & Proukakis, C. (1990). Bone mineral content of junior competitive weightlifters. *International Journal of Sports Medicine, 11*, 244–246.

Vrijens, F. (1978). Muscle strength development in the pre- and post-pubescent age. *Medicine and Sport, 11*, 152–158.

Webb, D. (1990). Strength training in children and adolescents. *Pediatric Clinics of North America, 37*, 1187–1210.

Weltman, A, Janney, C., Rians, C., Strand, K., Berg, B., Tippit, S., Wise, J., Cahill, B., & Katch, F. (1986). The effects of hydraulic resistance strength training in pre-pubertal males. *Medicine and Science in Sports and Exercise, 18*, 629–638.

Weltman, A., Janney, C., Rians, C., Strand, K., & Katch, F. (1987). Effects of hydraulic-resistance strength training on serum lipid levels in prepubertal boys. *American Journal of Diseases in Children, 141*, 777–780.

Westcott, W. (1979). Female response to weight lifting. *Journal of Physical Education, 77*, 31–33.

Westcott, W. (1992). A new look at youth fitness. *American Fitness Quarterly, 11*, 16–19.

Williams, D. (1991). The effect of weight training on performance in selected motor activities for preadolescent males. *Journal of Applied Sport Science Research, 5*, 170.

Zahka, K. (1987). Adolescent hypertension update. *Maryland Medical Journal, 36*, 413–414.

Zaichkowsky, L., & Larson, J. (1995). Physical, motor, and fitness development in children and adolescents. *Journal of Education, 177*(2), 55–79.

Zaricznyj, B., Shattuck, L., Mast, T., Robertson, R., & D'Elia, G. (1980). Sports-related injuries in school-aged children. *The American Journal of Sports Medicine, 8*, 318–324.

11
Physiological and Psychological Benefits of Strength Training in Older Adults

Toshihiko Tsutsumi

Introduction

Although physical activity has long been recognized as an important element for health, new evidence of the effects of an active lifestyle has reinforced this impression (Bouchard, Shephard, Stephens, Sutton, & McPherson, 1990). An increasing number of epidemiological and experimental studies have demonstrated that exercise, a planned, structured, and repetitive physical activity for the purpose of improving and maintaining health (Caspersen, Powell, & Christenson, 1985), reduces the risk for various chronic diseases, including heart disease (Paffenbarger, Hyde, Wing, & Hsieh, 1986), hypertension (Blair, Goodyear, & Cooper, 1984), non-insulin-dependent diabetes mellitus (Helmrich, Ragland, Leung, & Paffenbarger, 1991), osteoporosis (Snow-Harter, & Marcus, 1991), colon cancer (Lee, Paffenbarger, & Hsieh, 1991), and problems with anxiety and depression (Taylor, Sallis, & Needle, 1985). Despite the overwhelming evidence of these health benefits, most adults in the United States remain sedentary (U.S. Department of Health and Human Services [USDHHS], 1991). Of particular concern is the older population, a group in which physical inactivity is particularly prevalent and a group that, therefore, could benefit most from adopting an active lifestyle.

Currently, life expectancy in the United States is at a record 75.8 years, and the overall mortality rate continues to decline (McGinnis & Lee, 1995). However, successful aging would not be just living longer, but taking control and living with less disability. Approximately 80% of individuals 65 years and over are reported to experience at least one age-related chronic health condition such as arthritis, heart disease, hypertension, or diabetes (USDHHS, 1984), and these health problems are leading many older adults to a substantial degree of disability. As more individuals live longer, the issue of disease prevention and/or health promotion is of growing importance. Because chronic conditions suffered by the elderly are closely related to their having led many years of a sedentary lifestyle (Danner & Edwards, 1992), the effort to promote a physically active lifestyle is of growing importance for prolonging the active life span and making the last stage of life more worth living.

In recent years, we have learned much about the beneficial effects of rebuilding muscle strength in older adults. There is clear evidence that physiological performance capacities can be significantly improved through strength training and, therefore, increasing the level of physical activity in an aging population. In addition, strength training reduces risk of various conditions that accompany the aging process. Research also suggests that strength training for the elderly may have psychological benefits that include relieving depressive syndrome as well as improving mood and personal control. This chapter will review recent studies that examine the effects of strength training in functional capacity among the elderly and focus further on psychological benefits, in relation to physical self-efficacy, a proposed cognitive and behavioral mechanism that may play an important role in improving psychological well-being following strength training.

Modification of Age-Related Changes in Functional Capacity

Aging is accompanied by numerous changes in metabolic and physiological function. Maximal oxygen consumption (VO2max) that represents cardiovascular function decreases 5 to 15% after age 25 (Heath, Hagberg, Ehsani, & Holloszy, 1981). Decreases in cardiac output and maximal arteriovenous VO2 difference are responsible for the declines in cardiovascular function (Fisher, Pendergast, & Calkins, 1991; Ogawa et al., 1992; Rodeheffer et al., 1984). A reduction of muscle strength is also seen as a major part of functional loss of normal aging (Mazzeo et al., 1998).

Among the numerous age-related changes in functional capacity, the most noticeable change may be the loss of muscle mass. Resulting declines in muscle strength can lead older adults to substantial degrees of impairment in physical function (Aniansson & Gustafsson, 1981; Fisher et al., 1990; L. G. Larsson, Grimby, & Karlsson, 1979). It has

been reported that approximately 15% of muscle strength is lost between the sixth and seventh decades and then 30% towards the end of life (Donneskoild-Samsore, Kofod, Munter, & Schnohr, 1984; Harries & Bassey, 1990; L. Larsson, 1978; Murray, Duthie, Gambert, Sepic, & Mollinger, 1985). These losses may be due to muscle atrophy resulting from a gradual loss of muscle fibers (Lexell, Henriksson-Larsen, Wimblod, & Sjostrm, 1983). Concurrent with the decrease in muscle mass, fat mass progressively increases after the third decade (Cohn et al., 1980). Subsequent decrease in metabolic rate may lead individuals to a gradual weight gain, and the resulting obesity makes them susceptible to chronic diseases, such as diabetes and hypertension.

The loss of muscle strength appears to be most pronounced in older women. In the Framingham study, collecting data of 2,654 individuals aged 55 to 84, 40% of women aged 55 to 64, 45% of women aged 65 to 74, and 65% of women aged 75 to 85 could not lift a 4.5 kg object (Jette & Branch, 1981). Similarly high percentages of women in this population were also unable to perform some household work. Importantly, the aging-associated muscle loss is considered as a progressive neuromuscular syndrome that lowers functional ability in daily performance and increases the risk of injuries caused by falling. Those who have experienced a fall suffer from serious injuries that can lead to functional disabilities and force them to face greater risk of institutionalization (Tinetti, Liu, & Clause, 1993).

Although biological aging is inevitable, at least a portion of the decline caused by disuse can be reversed by increasing the level of physical activity. For example, despite some negative findings in very early reports, recent investigation has clearly demonstrated that decline in the cardiovascular system can be modified by regular aerobic exercise. Studies have revealed that older adults can improve VO2max by 10 to 30%, and the magnitude of the increase in VO2max is comparable to that of young adults (Hagberg, Allen, et al., 1985; Seals, Hurley, Schultz, & Hagberg, 1984). Further evidence indicates that the rate of age-related loss of aerobic capacity may be slowed by engaging in endurance training (Kasch, Boyer, van Camp, Verity, & Wallace, 1993; Rogers, Hagberg, Martin, Ehsani, & Holloszy, 1990; Spina, Miller, Bogenhagen, & Schechtman, 1996).

Improvements in aerobic capacity can run counter to the declines accompanying age and be very important for reducing the risk of cardiovascular disease. However, aerobic exercise generally contributes to a relatively small functional benefit in muscular fitness (Fiatarone, O'Neill, et al., 1994). Klitgaard et al. (1990) compared leg and arm strength in young and elderly sedentary subjects and in elderly swimmers, runners, and strength-trained subjects trained 12 to 17 years. The researchers found that subjects who had been involved in strength training exhibited significantly greater maximal isometric torque and upper arm and mid-thigh muscle mass than did the swimmers and runners. In addition, only the strength-trained older subjects had muscle strength and muscle cross-sectional areas comparable to those of the younger control subjects. Although these findings suggest that endurance types of exercise are not effective in preventing deterioration of the muscle system, strength training effectively helped older individuals to maintain muscle mass and muscle strength, and the capacity of improvements in muscle strength is preserved regardless of age.

Safety and Efficacy of Strength Training in the Elderly

A decade ago, physical activity or exercise for older adults normally meant aerobic ac-

tivities such as walking, swimming, and cycling, but the importance of strength training is increasingly being recognized as a means to maintain independence by preserving and enhancing muscle strength and endurance. Although there is no doubt that aerobic fitness is very important for older adults to perform daily activities, recent investigation has revealed a critical association between muscle strength and functional impairments in daily activities. For example, walking was generally thought of as aerobic activity, but recent findings reveal that self-selected walking speed is associated with leg-muscle strength (Bassey, Bendall, & Pearson, 1988; W. R. Frontera, Meredith, O'Reilly, & Evans, 1990). In other research, leg-muscle power was found to explain 86% of the variance in walking speed (Bassey, Fiatarone, et al., 1992).

The past decade has seen an accumulation of evidence of the benefits of rebuilding muscle strength in the elderly (Fiatarone, Marks, Ryan, et al., 1990; W. R. Frontera, Meredith, O'Reilly, & Knuttgen, 1988; Tsutsumi, Don, Zaichkowsky & Delizonna, 1997). Until recently, however, researchers and exercise practitioners were reluctant to use strength training for the aging population because of feared risks such as from sharp increases in blood pressure or too much stress on aged joints. They were also skeptical about the trainability of aged musculoskeletal systems.

Given adequate instruction and supervision, safety of resistance training has been proven by a number of studies in which participants completed strength-training intervention without injury. One study indicates that strength training may be even safer than low-intensity aerobic exercise for older adults to perform. Pollock et al. (1989) conducted a 6-month exercise intervention study with men and women, aged 70 to 79 years, who were previously sedentary. The participants were divided into three groups: strength training, walk/jogging exercise, and nonexercising control group. The participants in the strength-training program significantly improved muscle strength whereas the participants in the aerobic exercise group improved aerobic capacity compared to the control group. Thus, both intervention programs were successful in improving physical fitness. However, although no injuries were reported by participants in the strength-training program, many participants in the walk/jog group reported injuries despite the fact that participants performed a walking program for 3 months before they started jogging. These findings suggest that strength training can be a safer exercise modality than jogging in older adults.

However, strength training is not magic. Conservative or unsophisticated methods such as too low intensity or lack of progressive intensity, have failed to produce significant improvements in muscular fitness (Aniansson & Gustafson, 1981; Hagberg, Graves, et al., 1989; L. Larsson, 1982). Nevertheless, when given adequate training intensity and methodology, older men and women gain marked strength that is comparable to that of young individuals in a relatively short time. In an earlier study, Moritani and DeVries (1980) trained five older men whose mean age was 70 and five young men with moderate-intensity strength training at 66% of the one-repetition maximum (1 RM) during the course of 8 weeks of progressive strength training. After the training period, older men improved isometric arm strength of the muscle flexors by 23%, and the percentage increases in strength were similar to those of young men. The researchers concluded that changes in neural factors were responsible for the increased isometric strength in older adults.

More recently, W. R. Frontera at al. (1988) examined the effects of high-intensity strength-training program for extensors and flexors of both knee joints at 80% of the 1 RM in 12 healthy but untrained sedentary older men whose average age was 64 years.

The results showed that the older men significantly improved strength 107% in knee extensors and 227% in knee flexors. Isokinetic peak torque of extensors and flexors measured was also increased 10.0 and 18.5% at 60 degrees/s and 16.7 and 14.7% at 240 degrees/s. In this study, mid-thigh composition was analyzed by using computer tomographic scans, a more sophisticated technique compared to the method used in Moritani and DeVries's (1980) study. The researchers found that their older subjects increased the total mid-thigh cross-section area by 11% and quadriceps area by 9.3%. Thus, this study found evidence that muscle hypertrophy could occur in older adults following strength training.

Fiatarone, Marks, et al. (1990) found that muscle hypertrophy was seen even in the oldest. They trained 10 frail, institutionalized men and women aged from 87 to 96, with a mean age of 90, to perform progressive resistance training three times per week with knee extension at high intensity (80% of 1 RM) under close supervision for 8 weeks. The subjects experienced marked strength gain in the knee extensors, averaging by 174%, as well as 16% in walking performance measured in gait speed. This study also reported that the subjects increased 9% in mid-thigh muscle cross-sectional area. Researchers concluded that frail residents of nursing homes at ages up to 96 years significantly gained muscle strength, muscle size, and functional mobility. Perhaps, the most outstanding outcome of participation in the strength-training program in this study was that two frail, institutionalized subjects who had needed canes were able to walk without them, and one subject who needed to use his arm in order to rise from a chair became able to do so without leaning on anything. These findings indicate that strength training was effective to minimize and/or reverse the syndrome of physical frailty that is so prevalent among older adults. Further, throughout the 8 weeks of the training period, none of the participants reported any musculoskeletal injuries. Because muscle weakness and associated mobility impairment increase the risk of falls, reversing muscle atrophy can probably be the most functionally important factor for frail older adults to avoid functional dependency.

In addition to improvements in functional capacity, strength training seems to have important therapeutic effects for many geriatric syndromes common to this vulnerable population. Nelson et al. (1994) conducted a study to evaluate if multiple risk factors for osteoporotic fractures could be modified by strength training in postmenopausal, sedentary women between the ages of 50 and 70. During the course of this one-year intervention study, the subjects performed high-intensity strength training (75–85% of 1 RM) with five different exercises. The strength-trained women increased femoral neck bone mineral density and lumbar spine bone mineral whereas the control group decreased in these variables. Total body bone mineral content was preserved in the strength-training group but decreased in the control group. Menkes et al. (1993) found that strength training increased regional bone mineral density in middle-aged and older men as well. These effects are expected to offset the typical age-associated declines in bone health.

Further, strength training improves insulin sensitivity and gastrointestinal transit time, decreases pain and disability from arthritis, reduces body fat and central adiposity, and improves sleep quality (Mazzeo et al., 1998). Strength training also seems to be effective in reducing weight by increasing in resting metabolic rate in older adults (Campbell, Crim, Dallal, Young, & Evans, 1994). Thus, although strength training is an effective way to reduce the risk of a sedentary lifestyle by improving functional capacity, these preven-

tive and/or therapeutic benefits can contribute to an increase in active life expectancy; a subsequent increase in the level of physical activity can substantially influence quality of life.

Physical Activity and Depressive Symptoms

Although strength training influences older adults' quality of daily life by improving functional capacity, recent studies indicate that it may also be able to contribute to their quality of life by enhancing psychological health. Similar to physiological function, psychological function declines as individuals age. It has been reported that older adults with no apparent physical or mental illness are more prone to dysphoric mood states than younger persons are (Blazer, 1980). Declines in cognitive functions such as problem-solving skills and the ability to integrate new information have also been observed in healthy older adults (Emery & Blumenthal, 1991). With increasing age, both physiological and psychological ability to cope with stressful events may change. After long years of exposure to various stressors, aged organisms may become less capable of adapting to life stress compared to when they were young. Also, daily activities once easily performed, such as moving objects, walking, and climbing stairs, may become sources of excessive and chronic distress.

Perhaps the most frequently reported dysphoric condition among the elderly is depression (Blazer, 1989; Buschmann, Dixon, & Tichy, 1995). It is estimated that about 15% of the older population suffers from depressive symptoms (Koenig & Blazer, 1992), and the prevalence of depression may increase as individuals age (Wallace & O'Hara, 1992). Depression in later life may be caused by the multiple losses of aging. Although significant losses in functional capacity can lead older adults to depressive symptoms, loss of friends, loved ones, and social status may lead them to have transient negative mood states. Depressed individuals typically suffer from symptoms such as lethargy, lack of vigor, slowing of the thought processes, loss of appetite, confused mental and physical function, memory loss, and lack of interest in living. These conditions can severely impair the quality of individuals' lives.

However, as people grow older, too often they accept changes in health as the results of increasing age rather than of sedentary lifestyle. Because many psychological phenomena and physiological conditions can have a reciprocal relationship, it is no surprise that these psychological declines occur sooner if an individual is sedentary. Although a causal relationship is yet to be established, many researchers have demonstrated that sedentary older adults will be less likely to experience depressive symptoms when they adopt a physically active lifestyle (e.g., Camacho, Roberts, Lazarus, Kaplan, & Cohen, 1991; Mobily, Rubenstein, Lemke, O'Hara, & Wallace, 1996). However, these reports are inconclusive due to many measurement and methodological problems, such as cross-sectional design, small sample size, inadequate control, and limited fitness measures (Dunn & Dishman, 1991). Nevertheless, the fact that there is fairly consistent experimental evidence to support the inverse relation should certainly encourage older adults to adopt a more active lifestyle.

In a longitudinal cohort study spanning 20 years, Camacho et al. (1991), reported that men and women who were inactive in 1965 when baseline measurements were taken were associated with greater risk of depression at followup than were those who were active, but for those inactive men and women, subsequent increase in physical activity reduced the risk of future depression to the same level as that of those who had been active throughout the period under study ac-

tive. Another cohort study, by Mobily et al. (1996), reported that if subjects with more depressive symptoms had daily walking habits at baseline, they later had greater odds for improvement in the symptoms. Findings in other studies also suggest that older adults will be less likely to suffer from depressive symptoms if they alter their lifestyle from a completely sedentary one to one of minimal physical activity.

Strength Training in Clinical Depression

Because most obvious causes of decreasing physical activity are physical limitations, strength training can help minimize the risk of depression by simply increasing the level of physical activity through improvements in functional capacity. On the other hand, therapeutic use of strength training as a nonmedical treatment for depression has also been documented. Although reports on this effect focus largely on aerobic exercise, the empirical evidence for a link between exercise and depression indicates that strength training has therapeutic effects similar to those of aerobic exercise. Two studies with younger patients and one with older patients have been published. In a younger population of mixed major and minor clinically depressed women, Doyne et al. (1987) compared the effects of aerobic exercise to those of strength training. After the 8-week training period, patients in both training programs significantly reduced depression scores assessed by the Beck Inventory, Lubin's Depression Adjective List, and the Hamilton Rating Scale for Depression. In addition, both exercise programs were found to be equally effective in decreasing depression.

Martinsen, Hoffart, and Solberg (1989) conducted a similar study. Ninety-nine patients with major depression, dysthymic disorder, or depressive disorder were assigned either aerobic exercise or strength training and trained three times a week for 8 weeks. After the training period, depression scores were significantly reduced in both groups, and no significant difference were found between the groups. A significant increase in aerobic fitness in the aerobic group was weakly associated with reduction in depression. As expected, no improvement in aerobic fitness was observed in the strength-training group. This suggests that although exercise is associated with an antidepressive effect in patients with mild to moderate depressive disorders, aerobic fitness does not seem to be a factor for the antidepressive effect. These studies thus demonstrate the efficacy of both strength training and aerobic exercise in treating depression.

A study with depressive older adults conducted by Singh, Clements, and Fiatarone (1997) also reported significant effects. In this study, the researchers trained 32 older adults (average age 71) with major or minor depression or dysthymia. The subjects performed closely supervised high-intensity (80% of 1 RM) progressive resistance training for 10 weeks. After completing the program, depressed older subjects experienced a significant reduction of both self-reported and therapist-rated depression scores. It was further reported that 14 of 16 subjects no longer met the criteria for clinical depression. It should be noted that the subjects also reported significant improvements in quality-of-life scores, measured by the Medical Outcome Survey Short Form (SF-36). They improved physical functioning, vitality, social functioning, emotional, and mental health subscales significantly, compared to baseline measurements. Further, they also improved scores of vitality, bodily pain, emotional and social functioning significantly more than did the control group in a health education program. Scores of these subscales of quality of life for the strength group approximated or exceeded those of age-matched norms,

whereas controls remained lower than these scores. These findings suggest that whereas strength training is an effective treatment modality for clinically depressed older adults, it also improves their quality of life by influencing a variety of emotional and social health aspects.

Mood, Emotional Well-Being, and Stress Reduction

Although it is important to know that the effects of strength training appear positive in many ways in older clinical populations, generalization of these gains in emotional health to the nonclinical population should also be important because the majority of community-dwelling elderly are not likely to be mentally ill. During the past decade, a considerable number of studies have demonstrated that exercise is associated with psychological health (Brown, 1992; Folkins, & Sime, 1981; McAuley & Rudolph, 1995; Sonstroem & Morgan, 1989). Although there is no conclusive evidence that one form of exercise may be superior to others, strength training appears to be uniquely specific in enhancing psychological health.

Tsutsumi, Don, Zaichkowsky, Takenaka, et al. (1998) conducted a study that examined the effects of strength training on mood and anxiety in older women. In this study, healthy but sedentary older women were trained with moderate- to high-intensity strength training. Older women whose average age was 69 years were assigned to perform high-intensity (75 to 85% of 1 RM) or a moderate-intensity strength training (55 to 65% of 1 RM) or were assigned to a nonexercise control program. Strength training was performed 3 days a week for 12 weeks. After the training period, both high and moderate strength-training programs produced significant improvements in muscle strength and body composition compared to muscle strength and body composition of the control subjects.

Older women in both training groups significantly improved positive mood, and the moderate-intensity group significantly reduced trait anxiety compared to the control group. Although these findings provide evidence for the effectiveness of strength training to enhance mood states in older women, both moderate- and high-intensity training are beneficial for older women to improve psychological health, with moderate-intensity rather than high-intensity training tending to be more effective for older women to improve psychological health.

In examining the effects of strength training, Norvell and Belles (1993) found that psychological benefits of strength training generalize beyond measures of mood states and include stress-reducing effects. The investigators assigned male police officers to either circuit strength training (70 to 80% of 1 RM) or a control group. After completing 16 weeks of the intervention program, the officers in the strength-training program significantly improved self-reported measures of depression, anxiety, and hostility with reducing perceived stress. Because these law enforcement personnel are often described as having one of the most stressful occupations, they are frequently targeted for stress management intervention (Malloy & Mays, 1984). The researchers speculate that improvements in mood states following strength training may be related to the reduction of their stress. Therefore, they recommended the inclusion of strength training in stress-management intervention programs for individuals who are exposed to high occupational stress.

We now know that strength training reduces cardiovascular reactivity during stressful situations (Tsusumi, Don, & Zaichowsky, 1999). In the past researchers thought that it was aerobic conditioning that allowed individuals to reduce cardiovascular reactivity to psychological stress. The hypothesized mechanism was that because fitter individuals' sympathetic responses to physiological load were lower, they might also be less responsive to psychological stress. Although the effectiveness of aerobic adaptation to stress has been demonstrated by some investigators (Blumenthal, Emery, et al., 1988; Blumenthal, Fredrickson, et al., 1990; Takenaka & Zaichkowsky, 1990), others have reported either equivocal results or no effects (De Geus, van Doornen, de Visser, & Orlebeke, 1990; Roskies et al., 1986). Although results of studies examining the effects of aerobic exercise on stress reactivity are ambiguous, some researchers have found that nonaerobic forms of exercise, in particular strength training, may also reduce cardiovascular reactivity to stress.

Don, Zaichkowsky, and Tsutsumi (1996) investigated the effects of a strength-training program on cardiovascular reactivity to psychological stress in college women. Thirty-five female students were randomly assigned to either high-intensity strength training (80% of 1 RM), moderate-intensity strength training (65% of 1 RM), or a health education control group. Subjects in the strength-training groups performed progressive resistance training with close supervision. Before and after 10 weeks of training, all subjects underwent measurements of muscle strength, muscular endurance, body composition, aerobic capacity, and heart rate and blood pressure responses to stress. Results demonstrate that both intensity strength programs significantly improved all measurements in physical fitness except for aerobic capacity. In addition, both experimental groups significantly reduced heart rate and blood pressure reactivity during various psychological stressors compared to that of the control subjects. This study clearly demonstrated that nonaerobic strength training may also have potential to reduce cardiovascular reactivity to stress.

To study the relevance of Don et al.'s (1996) findings for older adults, Tsutsumi,

Don, and Zaichkowsky (1999) conducted a study that examined the effects of strength training on cardiovascular stress reactivity in older adults. Healthy but sedentary senior citizens (60–84 years) were recruited and randomly assigned to high-intensity (80% of 1RM), moderate-intensity (60% of 1RM), or nonexercise (control) groups. Subjects in the exercise groups performed progressive strength-training programs three sessions a week for 12 weeks. These subjects were closely supervised. Measurements of physical fitness included arm and leg muscle strength, aerobic capacity, body composition, heart rate, and blood pressure reactivity to various psychosocial stressors. Results of this study generally supported Don et al.'s findings. Both strength-training paradigms produced equally significant improvements in all the physiological measures, whereas aerobic capacity remained constant. Older adults in strength-training groups exhibited a significant reduction in both systolic and diastolic blood pressure reactivity on various tasks compared to that of the control group. Thus, findings in this study showed that the elderly who participate in strength training significantly reduce cardiovascular responses to stress, which indicates that strength conditioning can influence older adults' mental health by protecting them against stress.

These findings may have important implications. Reduction of physiological responses to stress, possibly because strength training can greatly contribute to older adults' quality of life by reducing psychosomatic distress. In addition, the physiological adaptations to stress may also help place older adults at lower risk of cardiac events because stress is considered an important risk factor. Cardiovascular disease is responsible for 70% of all deaths in individuals aged over 75 years (Kannel, 1995); it is also a major cause of physical disabilities (Kannel). The relationship between exercise training and stress re-

activity should be investigated further in order to find more evidence of its efficacy in modifying stress responses. Nonetheless, findings from these studies offer additional reasons to encourage older adults to participate in strength training.

Strength Training and Physical Self-Efficacy

Despite evidence of potential psychological benefits, information on how strength training enhances psychological function remains unclear. Many researchers used to think that negative psychological states were associated with low levels of aerobic fitness, and therefore, the effects of aerobic exercise on psychological health have been studied with great interest. One reason for this is the fact that most psychologically disturbed individuals appear to be unfit. However, positive effects have also been found in a wide range of exercise modalities from aerobic exercise to nonaerobic strength training or flexibility exercise such as yoga. This indicates that aerobic fitness is not necessary for causing psychological change, and this makes it difficult to identify the specific mechanisms that are responsible for psychological changes.

To date, one of the most frequently reported aspects of psychological function in exercise literature is the role of a sense of personal control in physical tasks, or physical self-efficacy. Self-efficacy theory, a fundamental component of social cognitive theory developed by Bandura (1977a,b; 1986), explains the individual's perception of ability to perform a specific behavioral task. Efficacy of personal control can be defined as the individual's perceived ability to execute a given behavioral task (Ewart, 1989). Its striking psychological power has been applied to diverse psychological functions of all ages, including exercise behavior in older adults (McAuley, Sheaffer, & Rudolph, 1995), and phobias, smoking cessation, career development in adults (Bandura, Adams, & Beyer, 1977; Condiotte & Lichtenstein, 1981; Hackett, & Betz, 1981), and educational achievement in children (Schunk, 1982).

In a series of studies with cardiac patients, Ewart (1989) maintains that efficacy of personal control for physical activities plays a major role in recovery of a normal life and that strength training may uniquely enhance patients' physical self-efficacy and related emotional well-being during cardiac rehabilitation. It is believed that cardiac patients who experience sudden and frightening heart attacks are often limited more by their sense of lessened self-control than they are by any real physical limitations and that they consequently develop inappropriate perceptions of their personal capabilities (McCartney & McKelvie, 1996). These misperceptions may force them to experience difficulty in resuming daily routines, which may result in mood disturbance and inactivity. A sense of personal control may thus be an important factor for cardiac patients. Strength training appears to help these patients regain confidence in their physical abilities through a greater sense of reward from improvements in physique and strength gains. It can also act as strong positive feedback and have a greater impact on emotional well-being. Further, somatic indicators of personal efficacy are particularly relevant in domains that involve physical achievements; strength training "is uniquely variable in its ability to provide direct, varied, and highly reliable information concerning patients' physical capabilities" (Ewart, 1989, p. 683).

Kelemen et al. (1986) studied the effects of strength training on self-efficacy in cardiac patients enrolled in a rehabilitation program. They assigned 40 patients to either a strength-training or traditional rehabilitation program that included aerobic activities (walking and jogging) and recreational volleyball. The strength-training group performed the same aerobic activities and low-impact (40% of 1RM) circuit weight training. After 10 weeks, strength-trained patients showed significant gains in muscle strength, whereas the control patients had little. The experimental group also exhibited significant increases in self-efficacy for activities requiring arm or leg strength, but the control group did not change in these variables.

In a followup study, Stewart, Kelemen, and Ewart (1994) assessed the effects of a 3-year strength-training program on physical self-efficacy in cardiac rehabilitation patients. Seventeen patients who attended more than 50% of the sessions during the training period were compared to 8 patients who completed a conventional rehabilitation program. Compared to the baseline value measured 3 years earlier, patients in the strength-training group increased strength by 13% in arm strength and 40% in leg strength, and 16% in arm self-efficacy and 6% in leg self-efficacy. It should be noted that control patients decreased 11% in arm and 20% in leg self-efficacy. Findings in these studies with cardiac patients indicate that only strength training could enhance self-efficacy for activities similar to the training tasks. This suggests that cardiac rehabilitation programs including strength training would be more effective than those comprising aerobic exercise alone.

In addition to influencing involvement in behavioral tasks, strength training appears to play an important role in enhancing physical self-efficacy as well as emotional well-being. Recently, Stewart, Kelemen, and Ewart (1994) applied strength training for 41 men (25 to 59 years) with mild hypertension concurrently in drug therapy. The subjects were randomized to beta-blocker, calcium-channel blocker, or placebo medications, and assigned to 10 weeks of low-intensity (40% of 1 RM) circuit strength training and moderate-intensity aerobic activities. A beta-blocker was used to prevent the aerobic conditioning effects. As expected, exercise training significantly increased aerobic capacity in the calcium-channel blocker and placebo groups, but not in the beta-blocker group. All three treatment groups had significant increases in self-efficacy in arm and leg strength, and these gains were associated with improved mood. All subjects exhibited an increase in vigor and decreases in tension and total mood disturbance. However, gains in either muscle strength or aerobic capacity were not related to mood states. These findings indicate that changes in emotional well-being were not solely dependent on the physiological changes; rather, enhanced perception of self-control was more favorably related to the mood improvements.

Given the findings with cardiac patients, the notion of physical self-efficacy may also be applied effectively to the older population. With age, promotion of a sense of personal control becomes vital to both physical and psychological health (Hickey, Owen, & Froman, 1992) because declines in physical, sensory, and cognitive function generate the feeling of substantial loss of personal control. Just as in cardiac patients, in older adults, resulting perception of the substantial loss and self-doubt in functional capacity can limit performance in daily activities, and older adults may easily develop lower levels of confidence than their actual capabilities warrant. As is evident in cardiac rehabilitation patients, strength training may modify older adults' feeling of competence by improving the perceived capability to perform daily activities in older adults who could also be suffering from functional limitations.

Despite the extensive literature, because application of self-efficacy theory to older adults is fairly recent, little is currently known about how strength training effects self-efficacy in older adults. However, one study showed that strength-training intervention effectively improved mood and physical self-efficacy. Tsutsumi, Don, Zaichkowsky, and Delizonna (1997) investigated psychological adaptations in response to 12 weeks of strength training in healthy but sedentary older men and women whose average age was 68. The researchers evaluated the effects of moderate- to high-intensity (55 to 85% of 1 RM) progressive resistance training on muscular strength, body composition, mood, and physical self-efficacy. Following the 12-week intervention program, older adults in strength programs showed marked muscle strengthening, improved mood, decreased anxiety, and increased physical self-efficacy. Participation in 12 weeks of moderate- to high-intensity strength training helped older adults improve physical self-efficacy and mood with improving muscle strength and body composition.

Thus, strength training appears to be effective in improving physical self-efficacy. Improvements in muscle strength and function may strongly influence older adults' perceived control in physical tasks. In addition, during judgment of their capabilities, people rely partly on somatic information conveyed by physiological and emotional states (Bandura, 1997). With gains in strength, muscle mass, and functional capacity, direct, varied, and highly reliable somatic sensations through impact of resistance training (Ewart, 1989) may also have helped older adults to develop more confidence in their own functional capabilities. Strength training can be uniquely valuable in its ability to provide a new experience with graduated performance goals. This may provide an exerciser with continuous challenge for increasing resistance and the resulting feeling of success and mastery. Finally, psychosocial aspects of strength training such as positive feedback received from their instructors, peers, children, and even grandchildren may promote feelings of success and achievement (Faigenbaum, 1995). These experiences may lead older adults to perceive themselves as having more control in daily life and emotional well-being.

Conclusion

Strength training has considerable potential to promote human health. Importantly, this form of exercise training is unequally variable for helping older individuals who are likely to suffer from loss in functional capacity. Studies have demonstrated that strength training is associated with gains in strength, muscle mass, and functional capacity in older adults. These benefits have also been documented for very old and frail individuals. In addition, recent research suggests that strength training may be helpful in buffering the effects of stress, depression, and anxiety and in improving emotional well-being. In addition, its application to the theory of self-efficacy has important implications in the case of many adults who are suffering from loss in functional capacity and, therefore, perceived control for daily activities. Older adults with strong self-efficacy can protect themselves against the variety of adverse effects of disabilities and successfully manage health-related behavior (Bandura, 1997). Promoting health status in older adults is of special importance because health problems create loss of autonomy and severely impair quality of life. Even with physical limitation, a strong sense of personal efficacy increases the ability to cope with stressors or enjoy greater autonomy and emotional-well being. Strength training appears to improve physical self-efficacy for older adults.

The combination of these physiological and psychological benefits should greatly influence health variables and play a critical role in maintaining an independent lifestyle in the final stage of human life. However, application of the effects of strength training and improved physical self-efficacy to mental health in older populations is fairly re-

cent. Further studies are expected to elucidate clearer explanations of the psychological benefits of strength training and the ways in which self-efficacy is involved in strength training and changes in psychological and behavioral function in older adults.

References

Aniansson, A., & Gustafsson, E. (1981). Physical training in elderly men. *Clinical Physiology, 1*, 87–98.

Bandura, A. (1986). *Social foundations of thought and action*. Englewood Cliffs, NJ: Prentice Hall.

Bandura, A. (1977). Self-efficacy: Toward a unifying theory of behavioral change. *Psychological Review, 84*, 191–215.

Bandura, A. (1997). *Self-efficacy: The exercise of control*. New York: B. H. Freeman and Company.

Bandura, A., Adams, N. E., & Beyer, J. (1977). Cognitive processes mediating behavioral change. *Journal of Personality and Social Psychology, 35*, 125–139.

Bassey, E. J., Bendall, M. J., & Pearson, M. (1988). Muscle strength in the triceps surae and objectively measured customary walking activity in men and women over 65 years of age. *Clinical Science, 74*, 85–89.

Bassey, E. J., Fiatarone, W. A., O'Neill, E. F., Kelly, M., Evans, W. J., & Lipsitz, L. A. (1992). Leg extensor power and functional performance in very old men and women. *Clinical Science, 82*, 321–327.

Blair, S. N., Goodyear, N. N., & Cooper, K. H. (1984). Physical fitness and incidence of hypertension in healthy normotensive men and women. *The Journal of American Medical Association, 252*, 487–490.

Blazer, D. (1989). Current concepts: Depression in the elderly. *New England Journal of Medicine, 320*, 164–166.

Blazer, D. (1980). The epidemiology of mental illness in late life. In E. W. Busse & D. G. Blazer (Eds.), *Handbook of geriatric psychiatry* (pp. 142–157). New York: Van Nostrand.

Blumenthal, J. A., Emery, C. F., Walsh, M. A. Cox, D. R., Kuhn, C. M., Williams, R. B., & Williams, R. S. (1988). Exercise training in healthy Type A middle-aged men: Effects on behavioral and cardiovascular responses. *Psychosomatic Medicine, 50*, 418–433.

Blumenthal, J. A., Fredrickson, M., Kuhn, C. M., Ulmer, R. L., Walsh-Riddle, M., & Appelbaum, M. (1990). Aerobic exercise reduced levels of cardiovascular and sympathoadrenal responses to mental stress in subjects without prior evidence of myocardial ischemia. *American Journal of Cardiology, 65*, 93–98.

Bouchard, C., Shepherd, R. J., Stephens, T., Sutton J. R., & McPherson, B. U. (Eds.). (1990). *Exercise, fitness, and health: A consensus of current knowledge*. Champaign, IL: Human Kinetics.

Brown, D. R. (1992). Physical activity, ageing, and psychological well-being. *Canadian Journal of Sports Science, 17,* 185–193.

Buschmann, M. T., Dixon, M. A., & Tichy, A. M. (1995). Geriatric depression. *Home Healthcare Nurse, 13*(3), 47–56.

Camacho, T. C., Roberts R. E., Lazarus, N. B., Kaplan, G. A., & Cohen, R. D. (1991). Physical activity and depression: Evidence from the Alameda County Study. *American Journal of Epidemiology, 134,* 220–231.

Campbell, W. W., Crim, M. C., Dallal, G. E., Young, V. R., & Evans, W. J. (1994). Increased protein requirements in the elderly: New data and retrospective reassessments. *American Journal of Clinical Nutrition, 60,* 167–175.

Caspersen, C. J., Powell, K. E., & Christenson, G. M. (1985). Physical activity, exercise, and physical fitness: Definitions and distinctions for health-related research. *Public Health Reports, 100,* 126–131.

Cohn, S. H., Vartsky, D., Yasumura, S., Savitsky, A., Zanzi, I., Vaswani, A., & Ellis, K. J. (1980). Compartmental body composition based on total-body potassium and calcium. *American Journal of Physiology, 239,* E524–E530.

Condiotte, M. M., & Lichtenstein, E. (1981). Self-efficacy and relapse in smoking cessation programs. *Journal of Consulting and Clinical Psychology, 49,* 648–658.

Danner, R., & Edwards, D. (1992). Life is movement: Exercise for the older adult. *Activities Adaptation & Aging, 16,* 15–26.

De Geus, E. J. C., van Doornen L. J. P., de Visser, A. C., & Orlebeke, J. F. (1990). Existing and training induced differences in aerobic fitness: Their relationship to physiological response patterns during different types of stress. *Psychophysiology, 27*(4), 457–478.

Don, B. M., Zaichkowsky, L. D., & Tsutsumi, T. (1996). Effects of strength training on cardiovascular reactivity to stress and psychological well-being in college women. *The Journal of Applied Sport Psychology, 9,* S20.

Donneskoild-Samsore, B., Kofod, V., Munter, J., Grimby, G., & Schnohr, P. (1984). Muscle strength and functional capacity in 77–81 year old men and women. *European Journal of Applied Physiology, 52,* 123–135.

Doyne, E. J., Ossip-Klein, D. J., Bowman, E. D. Osborn, K. M., McDougall-Wilson, I. B., & Neimeyer, R. A. (1987). Running versus weight lifting in the treatment of depression. *Journal of Consulting and Clinical Psychology, 55, 748–754.*

Dunn, A. L., & Dishman, R. K. (1991). Exercise and the neurobiology of depression. *Exercise and Sport Science Review, 19,* 41–98.

Emery, C. F., & Blumenthal, J. A. (1991). Effects of physical exercise on psychological and cognitive functioning of older adults. *Annals of Behavioral Medicine, 13,* 99–107.

Ewart, C. K. (1989). Psychological effects of resistive weight training: Implication for cardiac patients. *Medicine and Science in Sports and Exercise, 21,* 683–688.

Faigenbaum, A. D. (1995). Psychosocial benefits of prepubescent strength training. *Strength and Conditioning, 17,* 28–32.

Fiatarone, M. A., Marks, E. C., Ryan, N. D., Meredith, C. N., Lipsitz, L. A., & Evans, W. J. (1990). High-intensity strength training in nonagenarians: Effects on skeletal muscle. *The Journal of American Medical Association, 263,* 3029–3034.

Fiatarone, M. A., O'Neill, E. F., Ryan, N. D., Clements, K. M., Solares, G. R., Nelson, M. E., Roberts, S. B., Kehayias, J. J., Lipsitz, L. A., & Evans, W. J. (1994). Exercise training and nutritional supplementation for physical frailty in very elderly people. *New England Journal of Medicine, 330,* 1769–1775.

Fisher, N., Pendergast, D., & Calkins, E. (1991). Muscle rehabilitation in impaired elderly nursing home residents. *Archives of Physical Medicine and Rehabilitation, 72,* 181–185.

Folkins, C. H., & Sime, W. E. (1981). Physical fitness training and mental health. *American Psychologist, 36,* 373–389.

Frontera, W. R., Meredith, C. N., O'Reilly, K. P., & Knuttgen, H. G. (1988). Strength conditioning in older men: Skeletal muscle hypertrophy and improved function. *Journal of Applied Physiology, 64,* 1038–1044.

Frontera, W. R., Meredith, C. N., O'Reilly, K. P., & Evans, W. J. (1990). Strength training and determinants of VO2max in older men. *Journal of Applied Physiology, 68,* 329–333.

Hackett, G., & Betz, N. (1981). A self-efficacy approach to the career development of women. *Journal of Vocational Behavior, 18,* 326–339.

Hagberg, J. M., Allen, W. K., Seals, D. R., Hurley, B. F., Ehsani, A. A., & Holloszy, J. O. (1985). A hemodynamic comparison of young and older endurance athletes during exercise. *Journal of Applied Physiology, 58,* 2041–2046.

Hagberg, J. M., Graves, J. E., Limacher, M., Woods, D., Cononie, C., Leggett, S., Gruber, J., & Pollock, M. (1989). Cardiovascular responses of 70- to 79-year-old men and women to exercise training. *Journal of Applied Physiology, 66,* 2589–2594.

Harries, U. J., & Bassey, E. J. (1990). Torque-velocity relationships for the knee extensors in women in their 3rd and 7th decades. *European Journal of Applied Physiology and Occupational Physiology, 60,* 187–190.

Heath, G., Hagberg, J., Ehsani, A., & Holloszy, J. (1981). A physiological comparison of young and older endurance athletes. *Journal of Applied Physiology, 51,* 634–640.

Helmrich, S. P., Ragland, D. R., Leung, R. W., & Paffenbarger, R. S. (1991). Physical activity and reduced occurrence of non-insulin-dependent diabetes mellitus. *New England Journal of Medicine, 325,* 147–152.

Hickey, M. L., Owen, S. V., & Froman, R. D. (1992). Instrument development: Cardiac diet and exercise self-efficacy. *Nursing Research, 41,* 347–351.

Jette, A. M., & Branch, L. G. (1981). The Framingham disability study: II—Physical disability among the aging. *American Journal of Public Health, 71,* 1211–1216.

Kannel, W. B. (1995). Epidemiological insights into

atherosclerotic cardiovascular disease—From the Framingham Study. In M. L. Pollock, & D. H. Schmidt (Eds.), *Heart disease and rehabilitation* (pp. 3–16). Champaign, IL: Human Kinetics.

Kasch, F., Boyer, J., Van Camp, S., Verity, L., & Wallace, J. P. (1993). Effect of exercise on cardiovascular ageing. *Age and Ageing, 22*, 5–10.

Kelemen, M. H., Stewart, K. J., Gillian, R. E., Ewart, C. K., Valenti, S. A., Manley, J. D., & Kelemen, M. D. (1986). Circuit weight training in cardiac patients. *Journal of the American College of Cardiology, 7*, 38–42.

Klitgaard, H., Mantoni, M., Schiaffino, S., Ausoni, S., Gorza, L., Laurent-Winter, C., Schnohr, P., & Saltin, B. (1990). Function, morphology and protein expression of aging skeletal muscle: A cross-sectional study of elderly men with different training backgrounds. *Acta Physiologica Scandinavica, 140*, 41–54.

Koenig, H. G., & Blazer, D. G., (1992). Epidemiology of geriatric affective disorders. In G. S. Alexopoulos (Ed.), *Clinics in geriatric medicine* (pp. 235–252). Philadelphia: Saunders.

Larsson, L. (1978). Morphological and functional characteristics of the aging skeletal muscle in man. *Acta Physiologica Scandinavica, 457* (Suppl), 1–36.

Larsson, L. (1982). Physical training effects on muscle morphology in sedentary males at different ages. *Medicine and Science in Sports and Exercise, 14*, 203–206.

Larsson, L. G., Grimby, G, & Karlsson, J. (1979). Muscle strength and speed of movement in relation to age and muscle morphology. *Journal of Applied Physiology, 46*, 451–456.

Lee, I., Paffenbarger, R. S., & Hsieh, C. (1991). Physical activity and risk of developing colorectal cancer among college alumni. *Journal of the National Cancer Institute, 83*, 1324–1329.

Lexell, J., Henriksson-Larsen, K., Wimblod, B., & Sjostrom, M. (1983). Distribution of different fiber types in human skeletal muscles: effects of aging studied in whole muscle cross sections. *Muscle and Nerve, 6*, 588–595.

Malloy, T. E., & Mays, G. L. (1984). The police stress hypothesis: A critical examination. *Criminal Justice and Behavior, 11*, 197–224.

Martinsen, E. W., Hoffart, A., & Solberg, O. (1989). Comparing aerobic and non-aerobic forms of exercise in the treatment of clinical depression: A randomized trial. *Comprehensive Psychiatry, 30*, 324–31.

Mazzeo, R. S., Cavanagh, P., Evans, W. J., Fiatarone, M., Hagberg, J., McAuley, E., & Startzell, J. (1998). Exercise and physical activity for older adults. *Medicine & Science in Sports & Exercise, 30*, 992–1009.

McAuley, E., & Rudolph, D. (1995). Physical activity aging, and psychological well-being. *Journal of Aging and Physical Activity, 3*, 67–96.

McAuley, E., Shaffer, S., & Rudolph, D. (1995). Affective responses to acute exercise in elderly impaired males: The moderating effects of self-efficacy and age. *International Journal of Aging and Human Development, 41*, 13–27.

McCartney, N., & McKelvie, R. S. (1996). The role of resistance training in patients with cardiac disease, *Journal of Cardiovascular Risk, 3*, 160–166.

McGinnis, J. M., & Lee, P. R. (1995). Healthy people 2000 at mid decade. *The Journal of the American Medical Association, 275*, 1123–1129.

Menkes, J. Mazel, D. & Redmond, C. (1993). Strength training increases regional bone mineral density and bone remodeling in middle-aged and older men. *Journal of Applied Physiology, 74*, 2478–2484.

Mobily, K. E., Rubenstein, L. M., Lemke, J. H., O'Hara, W., & Wallace, R. B. (1996). Walking and depression in a cohort of older adults: The Iowa 65+ rural health study. *Journal of Aging and Physical Activity, 4*, 119–135.

Moritani, T., & DeVries, H. (1980). Potential for gross muscle hypertrophy in older men. *Journal of Gerontology, 35*, 672–682.

Murray, M. P., Duthie, E. H., Gambert, S. T., Sepic, S. B., & Mollinger, L. A. (1985). Age-related differences in knee muscle strength in normal women. *Journal of Gerontology, 40*, 275–280.

Nelson, M. E., Fiatarone, M. A., Morganti, C. M., Trice, R. A., Greenberg, R. A., & Evance, W. J. (1994). Effects of high-intensity strength training on multiple risk factors for osteoporotic fractures. *The Journal of the American Medical Association, 272*, 1909–1914.

Norvell, N., & Belles, D. (1993). Psychological and physical benefits of circuit weight training in law enforcement personnel. *Journal of Consulting and Clinical Psychology, 61*, 520–527.

Ogawa, T., Spine, R., Martin III, W., Kohrt, W. Schechtman, K., Holloszy, J., & Ehsani, A. (1992). Effects of aging, sex and physical training on cardiovascular responses to exercise. *Circulation, 86*, 494–503.

Paffenbarger, R. S., Hyde, R. T., Wing, A. L., & Hsieh, C-C. (1986). Physical activity, all-cause mortality, and longevity of college alumni. *New England Journal of Medicine, 314*, 605–613.

Pollock, J. L., Graves, J. E., Leggett, S., Jones, A. E., & Colvin, A. B. (1989, May). *Injuries and adherence to aerobic and strength training exercise programs for the elderly*. Paper presented at the annual meeting of the American College of Sports Medicine, Baltimore.

Rodeheffer, R., Gerstenblith, G., Becker, L., Fleg, J., Weisfeldt, M., & Lakatta, E. (1984). Exercise cardiac output is maintained with advancing age in healthy human subjects: Cardiac dilatation and increased stroke volume compensate for a diminished heart rate. *Circulation, 69*, 203–213.

Rogers, M., Hagberg, J., Martin, W., Ehsani, A., & Holloszy, J. (1990). Decline in VO2max with aging in master athletes and sedentary men. *Journal of Applied Physiology, 68*, 2195–2199.

Roskies, E., Seraganian, P., Oseasohrn, R., et al. (1986). The Montreal Type A intervention project: Major findings. *Health Psychology, 5*, 45–69.

Schunk, D. (1982). Effects of effort attributional feedback on children's perceived self-efficacy and achievement. *Journal of Educational Psychology, 74*, 548–556.

Seals, D. R., Hurley, B. F., Schultz, J., & Hagberg, J. M. (1984). Endurance training in older men and women: I. Cardiovascular responses to exercise. *Journal of Applied Physiology, 57*, 1024–1029.

Singh, N. A., Clements, K. M., & Fiataron, M. A. (1997). A randomized controlled trial of progressive resistance training in depressed elders. *Journal of Gerontology, 52*, M27–M35.

Snow-Harter, C., & Marcus, R. (1991). Exercise, bone mineral density, and osteoporosis. *Exercise and Sports Science Review, 19*, 351–388.

Sonstroem, R. J., & Morgan, W. P. (1989). Exercise and self-esteem: Rationale and model. *Medicine and Science in Sports and Exercise, 21*, 329–337.

Spina, R. J., Miller, T. R., Bogenhagen, W. H., & Schechtman, K. B. (1996). Light training improves muscular strength and self-efficacy in cardiac patients. *Journal of Cardiopulmonary Rehabilitation, 8*, 292–296.

Takenaka, K., & Zaichkowsky, L. D. (1990). Physiological reactivity in acculturation: A study of female Japanese students. *Perceptual and Motor Skills, 70*, 503–513.

Taylor, C. B., Sallis, J., & Needle, R. (1985). The relationship of physical activity and exercise to mental health. *Public Health Reports, 100*, 195–202.

Tinetti, M. E., Liu, W. L., & Clause, E. (1993). Predictors and prognosis of inability to get up after falls among elderly persons. *The American Journal of Medical Association, 269*, 65–70.

Tsutsumi, T., Don, B. M., & Zaichkowsky, L. D. (1999). Psychophysiological effects of strength training on cardiovascular stress reactivity in older adults. In M. Sato, H. Tokura, & S. Watanuki (Eds.), *Recent advances in physiological anthropology* (pp. 329–338). Fukuoka: Kitakyushu University Press.

Tsutsumi, T., Don, B. M., Zaichkowsky, L. D., & Delizonna, L. L. (1997). Physical fitness and psychological benefits of strength training in community dwelling older adults. *Applied Human Science, 16*, 257–266.

Tsutsumi, T., Don, B. M., & Zaichkowsky, L. D., Takenaka, K., Oka, K., & Ohno, T. (1999). Comparison of high and moderate intensity of strength training on mood and anxiety, in older adults. *Perceptual and Motor Skills, 87*, 1003–1011.

U.S. Department of Health and Human Services. (1984). *Executive summary: Aging and health promotion: Market research for public education.* Washington, DC: U.S. Government Printing Office.

U.S. Department of Health and Human Services. (1991). *Healthy people 2000: Summary report.* Boston: Jones and Bartlett Publishers.

Wallace, J., & O'Hara, M. W. (1992). Increases in depressive symptomatology in the rural elderly: Results from a cross-sectional and longitudinal study. *Journal of Abnormal Psychology, 101*, 398–404.

12
Physical Exercise and Epilepsy

Hege R. Eriksen

Bjørn Ellertsen

Knut A. Hestad

Physical exercise is becoming increasingly important in modern society. The reason for this is that there has been a general decrease in physical activity amongst most individuals, which at least partly is due to reduced physical demands from the society. This fact makes leisure-time physical exercise even more important than it was in earlier times. Although engagement in physical exercise during leisure time seems to increase, about one third of the population of the United States, England, and Australia engage in activities of a frequency and intensity insufficient to obtain cardiorespiratory fitness (Stephens & Caspersen, 1994).

Physical exercise is by now often offered in working life in order to prevent or reduce health problems, among "healthy individuals." There is also an increase in adapted physical activity for individuals with disabilities. Thus, physical exercise is recommended for individuals with a variety of different medical conditions, such as coronary heart disease and diabetes (Andersen et al., 1995) and low back pain (Biering Sorensen, Bendix, Jorgensen, Manniche & Nielsen, 1994). The number of conditions that traditionally have led to expert recommendation to refrain from participation in sport and exercise has been reduced. However, the reduction in warnings seems to remain unknown to many practitioners. The traditional approach to exercise in patients with epilepsy has been to be cautious and at least not to be involved in exercise that could provoke seizures or lead to an increased risk of accidents. In 1960, Lennox wrote that patients with epilepsy could be described in one word: stagnation. They were, according to him, slow in movement, thought, communication, and bowel movement. A number of possible causes were indicated, among which were the epileptic problem itself, side effects of pharmacological treatment, general treatment policy, and lack of physical activity. The consequence in clinical practice was often that the patients with epilepsy were recommended not to be involved in any kind of exercise at all. Our present approach and recommendations are the opposite.

Recommendations have often been made on the basis of clinical experience and anecdotal data. Thus, Mendell (1984) stated that seizures seldom seem to occur in connection with physical activity and that available research is sparse. The literature is, however, characterized by reservations and rules of caution regarding participation in physical activities, in spite of the fact that few methodologically sound empirical studies are available. This chapter discusses the relationship between exercise and epilepsy, dangers and benefits, and how new knowledge may be implemented. There is very little in the literature indicating that patients with epilepsy who exercise or are physically active have more seizures than do patients who are inactive or not involved in physical exercise (Ellertsen, Eriksen, Mostofsky, & Ursin, 1993). Nevertheless, many individuals with epilepsy are excluded from or restricted in their activities due to fear of injuries (Bjørholt, Nakken, Roehme, & Hansen, 1990) or fear of exercise eliciting seizures (Williams, Roth, & Ruiz, 1991). In general, most publications recommend that both children and adults with epilepsy participate in physical activities (Gates, 1991; van Linschoten, Back, Mulder, & Meinardi, 1990; Livingstone, 1971). According to Livingstone (1971), children with epilepsy should be allowed to participate in physical activities on equal terms with their peers, provided that the seizures are controlled. In fact, the consequences of restrained physical activity may represent more serious problems than the possible negative consequences of seizures. Important keywords in this connection are overprotection, psychosocial problems, negative self-image, stigma (American Academy of Pediatrics, 1983; Freeman, 1985; Livingstone, 1971), anxiety/frustrations (Gates, 1991), and lack of positive physiological effects from physical activity (van Linschoten et al., 1990).

Epilepsy

Lennox (1960) defined five features of epileptic seizures: (a) loss or derangement of consciousness or remembrance (amnesia); (b) excess or loss of muscle tone or movement; (c) alternation of sensation, including hallucinations of special senses; (d) disturbance of the autonomic nervous system with resulting vegetative and visceral phenomena of various sorts; and (e) other psychic manifestations, abnormal thought process, or moods.

In other words, epilepsy may present itself with a variety of symptoms ranging from short absences to major convolutions. The epileptic seizures may be generalized without focal symptoms and with EEG changes in both cerebral hemispheres. These attacks are divided into primary and secondary generalized epilepsies. In primary generalized epilepsy, the patient is neurologically "healthy," the background activity of the EEG is normal, and magnetic resonance imaging or computer tomography yield normal findings. In secondary generalized epilepsy, clinical or laboratory findings, or both, confirm illness or damage in the central nervous system. Focal or partial epileptic attacks may present themselves in a number of ways such as minor focal convolutions, numbness in a hand, perspiration, turning of the head, or eye deviation towards one side.

The attacks may also be of a subclinical type in which no clinical symptoms are seen whereas EEG recordings show epileptic activity. In these cases, neuropsychological testing may reveal cognitive impairments during the abnormal EEG activity such as delayed reaction time or difficulties in discrimination between stimuli or signals (Rugland, 1990). Other conditions than epilepsy may produce similar symptoms. It has been maintained that about one fifth of patients with "intractable epilepsy" do not have epilepsy and that most of these patients have psychogenic attacks (Lesser, 1996), panic attacks with hyperventilation, migraine equivalents (Cordova, 1993), or that they present a variety of vasovagal syncope symptoms (Sander & O'Donoghue, 1997). Examples of the latter are bradycardia with vasovagal syncope and cardiogenic syncope. Among the cardiovascular syncopes, special attention has been directed to a long Q—T syndrome, characterized by a prolongation of the Q—T—interval in the electrocardiogram, which may lead to seizures (Gordon, 1994). This condition may be treated with beta-blockers and should not be confused with epilepsy. The physician must also consider hypoglycemia and changes in blood pH levels, which often are related to hyperventilation. Accordingly, diagnostic accuracy is of crucial importance (Sander & O'Donoghue, 1997). Epileptic seizures affecting the level of consciousness are obviously more problematic with reference to physical activities than are the focal epilepsies.

Exercise and Epilepsy

All changes in the homeostatic balance in biological variables may be risk factors for epileptic seizures. Thus, intense emotional responses have been reported as one of the most common seizure-eliciting factors (Aird, 1983). However, the situations studied were often linked to sleep deprivation, which is commonly reported as seizure inducing in itself (Aird, 1983). Seizures during physical exercise are not frequent, but may occur (Eriksen et al., 1994; Korczyn, 1979; Ogunyemi, Gomez, & Klass, 1988). The reason for the concern with regard to these relatively few cases is the risk involved in some types of sports, both for the patient and for the others engaged in the activity. Another and more generally important factor is the effect the occasional seizure during a sport activity may have for the future participation in that sport for the group of patients with epilepsy as such. There are no comprehensive data on the exact frequency of epileptic attacks in sports. The provoking factors may be related to any of the acute physiological changes taking place during exercise or to the psychological factors involved in the exercise. Ex-

ercise produces changes in the EEG and may also affect the epileptiform activity in the EEG. However, evidence also suggests that exercise (knee bends and ergometer cycling) may lead to decreased epileptiform activity in both adults and children (Götze, Kubicki, Munter, & Teichman, 1967; Horyd, Gryziak, Niedzielska, & Zielinski, 1981; Nakken, Løyning, Løying, Gløersen, & Larsson, 1997). The picture is, however, even more complicated because a rebound increase in epileptiform activity has been demonstrated after exercise in some individuals (Berney, Osselton, Kolvin, & Day, 1981; Götze et al., 1967; Horyd et al., 1981; Kuijer, 1978). This postexercise increase in epileptiform activity has been related to low blood pH values (Esquivel, Chaussain, Plouin, Ponsot, & Arthuis, 1991). A case study of two children with exercise-induced seizures did, however, not identify any obvious pathophysiological mechanisms (Schmitt, Thun Hohenstein, Vontobel, & Boltshauser, 1994).

Physical Exercise and Seizure Control

As stated earlier, there does not seem to be evidence supporting the notion that physical exercise in itself increases the incidence of seizures. The consensus seems to be contrary as most or all authors recommend at least some type of physical exercise for all patients with epilepsy. However, there are no acceptable randomized controlled studies on the effect of physical exercise on epilepsy in the literature. The variability in pathology and seizure risk and seizure frequency requires large groups and strict selection criteria in such studies. It is also difficult to perform such studies because most patients with epilepsy are clinically well controlled with few, if any epileptic seizures. Patients with more serious, intractable seizures are actually relatively few.

There are several examples of smaller pre-post follow-up designed studies, including patients with intractable epilepsy (Eriksen et al., 1994) or less serious epilepsy (Nakken, Bjørholt, Johannessen, Løyning, & Lind, 1990) demonstrating a reduced number of seizures in the periods when the patients were involved in aerobic training. This training also had a beneficial effect on muscle pain, sleep problems, and fatigue (Eriksen et al. 1994).

These secondary gains on life quality and subjective health have been ascribed to general psychobiological aspects of exercise, which also may be related to reduction in seizure incidences (Eriksen et al., 1994). The subjective experience of being able to gain control over the personal life situation and the challenges confronting the person reduce the stress response (Levine & Ursin, 1991). Thus, the expectancy to be able to handle challenges and stressors is referred to as coping (Levine & Ursin, 1991), and individuals with such expectancies show significantly less response to stressors and significantly better subjective health (Ursin, 1998). The pathophysiological mechanisms for the effects on seizure threshold remain speculative (Götze et al., 1967), but they are compatible with the general principle of seizures being elicited by homeostatic imbalance, and therefore, also dampened by any event that stabilizes this balance. Because physically fit persons in general are better able to handle stress, it may be hypothesized that the physically fit patient with epilepsy stands a better chance of avoiding seizures.

Emotional Disturbances and Epilepsy

Many patients with epilepsy report a feeling of being externally controlled and obtain notoriously high scores on checklists related to depression and anxiety (Ettinger et al., 1998). Several studies indicate that physical exercise has beneficial effects in reducing symptoms of depression and anxiety among patients and in general (Martinsen, Hofart, &

Solberg, 1989; Martinsen, Medhus, & Sandvik, 1985; Martinsen, Strand, Paulsson, & Kaggestad, 1989; Morgan & Goldstone, 1987; Steptoe, Edwards, Moses, & Mathews, 1989). According to the reasoning presented above, this is important for patients with epilepsy. There is no reason to believe that patients with epilepsy and symptoms of depression or anxiety should gain fewer benefits from physical exercise than other people. The patients may, however, need this benefit more than the average person because physical exercise may lead to reduced emotional problems, which in themselves may be a risk factor with regard to seizures.

Physical Performance in Athletes with Epilepsy

There is no reason to believe that epilepsy itself should affect performance in any form of physical exercise, but there are two factors that may hinder optimal performance. The first factor is the psychological and social barriers that the athlete with epilepsy meets in the environment. Some athletes have enough stamina and support to break through this barrier, and there are many examples of excellent performance in athletes with epilepsy. It is difficult to know the extent to which it matters for the athletes that they know that they have a condition that some may consider a handicap. It is, however, reasonable to assume that this awareness may play a role for at least some of these athletes in the final psychological buildup before an important competition. It may become necessary to fight fear of seizures or lack of self-confidence, or both, in the final psychological preparation before the competition (Pensgaard, Roberts, & Ursin, 1999). The second factor that may hamper optimal performance is interference by the antiepileptic medication; this, in turn, depends on dosage and tolerance of the drug, and the type of activity in which the athlete is involved.

Empirical Data—
Is It Really Dangerous?

The general recommendations regarding physical exercise and sport for individuals with epilepsy have changed substantially since the 1960s. In 1960, Lennox maintained that activity worked as an inhibitor for seizures, but in 1976, the American Medical Association Committee on the Medical Aspects of Sports stated that patients with intractable seizures should be excluded from a number of different sports. This view was highly criticized (Livingstone et al., 1978), and the recommendations were later revised. Today, there seems to be a general agreement in the literature that the recommendations regarding physical exercise for patients with epilepsy are too restrictive (Eriksen et al, 1994; Gates & Spiegel, 1993; van Linschoten et al., 1990). The former Swedish ski jumper Jan Boklöv became well known for his performance in the World Cup and his development of a new ski jumping technique (the "V" style), and for having epilepsy. However, for most individuals with epilepsy, activities like ski jumping, skydiving, or rock climbing are not recommended because of the fatal consequences even small or subclinical seizures may have (American Academy of Pediatrics, 1983; Spack, 1984).

The American Academy of Pediatrics (1983) stated that satisfactory seizure control and adequate counseling are important for children participating in physical activities involving risk of damage. It is now generally accepted that persons with frequent seizures, causing falling and damage, should be restricted in their activities (Cordova, 1993; Gates, 1991). Some authors do, however, contradict even this point of view, with possible exceptions regarding diving and climbing (Mendell, 1984). Greensher (1985) stated that the risk of drowning is four times higher in children with epilepsy, as compared to that of other children. Nonetheless, professional athletes with a history of epilepsy are engaged in the above sports without evidence of undesirable consequences.

The Barriers and How
to Overcome Them

Even if there seems to be a general agreement that individuals with epilepsy should live active lives and participate in sport and physical exercise (Eriksen et al. 1994; Gates & Spiegel, 1993; Nakken, Bjørholt, et al., 1990; Nakken & Kornstad, 1998; Nakken, Løyning, Løying, Gløersen, & Larsson, 1997), this is still far from being implemented in real life. Thus, Hanai (1996) reported that only 55% of the teachers and 60% of families of children with epilepsy responded positively to the statement "For participation in physical education and school events, if seizures can be controlled, children should participate in all activities under individual considerations" (p. 29). The response "regardless of whether seizures are controlled, children should participate in all activities under individual considerations" was given by more families than teachers, and this response was more frequent among teachers in schools for children with disabilities and for families with children in schools for students with disabilities.

It seems obvious that individuals who have experienced seizures while exercising would be more reluctant to exercise than would individuals who have not experienced seizures. Satisfactory implementation of our present knowledge requires a realistic approach to how patients with epilepsy can cope with an active lifestyle. The challenges should be identified and met. One important obstacle for obtaining an active lifestyle for patients with epilepsy is the lack of qualified supervisory personnel. Both active and inactive individuals with epilepsy report barriers to exercise. In a study by Roth, Goode, Williams, and Faught (1994), 38 % of the inactive and

18% of the active individuals reported fear of embarrassment caused by seizures while exercising. Further, 37% of the inactive and 21% of the active had no one to exercise with, and 34% of the inactive and 15% of the active were uncertain about how to begin or proceed an exercise program. Roth et al. (1994) reported that the inactive individuals had more fear and barriers related to epilepsy than the active individuals had. Inactive individuals were also more likely to have experienced seizures while exercising. However, the cause-effect relationships could not be determined in this study. The barriers may be overcome or at least reduced through supervision by qualified personnel. Thus, exercise for patients with intractable epilepsy seems to require support and supervision from, for example, physical therapists (Eriksen et al., 1994).

Recommendations

Before any advice is given regarding type of exercise, the type and frequency of seizures and the effects of and compliance with therapy should be considered for each patient. The advice given should be related to the risk of having seizures during exercise and the consequences of potential seizures for the particular sport discipline in question. The advice should also be directed toward the general effects of exercise and the general effects on seizure incidence, which, in general, are favorable. Other types of "fits" must also be excluded, for instance, bradycardia with vasovagal syncope, cardiogenic syncope, psychogenic seizures, panic attacks with hyperventilation, and migraine equivalents (Cordova, 1993).

There are certain types of sport that most patients with epilepsy should avoid or at least consider very carefully before becoming engaged. These are flying and parachuting, motor racing, mountain and rock climbing, high diving, scuba diving, underwater swimming, hang gliding, and abseiling. Cordova

(1993) considers these as absolute contraindications. He also considers the following sports as relative contraindications: aiming sports such as archery and shooting, contact sports (e.g., boxing), competitive cycling for children with absence epilepsy, swimming, and some aspects of gymnastics (e.g., trampoline). Being an Australian, he also warns against skiing and ice skating, but these restrictions would, for instance, be hard for the Nordic population to accept. Finally, he also warns against soccer where heading the ball is involved, as well as rugby and football. However, this may be an exaggerated precaution, when the data on concussive convulsions (McCrory, Bladin, & Berkovic, 1997) are considered.

Concussive convulsions occurring within seconds of an impact to the head have been widely assumed to represent a type of posttraumatic epileptic seizure. However, McCrory et al. (1997) questioned the classification of these convulsions as epilepsy. Their study was based on 22 Australian football players having experienced such attacks after minor head traumas. Their conclusion was that these attacks were benign, that recovery was quick, and that no subjects developed epilepsy. Jennett (1975) observed that seizures confined to the time of the head injury are not associated with subsequent epilepsy.

Conclusion

In general, epilepsy is not a contraindication of exercise. There is evidence suggesting the contrary as most individuals, individuals with epilepsy included, will benefit from physical exercise and sport activities. There is, however, a need for larger and better controlled studies than those available to date, studies in which the potential effects of exercise should be more closely investigated, depending on type of seizure and a number of other relevant factors. Satisfactory seizure control and adequate counseling are important for both children and adults participating in physical activities that involve risk of damage. It is generally accepted that persons with frequent seizures, causing falling and damage, should be restricted in their activities although some authors argue against this point of view, with possible exceptions regarding diving and climbing (Mendell, 1984). The consensus from recent reviews is that both the child and the adult with epilepsy should be encouraged and supported to engage in physical exercise. This is a way to break out of isolation and inactivity and to obtain the physiological and psychological advantages gained from exercise. Even if the activity itself may provoke seizures in certain persons, either during the exercise or after, the general effect on the seizure threshold appears to be favorable.

References

Aird, R. B. (1983). The importance of seizure inducing factors in the control of refractory forms of epilepsy. *Epilepsia*, 24, 567–583.

American Medical Association Committee on Medical Aspects of Sports of the American Medical Association. (1976). *Medical evaluation of the athlete: A guide*. Washington, DC: American Medical Association.

American Academy of Pediatrics. Committee on Children with Handicaps and Committee on Sports Medicine. (1983). Sports and the child with epilepsy. *Pediatrics*, 72(6), 884–885.

Andersen, S. A., Haaland, A., Hjermann, I., Urdal, P., Gjesdal, K., & Holme, I. (1995). Oslo diet and exercise study: A one year randomized intervention trial; effect on hemostatic variables and other coronary risk factors. *Nutrition, Metabolism and Cardiovascular Diseases*, 5, 189–200.

Berney, T. P., Osselton, J. W., Kolvin, I., & Day, M. J. (1981). Effects of discotheque environment on epileptic children. *British Medical Journal*, 282, 180–182.

Biering Sorensen, F., Bendix, T., Jorgensen, K., Manniche, C., & Nielsen, H. (1994). Physical activity, fitness, and back pain. In C. Bouchard, R. J. Shephard, & T. Stephens (Eds.), *Physical activity, fitness, and health: International proceedings and consensus statement* (pp. 737–748). Champaign, IL: Human Kinetics Publishers.

Bjørholt, P. G., Nakken, K. O., Roehme, K., & Hansen, H. (1990). Leisure time habits and physical fitness in adults with epilepsy. *Epilepsia*, 31, 83–87.

Cordova, F. (1993). Epilepsy and sport. *Australian Family Physician*, 22(4), 558–562.

Ellertsen, B., Eriksen, H. R., Mostofsky, D. I., & Ursin, H. (1993). Exercise and epilepsy. In D. I. Mostofsky & Y. Løyning (Eds.), *The neurobehavioral treatment of epilepsy* (pp. 107–122). Hillsdale: Lawrence Erlbaum Associates.

Eriksen, H. R., Ellertsen, B., Gronningsaeter, H., Nakken, K. O., Loyning, Y., & Ursin, H. (1994). Physical exercise in women with intractable epilepsy. *Epilepsia*, 35(6), 1256–1264.

Esquivel, E., Chaussain, M., Plouin, P., Ponsot, G., & Arthuis, M. (1991). Physical exercise and voluntary hyperventilation in childhood absence epilepsy. *Electroencephalography and Clinical Neurophysiology*, 79(2), 127–132.

Ettinger, A. B., Weisbrot, D. M., Nolan, E. E., Gadow, K. D., Vitale, S. A., Andriola, M. R. Lenn, N. I., Novak, G. P., & Hermann, B. P. (1998). Symptoms of depression and anxiety in pediatric epilepsy patients. *Epilepsia*, 39(6), 595–599.

Freeman, J. M. (1985). Epilepsy and swimming [Letter to the editor]. *Pediatrics*, 76(1), 139.

Gates, J. R. (1991). Epilepsy and sports participation. *The Physician and Sports Medicine*, 19(3), 98–104.

Gates, J. R., & Spiegel, R. H. (1993). Epilepsy, sports and exercise. *Sports Medicine*, 15(1), 1–5.

Gordon, N. (1994). The long Q-T syndromes. *Brain and Development*, 16(2), 153–155.

Greensher, J. (1985). Epilepsy and swimming [letter to the editor]. *Pediatrics*, 76(1), 139.

Götze, W., Kubicki, S., Munter, M., & Teichman, J. (1967). Effect of physical exercise on seizure threshold. *Diseases of the Nervous System*, 28(10), 664–667.

Hanai, T. (1996). Quality of life in children with epilepsy. *Epilepsia*, 37 (Suppl. 3), 28–32.

Horyd, W., Gryziak, J., Niedzielska, K., & Zielinski, J. J. (1981). Exercise effect on seizure discharges in epileptics. *Neurologia I Neurochirurgia Polska*, 5–6, 545–552.

Jennett, B. (1975). *Epilepsy after non missile head injuries* (2nd ed.). London: Heineman.

Korczyn, A. D. (1979). Participation of epileptics in sports. *Journal of Sports Medicine*, 19, 195–198.

Kuijer, A. (1978). *Epilepsy and exercise—an investigation into some physiological effects of exercise in people with epilepsy: Electroencephalographic and biochemical studies*. Academisch proefschrift, Universiteit van Amsterdam.

Lennox, W. G. (1960). *Epilepsy and related disorders*. London: J. & A. Churchill LTD.

Lesser, R. (1996). Psychogenic seizures. *Neurology*, 46, 1499–1507.

Levine, S., & Ursin, H. (1991). What is stress? In M. R. Brown, G. F. Koob, & C. Rivier (Eds.), *Stress, neurobiology and neuroendocrinology*. (pp. 3–21). New York: Marcel Dekker Inc.

van Linschoten, R., Back, F. J. G., Mulder, O. G. M., &

Meinardi, H. (1990). Epilepsy and sport [Review article]. *Sports Medicine, 10*(1), 9–19.

Livingstone, S. (1971). Should physical activity of the epileptic child be restricted? *Clinical Pediatrics, 10*(12), 694–696.

Livingstone, S., Pauli, L., & Pruce, I. (1978, January). Epilepsy and sports [Letter to the editor]. *Journal of American Medical Association, 239*(1), 22.

Martinsen, E. W., Hofart, A., & Solberg, Ø. (1989). Aerobic and non-aerobic forms of exercise in the treatment of anxiety disorders. *Stress Medicine, 5*, 115–120.

Martinsen, E. W., Medus, A., & Sandvik, L. (1985). Effects of aerobic exercise on depression: A controlled study. *British Medical Journal, 291*, 109.

Martinsen, E. W., Strand, J., Paulsson, G., & Kaggestad, J. (1989). Physical fitness level in patients with anxiety and depressive disorders. *International Journal of Sports Medicine, 10*, 58–61.

McCrory, P. R., Bladin, P. F., & Berkovic, S. F. (1997). Retrospective study of concussive convulsions in elite Australian rules and rugby league footballers: Phenomenology, aetiology, and outcome. *British Medical Journal, 314*, 171–174.

Mendell, J. R. (1984). The nervous system. In R. H. Strauss & W. B. Saunders (Eds.), *Sports medicine* (pp. 149–174). Philadelphia: Saunders.

Morgan, W. P., & Goldstone, S. E. (1987). *Exercise and mental health*. Washington, DC: Hemisphere.

Nakken, K. O., Bjørholt, P. G., Johannessen, S. I., Løyning, T., & Lind, E. (1990). Effect on physical training on aerobic capacity, seizure occurrence, and serum level on antiepileptic drugs in adults with epilepsy. *Epilepsia, 31*, 88–94.

Nakken, K. O., & Kornstad, S. (1998). Do males 30–50 years of age with chronic epilepsy and on long-term anticonvulsant medication have lower-than-expected risk of developing coronary heart disease? *Epilepsia, 39*(3), 326–330.

Nakken, K. O., Løyning, A., Løying, T., Gløersen, G., & Larsson, P. G. (1997). Does physical exercise influence the occurrence of epileptiform EEG discharges in children? *Epilepsia, 38*(3), 279–284.

Ogunyemi, A. O., Gomez, M. R., & Klass, D. W. (1988). Seizures induced by exercise. *Neurology, 38*, 633–634.

Pensgaard, A. M., Roberts, G. C., & Ursin, H. (1999). Motivational factors and coping strategies of Norwegian Paralympic and Olympic winter sport athletes. *Adapted Physical Activity Quarterly.*

Roth, D. L., Goode, K. T., Williams, V. L., & Faught, E. (1994). Physical exercise, stressful life experience, and depression in adults with epilepsy. *Epilepsia, 35*(6), 1248–1255.

Rugland, A. L. (1990). "Subclinical" epileptogenic activity. In M. Sillanpaa, S. I., Johannessen, G. Blennow, & M. Dam (Eds.). *Pediatric epilepsy* (pp. 217–224). Petersfild: Wrightson Biomedical Publ. Ltd.

Sander, J. W. A. S., & O'Donoghue, M. F. (1997). Epilepsy: Getting the diagnosis right. *British Medical Journal, 314*, 158.

Schmitt, B., Thun Hohenstein, L., Vontobel, H., & Boltshauser, E. (1994). Seizures induced by physical exercise: Report of two cases. *Neuropediatrics, 25*(1), 51–53.

Spack, N. P. (1984). Medical problem of exercising child: Asthma, diabetes, and epilepsy. In L. J. Micheli (Ed.), *Pediatric and adolescent sports medicine* (pp. 124–133). Boston: Little, Brown.

Stephens, T., & Caspersen, C. J. (1994). The demography of physical activity. In C. Bouchard, R. J. Shephard, & T. Stephens (Eds.), *Physical activity, fitness, and health: International proceedings and consensus statement* (pp. 204–213). Champaign, IL: Human Kinetics Publishers.

Steptoe, A., Edwards, S., Moses, J., & Mathews, A. (1989). The effects of exercise training on mood and perceived coping ability in anxious adults from the general population. *Journal of Psychosomatic Research, 5*, 537–547.

Ursin, H. (1988). Expectancy and activation: An attempt to systematize stress theory. In D. Hellhammer, I. Florin, & H. Weiner (Eds.), *Neurobiological approaches to human disease* (pp. 313–334). Toronto: Hans Huber.

Ursin, H. (1998). The psychology in psychoneuroendocrinology. *Psychoneuroendocrinology, 23*(6), 555–570.

Williams, V. L., Roth, D. L., & Ruiz, L. L. (1991, August). *Barriers to exercise in adults with epilepsy*. Poster session presented at the annual meeting of the American Psychological Association, San Francisco.

13
Physical Exercise in Pain Management

C. Zvi Fuchs

Kim Larsson

Leonard D. Zaichkowsky

It is well established that exercise and physical fitness play an important role in the maintenance and promotion of health. In addition, it seems that many health-related benefits are associated with physical activity. Exercise may attenuate the progression of and aid in the recovery from various cardiovascular disorders, as well as neurological and musculoskeletal diseases, most of which are associated with acute or chronic pain symptoms. These well-established clinical observations are supported by a substantial body of research. Indeed, the Centers for Disease Control and Prevention and the American College of Sports Medicine recently provide the following guidelines for exercise. They state that "every U.S. adult should accumulate 30 minutes or more of moderate intensity physical activity on most, preferably all, days of the week" (Pate et al., 1995, p. xx). These guidelines continue to specify that this activity can be of any sport, fitness, or recreational activity that resembles the intensity of walking two miles briskly per day. The activity can be continuous or intermittent and supervised if needed.

Ironically, most of the population, and especially patients who suffer from pain as part of their presenting symptomatology, associate an exercise program with the induction, rather than the elimination, of pain. It is no wonder that out of an average of 25% of the American population who exercise on a regular basis (Deuster, 1996), only about 4% exercise sufficiently to have a positive influence on chronic pain (Linchitz, 1987). It is common that even healthy nonexercisers who start an exercise program may experience an acute short-term pain, due to the increased accumulation of lactic acid in the blood and the exercised muscles. However, this short-term pain usually dissipates within one hour or less (Cailliet, 1995; Fox, 1979). A more common pain associated with the beginning of exercise, in nonexercisers, appears somewhat later and lasts usually between 24 and 72 hours after exercising. It is termed *delayed onset muscle soreness* (DOMS) and is perceived as a sensation of discomfort and soreness in the exercising muscle(s). This pain is most commonly felt after eccentric exercise (elongation of muscles while resisting increased weight) and is attributed to complex normal metabolic and micro injuries to the muscle tendon junction and the muscle cell connections (MacIntyre, Reid, & McKenzie, 1995). In some cases, when the postexercise pain continues longer than 72 hours, medical advice is essential because the pain may indicate an aggravation of a previously existing condition, such as inflammatory myopathies, metabolic irregularities, ischemic diseases, or a new injury (Bove, 1983).

Because the health benefits of exercising override the potential for increased pain and injury, it seems logical to incorporate an exercise regimen in any rehabilitation program. As a matter of fact, more than 20 years ago Fordyce (1976) noted that when exercise is the center of a behavioral pain-management program, exercise facilitates the decrease in pain behaviors and simultaneously builds a maintenance pattern for health-promoting behaviors after treatment. As clinicians, however, we often notice that pain patients' compliance and avoidance of exercise are firmly established across a range of pathologies. The fear of extended or newly evoked pain is evident despite emerging evidence that the increased release of endorphins during prolonged rhythmic exercise has the property of decreasing pain and depression (Lobstein, Rasmussen, Dunphy, & Dunphy, 1989; Thorén, Floras, Hoffman, & Seals, 1990). The fear of therapeutic exercise as a pain stimulator is often not even relieved by the therapist's reassurance, explanations, slow and gradual progression, and substitution of exercise regimens (Huyser, Buckeley, Hewett, & Johnson, 1997). Adherence to an exercise program is also a major problem, mainly because of the fear of increasing the pain.

This chapter attempts to summarize the clinical research findings concerning physical activities and regimented exercise routines in selective clinical pain syndromes,

which include chronic low back pain (CLBP), pain in the upper and lower extremities, arthritis, headaches, and fibromyalgia. Those are conditions and diseases that include pain as a prominent presentation in their symptomatology, diagnosis, and treatment. We will also attempt to discuss practical recommendations for implementing exercise programs as an integral component in a multidisciplinary pain-management approach. It is our belief that this knowledge will serve to promote health and especially to decrease pain that is associated with these major painful conditions and diseases.

Low Back Pain

Low back pain (LBP) is one of the leading reasons for visits to physicians, hospitalization, and disability. Statistically between 60 and 80% of the population in the industrialized nations suffer from LBP at some time or another. The pain may be acute, subacute, or chronic. Each year, about 5% of adult Americans experience an episode of LBP. About 5 million cases will be inflicted with partial disability, and about 2 million will remain totally disabled. These conditions have an estimated $25–50 billion impact on the U.S. economy annually (Cailliet, 1995; Carey et al., 1995; Deyo, 1998).

Acute LBP (ALBP) lasts from a few days up to about 6 weeks, and it seems that the mainstay of treatment is rest, gradual limited physical activities, and pharmacological therapy that consists usually of analgesics and, most often, mild antianxiety drugs. Narcotics are used rarely and when used, only for a very short time (National Institutes of Health [NIH], 1986). More active therapies, like exercise, for ALBP will be discussed later in details. Subacute pain lasts up to 3 months. It is usually treated by the same medications as ALBP and gradual return to normal activity. Pain is termed chronic if it persists for 3 to 6 months and longer. Chronicity is established not only as a function of time, but especially after various interventions have failed totally or have brought only minor pain relief. As a matter of fact, chronic low back pain (CLBP), with or without organic causes or objective findings (e.g., X-rays, CT, MRI, significant neurological deficits), is usually combined with insomnia, depression, and sometimes anxiety that is probably due to an avoidance response associated with fear of increased pain (McCracken, Zayfert, & Gross, 1992; Murphy, Lindsay, & Williams, 1997). Rest is an old remedy that is still used sometimes even today. However, exercise seems to be a major therapy modality. Drug therapy is usually limited to nonsteroidal anti-inflammatory drugs (NSAID), tricyclics, and antidepressants. Narcotics have a limited use, because the fear of developing tolerance and addiction is a major concern (NIH). Also, most clinicians seem to believe that in the majority of CLBP sufferers, the magnitude of the pain behaviors is disproportional to the initial injury or that "It's all in your head." This attitude implies that the pain complaints are exaggerated or even manufactured by the patient who is one who somatizes, maligns, or is being influenced by some secondary gains and/or by stress and tension that sustain the chronic pain (Sarno, 1998).

For many decades and for most patients and clinicians, it seemed intuitively right that exercise was the major, or even the only, conservative modality in the treatment and management of LBP. Some patients traced the onset of the pain to an abrupt or an extreme movement involving the back while lifting or doing other strenuous activity. This approach partially influenced the notion that what was caused by movement can be cured by exercise. The physical deconditioning of most of these patients is also "proof" that deconditioning might not be the result of CLBP but the cause for it. It seemed logical that ex-

ercise that strengthens the musculature around the spine, not only can reduce existing LBP, but also prevent or delay the onset or reoccurrence of another episode of pain. Indeed, numerous studies that involve exercise regimens are based directly or indirectly on the assumption that exercise can increase the preventative potential for the onset of LBP by helping to stabilize, strengthen, and improve the trunk's musculature capabilities of a deconditioned and/or painful back (De-Michele et al., 1997; Manniche, Hesselsøe, Bentzen, Christensen, & Lundberg, 1988; McGill, 1997; Nelson et al., 1995; Rainville, Sobel, Hartigan, Monlux, & Bean, 1997; Shields & Givens Heiss, 1997; Smidt, Blanpied, & White, 1989).

The exercise regimens are many and variable. We will only review samples of representative exercise regimens. For example, a popular book, *Backache: When Exercise Works*, by Sobel and Klein (1994) for home exercises, includes stretching, strengthening, and aerobic activities and is a good resource. This book can be used by the patient as a guide for prevention or maintenance. Its greatest asset is the clear and simple text and the illustrations of the exercises. However, for better clinical understanding of the role of physical medicine modalities, Soric (1989) and Revel (1995) briefly but precisely describe many exercise modalities. Passive modalities such as rest, therapeutic heat, and cold applications are discussed as well as active modalities such as William's flexion exercises, which supposedly relieve compression of the nerve root, or David's flexion method to increase intra-abdominal pressure in order to strengthen the abdominal muscles and decrease mechanical stress on the lumbar spine. McKenzie's most popular extension routine is explained as an effort to shift the nucleus pulposus array from the spinal nerve. Other proponents of extension regimens emphasize that extension exercises are essential to decreasing the axial compression on the spine. Soric also advocates aerobic exercise, such as walking, jogging, and swimming, especially for pain reduction. It seems that increasing the central release of beta endorphins to the peripheral circulation plays an important role in the modification of pain (Lobstein et al., 1989; Thorén et al., 1990). Soric also reviews postural adjustment exercises, mobilization, traction, manipulation, and other physical techniques. Another short but excellent source for back-to-work activities and exercises in LBP rehabilitation can be found in a paper by Hartigan, Miller, and Liewehr (1996).

For a good review of the "back school" in the management of LBP, we recommend Hall's (1989) chapter on the subject. Hall traces the origin of the back school to the early 1970s in Sweden. He emphasizes that the original intention was educational ergonomics, promotion of confidence in the back's natural ability for recovery, and encouragement to increase the level of physical activity. Only later on were specific back exercises that are usually an extension of physical therapy and low-impact aerobic exercises included in some back schools. This comprehensive approach is also recommended favorably by Nordin (1996), who summarized the findings of the Geneva (Switzerland) Conference on LBP patients' education.

Finally, chiropractic management of LBP is the most ambivalent exercise approach in the medical community, but increasingly popular with patients (Carey et al., 1995; Eisenberg et al., 1993). Burns and Mierau (1997) comprehensively describe chiropractic exercise interventions. They distinguish clearly between mobilization and manipulation exercises. Mobilization is usually gentle, oscillatory, high-amplitude, low-velocity maneuvers for stretching. Manipulation, on the other hand, is a quick, forceful, but controlled, thrust of the spine. Manipulation carries the

joint slightly beyond its normal physiological range of motion and usually results in a cracking noise that is associated with pain relief. The spectrum of chiropractic exercises, which are also used by osteopaths and some physical therapists, includes lumbar flexion rather than extension exercise and is usually followed by an exercise program to be executed by the patient at home (Shekelle, Adams, Chassin, Hurwitz, & Brook, 1992).

It is clear that most researchers and clinicians agree that LBP is a result of complex interactions among biological processes, mechanical malfunction of the spinal structures and supportive areas, emotional, behavioral, socioeconomic, and litigation status. It seems that also responses and reinforcement to the pain dynamics play a major role (Blake & Garrett, 1997; Fordyce, 1976; Sollner & Doering, 1997). It is, therefore, no wonder that most of the therapeutic interventions today apply multidisciplinary approaches to LBP rehabilitation (Altmaier, Lehmann, Russell, Weinstein, & Kao, 1992; Flavell, Carrafa, Thomas, & Disler, 1996; Gottleib et al., 1977; Nicholas, Wilson, & Goyen, 1992; Turner, Clancy, McQuade, & Cardenas, 1990).

In this section, we accept that all of the interventions are multidisciplinary, unless otherwise specified. However, despite the difficulty of sorting out the exact role of exercise in such regimens, we will try to review only studies with exercise as a dominant component. Last and most important, due to the large number of studies that involve exercise as a tool in LBP management, we will include only comprehensive review papers on the subject. Indeed, many review papers employ various prescreening procedures as criteria for inclusion and conclusions. This is a major factor in our decision to employ the review papers. Many individual papers were criticized for methodological flaws such as inadequate control groups, vague description, and/or insufficient standardization of the exercise intervention regimens (Koes, Bouter, & van der Heijden, 1995), as well as specific problems with design, execution, data analysis methods, and conclusion reporting (Van Tolder, Koes, & Bouter, 1997). We believe that we can extract a clear picture from these extensive reviews despite the apparent imperfection of their input. We will also make a major effort to give clear guidelines based on universal conclusions drawn from these review studies. However, the final part will also include several model individual studies in order to support or dispute some conclusions by the review studies.

In the early 1990s, the first serious attempt to evaluate the cumulative results of physiotherapy exercise for LBP in the previous 24 years (1966–1990) was made by Koes, Bouter, Beckerman, van der Heizden, and Knipschild (1991). Using a computer search (MEDLINE), they screened 23 randomized controlled studies. In a blind review, they scored the quality of the studies according to these categories: (a) study population, (b) the intervention, (c) measurement of effect, (d) data presentation, (e) statistical analysis, and (f) the main conclusions of the studies' author(s). Only 4 studies out of the original 23 scored over 50 points (out of 100). The other 19 studies were included but considered of inferior quality. Koes and his coauthors (1991) concluded that "no conclusion can be drawn about whether exercise therapy is better than other conservative treatments for back pain or whether a specific type of exercise is more effective" (p. 1572).

Using the same database and screening method, Faas (1996) continued where Koes et al. left off in 1991. Faas also divided the studies into acute, subacute, and chronic pain. In the period from 1991 to 1995, he identified and included only 11 studies for his review. Faas found that exercise therapy was ineffective in acute pain. In subacute pain, some exercise with a gradually increased ac-

tivity program seemed to be promising. However, in chronic pain, intensive exercise programs seemed to have the most promising results, but even these results disappeared after one year. No specific exercise program seemed to be superior, but he noted that McKenzie's method seemed to deserve more attention as a promising leading exercise method. Considering the small sample, this study can only be suggestive in two directions. First, it makes clear that active physical therapy exercises are contraindicated in acute pain. Second, intensive exercises are beneficial in chronic pain, but they have no lasting effect if the patient stops exercising after the therapy ends.

Lahad, Malter, Berg, and Deyo (1994) presented another MEDLINE review study that covers 27 years (1966–1993) and reviews 190 papers. Only 64 studies that contained primary data about clear methods for treatment of LBP were further critically reviewed, and of those, only 16 were primarily exercise studies. Besides using randomized studies only, the criteria for inclusion were very unimpressive for a review paper. For example, some reviewed studies included patients with or without prior back pain as one population. Lahad et al.'s conclusion is that various trunk-muscle exercises, including aerobic exercise, seem to be mildly protective against LBP and are associated with decreased frequency and duration of LBP when it happens. The use of asymptomatic subjects in these studies strengthens the first conclusion. However, poor selection criteria, the lack of a strong recommendation for exercise as a preventive measure, and the fact that the papers reviewed were primarily not clinical but studies conducted in the workplace makes these almost obvious conclusions merely superficial.

Scheer, Radack, and O'Brien (1995) attempted a more selective review. They reviewed 10 well-selected papers from 1975 to 1993 for their analysis and conclusions of industrial ALBP. The selection process started with 4,000 papers, of which only 35 met their methodological rigor of randomization, control, and outcome on a 26-point system for quality. They decided to concentrate on only 10 of these papers that included various exercise interventions. The interventions included spinal flexion, extension, isometric strengthening of the trunk musculature, aerobic exercise, pool exercise, stretching, manipulation, stabilization, posture improvement, and other active physical methods. Despite the array of exercise methods used, their conclusions seem to be extremely strong and unequivocal. First, short bed rest and no exercise are recommended for ALBP. Second, a generalized fitness program is highly recommended for long-term prevention. Third, Back School and spinal manipulation need more and better research in order to establish their efficacy in ALBP therapy. Surprisingly, in a continuation of this investigation, 2 years later, Scheer, Watanabe, and Radack (1997) could not find any acceptable studies to support clearly the use of exercise in subacute and CLBP.

Other review studies that examine the role of exercise intervention in ALBP demonstrate major methodological and decision-making flaws. However, their conclusions seem to be mostly in line with the previous reviews. Twomey and Taylor (1995), who used nonspecific criteria for the selection of the reviewed studies, found that passive manipulation and mobilization are extremely useful in speeding the recovery of ALBP episodes. However, the controls for spontaneous recovery were insufficient. Spontaneous recovery and not passive manipulation/mobilization exercise could probably be the main factor in these self-limiting episodes. Twomey and Taylor also conclude, without sufficient evidence for a review paper, that exercise and especially vigorous exercise programs have good to excellent outcome in

CLBP. Wheeler and Hanley (1995) and Wheeler (1995), in a similar general nondiscriminative review, concluded against active exercise in the acute phase. In the subacute and CLBP, gradually executed exercise against increased resistance was recommended. As for prevention, a multidisciplinary approach of general fitness (aerobic and anaerobic), as well as psychosocial intervention, seems to be supported in these two reviews. In a seemingly contrasting review, Mälkiä and Ljunggren (1996) concluded that exercise rehabilitation alone has a positive effect on the physical disability. However, exercise alone, which excludes a multidisciplinary approach, has no carryover to social and occupational activities.

Two parallel excellent reviews by Manniche (1995, 1996), based on his group work in Denmark, are interesting primarily for two reasons: the inclusion of some Scandinavian studies that do not always find their way to the dominant mainstream English language journals and the concentration on exercise as a treatment modality in pre- and postoperative disc patients. In his extensive description of a series of six studies that include a total of 555 CLBP patients, before and after disc surgery, Manniche (1995, 1996) showed that these subacute and CLBP patients can tolerate and benefit from back-to-work rehabilitation programs that included mainly high-intensity exercises with virtually no side effects. His studies are supported by some other lumbar disc/herniation studies that show similar beneficial effects of extensive exercise regimens even with post-surgery patients who still suffer from CLBP, sciatica, functional daily disabilities, and severe work limitations (Manniche, 1995, 1996; Saal, 1996). In contrast, a Canadian review (Teasell & Harth, 1996) of functional restoration programs that also included aggressive physical exercises showed similar results to nonexercise programs in the rate of returning to work. They criticized all but one study for serious methodological flaws and biases, and even this properly randomized trial with adequate controls failed to show any significant difference between the exercise group in returning to work as compared to controls (79% vs.78%). It is important to remember that the main goal of this review is very narrow, namely return to work.

Other review studies that evaluated exercise programs seem to help to settle the dispute over the cost-effectiveness of exercise in LBP rehabilitation in the workplace. Karas, Cohn, and Conrad (1996) used strict inclusion criteria for their review of LBP studies from 1987 to 1994. After choosing only 15 studies, they concluded that despite major methodological problems, exercise/flexibility programs and back school programs that include exercise demonstrate better outcomes than those of either immobilization (back belts) or educational classes alone. In an English publication that also included studies conducted in France, Revel (1995) reviewed physical therapy approaches to the treatment of LBP. His review selected only 30 studies, which met widely accepted validity and applicability criteria. Revel's conclusion was that most back-school programs, which excluded intensive exercise regimens or did not include any exercise, were unsuccessful. Even spinal flexion/extension exercise showed only short-term positive effects, regardless of the method used by the physical therapist. However, functional restoration programs that were based on graded exercise seemed to yield long-term physical and psychosocial benefits.

In another review, Campello, Nordin, and Weiser (1996) shared the same frustration concerning poor design/methodology of the LBP studies and the lack of precise reporting of the exercise method(s) used, their intensity, frequency, and duration. These flaws made it hard for them to decipher the unique contribution of exercise as compared to other therapies in LBP. However, their reviewed literature showed clearly that rest and inactivity are instrumental in deconditioning, leading to delay in return to normal activity and a host of other negative psychophysiological problems in LBP patients. Their logical conclusion is that physical reconditioning via exercise is probably the most effective management tool in subacute and CLBP.

It seems that with regard to ALBP and exercise therapy, the review findings are extremely clear. Short bed rest of 2–3 days, followed by continuing regular activities within the limits permitted by the pain (Malmivaara et al., 1995) and/or gentle passive manipulation, as practiced usually by osteopathic physicians, chiropractors, and some physical therapists, is probably the best approach to ALBP (Bronfort, Goldsmith, Nelson, Boline, & Anderson, 1996; Daniels, 1997; Shekelle et al., 1992). However, manipulation usually administered by chiropractors is the most expensive modality in ALBP intervention (Carey et al., 1995; Shekelle, Markovich, & Louie, 1995), and their outcomes are similar, or even inferior, to those of less costly interventions by primary care physicians, general practitioners, or a 15-minute educational session with a clinic nurse (Cherkin, Deyon, Street, Hunt, & Barlow, 1996; Deyo & Phillips, 1996, Faas et al., 1995). Again, these findings suggest strongly that no specific professional exercise intervention can modify the natural self-limiting history of ALBP.

Indeed, there is a unanimous agreement among most review studies that exercise has no value in most acute phases of LBP (Fass, 1996; Scheer et al., 1995; van Tulder, Koes, & Bouter, 1997; Wheeler 1995; Wheeler & Hanley, 1995). As a matter of fact, it seems that exercise at the acute phase may actually interfere with the recovery of the lumbar multifidus muscle and lead to a poor outcome and recurrence rate of symptoms (Hides, Richardson, & Jull, 1996), probably via the interference with the desirable increased collagen synthesis at the acute, but not chronic, phase (Hupli et al., 1997).

It is also quite clear from almost all of the studies and extensive reviews that, in CLBP, exercise programs are definitely beneficial, regardless of the regimen or mixture of exercise regimens. These universal agreements yield an array of very aggressive exercise interventions for therapy and preventions. Manniche, Lundberg, Christensen, Bentzen, and Hesselsøe (1991) studied the short-term effect of intensive dynamic back exercise on CLBP patients and, after 3 months, concluded that the higher the intensity the better are the results. However, this study excluded patients with lumbar nerve root compression and radiological signs of spondylolysis or halisteresis of the spine. More recently, Ljunggren, Weber, Kogstad, Thom, and Kirkesola (1997) completed a one-year exercise in which a home body weight resistance exercise instrument (TerapiMaster) was used successfully as measured by 75 to 80% less absenteeism at work. Another study (Bensen, Lindgärde, & Manthorpe, 1997) completed a 3-year followup study of a minimally supervised high-intensity rehabilitation of exercise for CLBP patients in a fitness center (gym). They reported good results and no side effects. Finally, Rainville et al. (1997) demonstrated successful results, with no risk, in a selected group of CLBP patients who went through an aggressive spine rehabilitation program including trunk strengthening against increased resistance (Cybex). It seems that current studies involve successfully more and more high resistance, intensity. and duration exercise with no regard to the pathophysiology of the CLBP and with minimal professional supervision. Based on these previous experiences in the United States and Scandinavia, the Labor Ministry of Japan issued mandatory guidelines for specific exercises before work at the workplace as a prevention measure against LBP (Yamamoto, 1997).

Even though an optional regimen(s) of exercises in CLBP is yet to be identified and will probably vary from patient to patient (Mälkiä & Kannus, 1996), extension exercises to strengthen the paravertebral musculature, isometric exercises to strengthen the abdominals, and stretching exercises for overall trunk flexibility, together with a general aerobic fitness program, seem to be essential in the therapy and prevention of recurrence episodes of CLBP (Sullivan, Kues, & Mayhew, 1996). The insufficient evidence to prefer one type of exercise over another could indicate that combination, individualization, and alternation of regimens are probably the best interventions. We hope that therapists, as well as patients, would accept these conclusions as an asset and not as a hindrance, because it enables them a variation and individualization that may increase adherence, which is a major problem in any exercise therapy and maintenance program (Pate et al., 1995). After the review of such strong and universal evidence for the inclusion of a comprehensive exercise program for CLBP, it is disappointing that a national survey of 1,200 physicians in the United States (U.S.) showed that many of them still continue to prescribe narcotics and bed rest for CLBP (Cherkin, Deyo, Wheeler, & Ciol, 1995). This practice is common despite the fact that 80% of the same physicians thought that physical therapy was the only effective treatment modality in CLBP. It seems that in spite of the current data, which suggest that exercise is extremely efficient in CLBP, physicians lack the persistence in conveying and imposing exercise therapy on reluctant and resistant patients.

When we consider all forms of LBP, van Tulder et al. (1997) produced the most updated systematic review of randomized control trials concerning the role of various exercise interventions in acute and chronic nonspecific pain. This excellent, comprehensive, and extremely well-documented study concluded that despite the majority of low-quality studies, a minority of 35% (28 studies) of ALBP and 25% (20 studies) of CLBP are of high quality. Based on these studies, their conclusions are firm. Strong evidence shows that exercise therapy is often contraindicated and definitely is not more effective than other conservative treatments for ALBP. However, in CLBP exercise and programs that include exercise as a major rehabilitation modality are very effective. This is true especially for short-term effects. They also emphasize that these positive effects can be extended and are long lasting for those patients who continue to exercise on their own.

In conclusion, the effectiveness of various exercise routines as a therapy for LBP seems to be clearer. Most review studies and our own reviewed individual, selected representative studies showing that active exercise is not recommended and even may be detrimental at the acute phases of LBP. Bed rest should be limited to 2 to 3 days and generally discouraged, in ALBP, for longer periods. In subacute LBP, gradual increased daily activities and a gradual introduction of a localized and generalized exercise/fitness program are highly recommended. Various active exercise and fitness routines are extremely beneficial in the treatment of CLBP. The modality of the exercise routine is not as important as the gradual increased duration, frequency, and intensity. No serious side effects are associated with such programs when proper precautions are taken. Also, the goal in all life phases, before and after the onset of LBP, is the establishment of a long-term individualized exercise program, which

can be practiced in a nonclinical setting. This lifetime activity is especially essential in the process of reconditioning and prevention of LBP relapse. Finally, only anecdotal indications from research findings could be found concerning the role of exercise regimens on depression, anxiety, and insomnia in LBP. This seems to be an important area to be clarified because CLBP symptomatology almost always includes these adjunct conditions (NIH Technology Assessment Panel, 1996), which also seem to be greatly alleviated by exercise (Fuchs & Zaichkowsky, 1997).

Upper and Lower Extremities

When talking about chronic pain disorders of the upper and lower extremities, it has been traditionally believed that these types of conditions are limited to the limbs of the body.

Repetitive motion injuries such as carpal tunnel syndrome, reflex sympathetic dystrophy syndrome, thoracic outlet syndrome, and chronic exertional compartment syndrome fit into these categories and reflect the more common types of chronic pain conditions of the upper and lower extremities. Even though ulnar nerve and median nerve disorders exist by themselves, these conditions are less common than those formerly mentioned. In addition, low back pain (LBP) has already been discussed in the preceding sections. Therefore this section shall focus on the more common types of chronic pain disorders of the upper and lower extremities, which will include chronic pain disorders of the neck/shoulder region, given that this latter domain is a growing area of research and of clinical complaints (Jordan & Ostergaard, 1996).

Repetitive motion injuries (RMI) are chronic pain conditions that result from the strain of soft tissue that is caused by repetitive actions. In general, these repetitive actions are due to either work-related or leisure activities like word processing or playing an instrument. Researchers find that RMI frequently occur while doing productivity work tasks where the body performs a job in which the body is required to maintain the same position for hours on end. Assembly-line factory workers often fit this profile and are known to report symptoms of a common RMI, namely, carpal tunnel syndrome (CT) (Accerro & Baggs, 1993). Given that CT is reported to be one of the more common types of RMI, CT shall be used as the example for describing the role that exercise plays in managing this type of chronic pain condition ("Repetitive Motion Injuries," 1998).

CT affects approximately 1% of the general population of the United States. Empirical studies estimate that up to 35% of certain types of productivity workers such as shellfish packers will suffer from some type of CT symptoms at some point during their lives (Heller, 1994). In addition, scientists find that women are more likely to work in occupations that require repetitive motions and, therefore, are at greater risk for developing chronic pain conditions like CT (Katz, 1994). CT is caused by pressure on the median nerve where it passes, along with the flexor tendons of the fingers, through the carpal tunnel to the dorsal side of the carpal bones and to the transverse carpal ligament on the volvar aspect (Heller, 1994). Repetitive motions like repeated flexion, pronation, and supination of the wrist, or any repeated position that causes constriction over the wrist and puts pressure on the base of the palm of the hand, can result in disabling conditions like CT.

The classic pain symptom of CT has an expression of deep and achy tooth-like pain that is associated with tingling sensations at night. Other common symptoms of CT include numbness of the palmar surface of the thumb, index, and middle finger. This numbness may also involve the entire hand except for the fifth finger. Sometimes, symptoms of

pain spread into the forearm, or even more rarely, as far as the shoulder and neck regions. Nonetheless, it is quite common that CT will progress from unilateral symptoms presentation to bilateral symptoms presentation (Szabo & Madison, 1992).

Experts now know that reflex sympathetic dystrophy syndrome (RSD) is a neuropathic process and a chronic pain condition that affects the distal portion of the extremities (Acccero & Braggs, 1993; Reflex Sympathetic Dystrophy Syndrome Association of America, 1998).

Even though the exact cause of RSD has yet to be determined, nearly 82% of the RSD cases result from brachial plexus and median nerve injuries in the upper extremity and sciatic and tibial nerve injuries in the lower extremity. Most RSD hand cases are due to blunt-trauma industrial injuries in men and fractured wrists with median nerve damage in women (Acerro & Braggs, 1993). Other forms of RSD may be due to ischemic heart disease, myocardial infarction, cervical spine or spinal cord disorders, or cerebral lesions (Reflex Sympathetic Dystrophy Syndrome Association of America).

RSD is a disabling condition that involves many systems of the body and usually affects more than extremity or part of the body. Pain is the first and primary complaint. Swelling, diminished motor functioning, tremor, skin changes, vasomotor instability, osteoporosis, and joint swelling and tenderness are other symptoms that ensue and tend to manifest throughout the three stages of the RSD disease process. These stages and their accompanying symptoms are as follows:

• Stage I exhibits symptoms of severe and burning pain that is often limited to the site of the injury. Next, symptoms like localized edema, hyperaesthesia, muscle spasms, stiffness, limited mobility, and vasospasms that change the skin from being warm, red, and dry to cold, cyanotic, and sweaty manifest. In general, these symptoms last for 1 to 3 months in duration.

- Stage II symptoms include more severe and diffuse expressions of pain. Localized edema spreads and changes in nature from a soft type to a more solid type of swelling. Hair loss occurs, and nails become brittle, cracked, or heavily grooved. Joints thicken, muscles waste away, and spotty osteoporosis occurs early and can spread both widely and rapidly. These symptoms last anywhere from 3 to 6 months in duration.

- Stage III brings about changes that may be irreversible. In particular, pain becomes intractable and may involve an entire limb. Muscles atrophy even further, and joints of the foot or hand can become extremely weak and have limited range of motion. Sometimes, joints become ankylosed, contraction of the flexor tendons occurs, subluxations are produced, and bone deossification has become marked and diffuse (Reflex Sympathetic Dystrophy Syndrome Association of America, 1998).

Thoracic outlet syndrome (TO) is a disorder of the upper extremity and of the chest, neck, head, and shoulder regions. This syndrome is a neurovascular disorder that results from pressure being exerted on the nerves and vessels in the thoracic outlet area. In particular, the brachial plexus artery, the subclavian artery and vein, and the vertebral artery along their accompanying nervous system innervations are involved (Physical Therapy Corner, 1998). Researchers believe that the causes of pressure or compression include the presence of a cervical rib or an abnormal first rib, the presence of fibrous bands, and anatomical variations of the scalene muscles that produce symptoms of pain, diminished mobility, or disability when trying to perform activities such as combing hair, working with

the arms overhead as mechanics often do, and carrying heavy shopping loads (Nasim, 1997).

Symptoms of this disorder are categorized as either vascular or neurological. Vascular symptoms include swelling or puffiness in the arm or hand; a blue-like discoloration of the hand; feelings of heaviness in the arm or hand; a deep, boring, and achy pain in the neck and shoulder region that seems to worsen at night; easily fatigued arms and hands; a pulsating lump above the clavicle; and superficial venous distension in the hand. Neurological symptoms include numbness along the inside of the forearm and the palm, which are enervated by the C8 and the T1 nerve roots; muscle weakness and atrophy of the long finger flexors (gripping muscles) and the thenar and intrinsic small muscles of the hand; difficulty with fine motor tasks of the hand; muscle cramps in the long finger flexor muscles; generalized pain in the arm and hand; and tingling sensations coupled with feelings of numbness in the neck and shoulder region as well as in the arm and hand (Physical Therapy Corner, 1998). The prevalence rate of this disorder has yet to be determined (National Institute of Neurological Disorders and Stroke, 1996).

Finally, more generalized disorders of the upper and lower extremities will briefly be reviewed here. Chronic exertional compartment syndrome (CEC), which is now a recognized exercise-induced chronic pain condition, was formerly called either shin splints, medial tibial syndrome, or anterior tibial syndrome (Schepsis, 1996). During CEC, there is an increase in the intracompartmental pressure, which is significant enough to cause diminished blood flow to lower extremity tissues that results in pain or sometimes temporary neurologic deficits (Schepsis & Lynch, 1996). Professional athletes and runners are particularly prone to suffer from this condition, which afflicts both men and women alike, and prevalence rates of this disorder have yet to be determined (Schepsis & Lynch, 1996).

The major symptoms of CEC include subjective reports of recurrent pain that spreads throughout the compartment of the lower leg and is triggered by sports activity. This pain increases as exercising continues and is described as being achy, cramp-like, or tight. Some athletes find that they experience temporary numbness or "foot drop" over the top of their foot that can be accompanied by feeling of weakness or giving way to the ankle or foot (Schepsis & Lynch, 1996).

Chronic and generalized pain complaints of the neck and shoulder region that result from trauma or chronic strain of the cervical musculature are now being classified as chronic pain disorders of the neck and shoulder region. Studies from Denmark show that generalized neck/shoulder pain is as prevalent as low back pain. Epidemiologically, more than 30% of the Danish population experience some form of neck/shoulder pain within a 12-month period, and pain in the neck/shoulder region is one of the leading causes for which patients seek chiropractic services (Jordan & Ostergaard, 1996). The impact of chronic neck/shoulder pain usually results in limited functional capacities of the cervical musculature. This means that the ability to perform strength, endurance, and range of movement skills is significantly limited. These symptoms appear to worsen with age and affect both men and women equally. Because chronic neck and shoulder pain is a growing concern, work absenteeism is predicted to increase and become an ever greater problem (Jordan & Ostergaard, 1996).

In general, exercise is recommended for the rehabilitation of the chronic pain disorders of the upper and lower extremities and is considered to be a first line of defense in the management of these chronic conditions (Accero & Braggs, 1993; Jordan & Oster-gaard, 1996; Lynch, 1996). Exercise regimens are recommended to be supervised by physicians at primary care clinics, and clinicians are being encouraged to offer on-site exercise rehabilitation programs for the treatment of chronic pain disorders (Allegrant, 1996; National Institute of Neurological Disorders & Stroke, 1998). Recent literature reviews also suggest the integration of a psychoeducational approach with any nonmalignant musculoskeletal pain exercise rehabilitation program. Specifically, some studies find that when chronic pain patients are taught how to effectively communicate, problem solve, and cope while learning how to exercise, they experience significant reductions in their pain and significant improvements in their functional status (Lane & Thompson, 1997). Because this chapter focuses on the role of exercise in the management of chronic pain conditions, this next section shall review relevant exercise research findings that are indicated for the management of the chronic pain disorders of the upper and lower extremities as previously defined. Yet, given the importance of including a psychoeducational approach with any exercise training program, it will be understood that this treatment modality will naturally be a part of any exercise regimens recommended.

For repetitive motion injuries (RMI), like carpal tunnel syndrome (CT), it is recommended that one start any rehabilitation program conservatively (Heller, 1994). This refers to implementing the least invasive therapeutic modalities at the onset of any pain-symptom manifestation, and interventions like 24- to 48-hour icing, followed by moist heat therapy plus splinting, are typically applied. Splints can be worn for up to 3 months at a time and are important because they provide additional support to the carpal tunnel area, which helps reduce the risk of further strain, especially when engaging in activities like sleep or work. Subsequent isotonic and isometric exercises are found to be useful and are recommended as part of early intervention strategies (National Institute of Neurological Disorders and Stroke, 1998). In particular, researchers find that strength-training exercises hasten recovery by building up the strength and flexibility of the tissues in and around the carpal tunnel area as well as by reducing the risk of stiffness and diminished mobility. Without strength-training exercises, at the early stages, the carpal tunnel region can easily develop a limited range of motion and become vulnerable to needing more aggressive types of interventions like steroid injections or surgery. Finally, if surgery is indicated, exercise would most likely be prescribed as part of any postsurgical rehabilitation program (Nasim, 1997).

Another area of importance to assess is body positioning. Improper body positioning can exacerbate RMI. A thorough evaluation of how a patient holds and moves his or her body, particularly while engaging in repetitive work-related activities, is necessary and can determine if a patient needs to either modify the usual body stance or abstain from a particular work-related tasks altogether. This prophylactic intervention can reduce the occurrence of RMI and is recommended to be a part of any exercise rehabilitation program. Still, RMI may require pain management interventions in order for patients to participate in an exercise rehabilitation. Evaluation for this possibility needs to occur when an exercise rehabilitation program is initially prescribed, and appropriate pain management interventions need to be determined before starting any exercise regimen (Ross, 1997).

Research shows that for reflex sympathetic dystrophy syndrome (RSD), physical therapy and regular exercise are important because maintaining normal physical activity is critical for being able to live with this chronic pain condition. Yet, research also finds that any exercise regimen needs to be carefully supervised because too much or too strenuous of an exercise program can be as debilitating as no exercise at all (Reflex Sympathetic Dystrophy Association, 1998). Furthermore, the stage of the RSD disease process determines which types of exercise are indicated. In general, any exercise program should be gentle, nonpainful, and include a variety of exercise modalities. Varying any exercise regimen optimizes functional capacities and can build strength, endurance, and range-of-motion abilities. Such activity enable RSD patients to engage in activities of daily living as well as keep their limbs moving. Exercise recommendations for the three stages of RSD are as follows and again are indicated only under the supervision of a physician:

- For Stage I, this level of disease is best treated with active range-of-motion (ROM) exercises, light tissue massage and stress-loading exercises that can build muscle strength and endurance. Pain management is recommended if pain interferes with the exercise regimen. Nonsteroidal anti-inflammatory drugs (NSAIDs) taken orally are commonly used and found to be effective because they reduce swelling, which, in turn, diminishes reports of pain.
- For Stage II disease symptoms, any exercise program requires more intensive management. Stage II patients can engage in exercise recommend for Stage I symptoms of disease. However, what becomes more complicated is coordinating any exercise program with pain-management interventions. At this level of symptomatology, more aggressive and invasive measure are often implemented like administering intramuscular or intravenous nerve blockage. Once the pain is managed, exercise regimens may begin.

- For Stage III of the disease, any exercise program is highly individualized and often includes the guidance of pain-management specialists. Given the increased risk for osteoporosis at this level of disease, supervised pool therapy is frequently recommended, given that it is less likely to stress and strain limbs and joints or exacerbate current pain symptoms.

Clearly, all three stages of disease process, and especially Stage III of the RSD disease process, require highly individualized care for providing routine exercise therapy (Reflex Sympathetic Dystrophy Association of America, 1998).

For thoracic outlet syndrome (TO), it is recommended that physical therapy and exercise be prescribed and started as soon as possible. Given that poor posture and weakened shoulder muscles can exacerbate TO symptoms, the goals of any exercise therapy program are to correct postural abnormalities and strengthen shoulder muscles. Other exercises, like aqua therapy, are recommended, given that aquatic exercise programs not only increase muscle strength, flexibility, and endurance, but they also offer relief from chronic pain symptoms as well as a chance to improve psychological well-being (Foltz-Gray, 1997). In fact, studies today now show that when successful rehabilitation occurs, patients demonstrate a significant cognitive shift by moving from a perception of helplessness and passivity to one of resourcefulness and ability to function in life despite their chronic pain condition (Gatchel & Turk, 1996). These findings reinforce the many benefits that exercise can offer patients who suffer from TO.

For chronic exertional compartment syndrome (CEC), treatment is generally limited to the two choices of either surgery or exercise in moderation (Schepsis & Lynch, 1996). Interventions like physical therapy, rest, or-

thotics, and medications are not recommended because they have not demonstrated any therapeutic value. Furthermore, athletes who refuse to curtail their level of activity soon discover that surgery frequently becomes the only pain-management option (Hutchinson & Ireland, 1994). Finally, moderate exercise is considered to be a conservative treatment for CEC, and many experts claim that CEC is most appropriately treated with surgery (Clanton & Solcher, 1994).

For neck/shoulder chronic pain conditions, physical exercise is prescribed. Yet, determining the adequate dose and duration of exercise is what makes this condition a challenge to treat. Fortunately, researchers can agree that dosage is determined by the number and frequency of training sessions conducted in combination with the amount of exercises done per session. Building up duration means achieving real gains in strength. Optimal endurance training occurs when exercises are supervised and occur at a rate of 2 to 3 sessions per week for a minimal time period of 2 months (Jordan & Ostegaard, 1996).

Obviously, exercise is a key component for managing chronic pain disorders of the upper and lower extremities. Successful rehabilitation depends upon integrating conditioning exercises in a safe and effective manner. Often, the balance between too much versus too little exercise in combination with patient adherence is what makes any rehabilitation program challenging. Once established, this balance can reduce pain, increase functionality, and improve quality of life significantly. However, what makes sense clinically is hardly supported by solid and adequate research findings, and our exercise recommendations are based mainly on anecdotal reports and studies with small sample size.

Arthritis

By definition, arthritis is an inflammation of the joints caused by infectious, metabolic, or other constitutional reasons (Fuchs & Zaichkowsky, 1997). Medically, arthritis is a term used to refer to a spectrum of over 100 different types of illnesses and conditions and is reported to be one of the most common chronic illnesses seen in primary care settings (Callahan, Rao, & Boutaugh, 1996; Ross, 1997). In 1990, an estimated 37.9 million individuals, or nearly 15% of the U.S. population, whose age averaged 60 years old or older, reported having some type of arthritic condition (Ross, 1997). In the United States, arthritis is the most prevalent chronic condition found in women. The prevalence rate of female self-reported cases in 1990 was 22.8 million. This figure is projected to increase to 36 million by the year 2020 (Callahan et al., 1996). In addition, arthritis is one of the leading causes of disability in the United States, and for women, arthritis is reported to be the leading cause of physical limitations in activities of daily living (Callahan et al.). Household chores, writing, typing, or lifting are tasks that become difficult to complete. For men, arthritis is problematic and can be a leading cause of disability (Buckwalter & Lane, 1997).

Because arthritis refers to a variety of chronic conditions, this chapter focuses on two of the more common type of arthritis, namely osteoarthritis and rheumatoid arthritis. After defining these types, the role that exercise can play in the treatment and management of these chronic conditions shall be discussed with an emphasis on recent literature findings and reviews.

Osteoarthritis (OA) is considered to be the most common form of arthritis. It is characterized by general, progressive destruction of the articular cartilage. This destruction is accompanied by changes in subchondral bone, which manifest as remodeling and sclerosis of this bone structure. In many cases, subchondral bone cysts and osetophytes are formed. In addition, the tissues that form the synovial joint, meaning the synovium, the bone, and the joint capsule, are involved at varying degrees of degeneration (Arthritis Foundation, 1998; Callahan et al., 1996; Schlike, Johnson, Housh, & O'Dell, 1996).

The earliest and most visible signs of degeneration occur in the articular cartilage. These signs manifest as fibrillation or disruption of the most superficial layers of the articular cartilage tissue and tend to be localized. The superficial fibrillation is associated with both an increased water concentration and a decreased proteoglycan concentration. As the disease progresses, the surface irregularities of the articular cartilage become clefts. With time, the articular cartilage surface becomes increasingly roughened and irregularly shaped. This enables the fibrillations to extend deeper into the cartilage until these fissures reach the subchondral bone. As these fissures grow deeper, the superficial tips of the cartilage tear. This tearing allows free fragments of cartilage to move into the joint space and thus decrease the cartilage thickness. Simultaneously, enzymes erode the cartilage matrix, which further decreases the cartilage volume. (Buckwalter & Lane, 1997; Schlike et al. 1996). The resulting weakening of the articular cartilage makes mobility difficult, and the formation of this condition is both painful and problematic.

Rheumatoid arthritis (RA) is a chronic and inflammatory, systemic musculoskeletal disease that results in symmetrical joint inflammation and is accompanied by symptoms of fatigue and weakness (Hakkinen et al., 1997; Ross, 1997; Stenstrom, Arge, & Sundbom, 1997). The degenerative disease activity of rheumatoid arthritis in combination with the inflammation and associated pain results in decreased muscle strength and disuse muscle atrophy. This can become a vicious cycle because painful joints make joint movement difficult; joints that do not move do not exercise their accompanying muscles. Muscles in disuse loss their cell body mass and degenerate. Given that muscle-cell body mass is a significant portion of general body mass, the pattern of decline in body strength, body function, and body mass continues.

For RA patients, the loss of cell body mass is referred to as *rheumatoid cachexia* and is believed to be related to several factors, including medication side effects, inadequate dietary intake, catabolic cytokine profile, and decreased physical activity. Even though the exact percentage of body cell mass loss in RA patients is unknown, studies on cancer, AIDS, and cell starvation have shown that when a loss of body cell mass reaches 40%, cell death occurs. Furthermore, a 25-year prospective study found that on average, men with rheumatoid arthritis lose 7 years of their life expectancy whereas women with RA lose 3 years. Clearly, this disease is not benign (Gremillion & Vollenhoven, 1998; Hakkinen et al., 1997; Rall, Meydani, Kehayias, Dawson-Huges, & Roubernoff, 1996; Stenstrom et al., 1997).

In fact, RA is considered to be the second leading cause of disability in the United States. This is largely due to the significant decline in functional status that occurs over time. A serious consequence of this decline is a loss of job function. Studies show that nearly 50% of RA suffers cannot function at their jobs within 10 years of their disease onset. Other studies show that nearly two thirds of the 4 million RA patients between the ages of 35 and 50 years old have significant functional impairment (Gremillion & Vollenhoven, 1998). Clearly, the defining characteristics of RA encompass both physical and occupational functioning. This, in turn, affects social functioning. The result is deterioration of functioning in all of these domains.

The empirical literature unanimously recommends regular exercise as part of the treatment, prevention, and management of OA (*Exercise and Arthritis*, 1994; Gremillion & Vollenhoven, 1998). When joints are damaged by the slow progression of aging, regular mild to moderate exercise can benefit these joints and actually improve the strength and mobility of their functioning without causing further joint damage (Allegrant, 1996). The types of exercises currently recommended for age-related OA include range-of-motion, strengthening, and endurance training. They are useful in treating acute symptoms of osteoarthritis as well as in preventing the onset of the disease and improving the status of the osteoarthritis sufferer (Arthritis Foundation, 1998).

Range-of-motion (ROM) exercises are generally referred to as warm-up or stretching exercises. With these exercises, a person moves a joint as comfortably as it will go and then stretches it a bit farther without causing joint distress. ROM exercises limber up muscles and joints, increase and maintain joint mobility, and decrease joint pain while improving joint function; they can improve an arthritis sufferer's functional status significantly (Schlike et al., 1996). Researchers are now using both warm-up and cooldown ROM exercises as part of either muscle-strengthening or muscle-endurance exercise programs (Ettinger et al., 1997). Their results demonstrate improved measures of physical ability as well as decreased reports of pain and physical disability. Although some studies do not research the impact of ROM exercises alone, the importance of stretching as part of any exercise regimen is well documented (Arthritis Foundation, 1998; Cooper et al., 1996; Marlowe, 1994).

Strengthening exercises are intended to strengthen muscles and help stabilize weaker joints. These exercises use the muscles that surround the joint but do not move the joint. In general, researchers who have studied patients with knee OA have found that any therapies that can increase the mobility and decrease the pain of joints are important for OA sufferers. For example, a study by Schlike and his colleagues (Schlike et al., 1997) reports that the experiences of pain, stiffness, and mobility improved quite significantly after participating in an 8-week isokinetic strength-training program. From these findings, it is possible to conclude that strengthening exercises matter because they can protect the joint, decrease the joint pain, strengthen para-arthritic structures, and provide additional support to the joint in distress (Schlike et al.). Similar findings have been confirmed by other research studies (Marks, 1994; Tan, Balci, Spici, & Gener, 1995). Evidently, strengthening exercises are beneficial largely because they can improve the functional status of the arthritis suffer.

Endurance exercises strengthen the cardiovascular system and increase stamina. Exercises like walking, swimming, and stationary cycling are endurance exercises that are recommended for osteoarthritis suffers. Currently, the American Arthritis Foundation recommends aquatic, joint, and other recreational programs that target endurance training. They emphasize that exercise regimens need to be tailored to an individual's needs and treatment goals. More important, they stress that regular exercise, whether structured or recreational, should be as pleasurable as possible. Adherence to any chronic pain condition treatment plan occurs when the participant finds value in intervention or outcome (Arthritis Foundation, 1998).

In various supervised trials of fitness walking, individuals with knee osteoarthritis were randomized into walking endurance-exercise groups. All results demonstrated that participation in a regular walking exercise program improves walking distance and functional status and decreases reports of pain and medication usage (Callahan et al., 1996; Ettinger et al., 1997; La Croix, New-town, Leville, & Wallace, 1997; Schlike et al., 1996). Moreover, conditions like obesity are considered to be significant risk factors for the development of knee OA (Dabis, Ettinger, & Neuhaus, 1990; Felson, Zhang, Anthony, Naimark, & Anderson, 1992) as well as hip OA (Cooper et al., 1998). Given that endurance exercises are aerobic and, therefore, play an important part in weight loss and weight maintenance (George, Creamer, & Dieppe, 1994; Marlowe, 1994), these are not only indicated for knee and possibly hip OA prevention, but they also can significantly improve the quality of life of OA sufferers (Lane & Thompson, 1997).

Exercise also seems to have an impact on OA progress and mortality. Several new studies show that individuals without OA who exercise regularly appear to develop functional disabilities (Buckwalter & Lane, 1997; Lane & Thompson, 1997) at a significantly slower rate than do individuals without OA who do not exercise regularly. These same regular exercisers without OA also appear to have a greater survival rate with comparison to the survival rate of the same nonregular exercisers who do not have OA.

Just as it does with OA, the current literature consistently supports using regular exercise as an integral part of care in treating RA (Hakkinen et al., 1997; Neuberger et al., 1997; Shepard & Shek, 1997, Stentrom et al., 1997). Exercise helps to manage chronic pain, control joint swelling, prevent limited range of motion, increase strength, improve musculoskeletal and cardiovascular conditioning, improve functional status, manage fatigue, and positively affect psychosocial factors in the lives of patients with RA. In fact, a 5-year followup study has shown that RA sufferers in a conditioning program that reported doing more than 5 hours of exercise per week showed less radiographic progression of joint damage and reported having fewer days of hospitalization and fewer incidences of work disability than did their peers who did not participate in the conditioning program (Callahan et. al., 1996). Other studies have examined the effects of muscular detraining or muscular inactivity following a 6-month muscular-training program in patients with RA. In particular, RA patients who participated in the muscular-training program for RA patients demonstrated muscular strength gains during the muscle-training period. This group was compared to RA patients who did not adhere to any type of muscle-training program but instead maintained their usual level of daily activities. All strengths gained during this training period for the muscle-training group of RA patients were lost during the muscle-detraining period. The RA patients who did not participate in the muscle-training program were measured for changes in muscular functioning and demonstrated significant losses in trunk flexion and extension movements. Obviously, exercise is critical for maintaining functional status of RA sufferers, and a lack of exercise appears to be related to disease progression (Rall et al., 1996).

As discussed, RA, like OA, benefits from ROM, strength-training, and endurance-training exercises. Yet, because of the nature of the disease process of RA, it is important to take into consideration the RA sufferer's disease state, degree of joint swelling, over functional capacities, and levels of activity tolerance. With these factors in mind, active ROM exercises are indicated in most RA exercise programs because they can help optimize strength training exercises (Newcomber & Jurisson, 1994). Passive ROM exercises tend not to be indicated because this type of motion may increase the intra-articular temperature and leukocyte count (Rall et al., 1996). However, with any type of ROM exercise, the literature claims that any RA patient should learn proper body positioning before engaging in any type of exercise regi-

men. If strengthening exercises are done improperly, the RA patient may inadvertently apply forces on the joints that promote subluxation (Rall et al., 1996).

Finally, ROM exercises are indicated before engaging in any type of strength-training program. Yet, any strength-training exercise program depends on a patient's current functional capacities and degree of joint swelling (Newcomber & Jurisson, 1994). In general, most researchers agree that isometric exercises are indicated if a patient is suffering from acute joint swelling (Gremillion & Vollenhoven, 1998). Once joint swelling has diminished, researchers generally agree that RA patients can begin to incorporate strength-training exercise into their daily exercise regimen. Yet, the start of any isotonic exercise program needs to begin by using low weights with few repetitions, and the goal of this type of exercise intervention is to gradually build up and maintain strength in a safe and effective manner. A word of caution, however, is that if pain persists for more than one hour after completion of an exercise regimen, particularly with ROM exercises, then the exercises were probably done in an excessive manner. Clearly, moving forward with any exercise regimen needs to occur gradually and with great care (Gremillion & Vollenhoven, 1998; Newcomber & Jurisson, 1994).

Endurance exercises benefit RA sufferers because this type of intervention improves cardiovascular functioning, psychosocial factors, and psychological well-being (Newcomber & Jurisson; 1994). Although many of the literature reviews studied addressed strength training and ROM exercises, it is unanimously understood that endurance training, if tolerated, plays an important role. For example, endurance-training exercises have been found to positively affect fatigue and psychosocial well-being (Dubbert, 1992), provided that any type of endurance training must take into consideration a patient's activity tolerance level and build from there. Incorporating periods of rest is indicated and in general does not seem to interfere with endurance-training goals (Haskell, 1994).

Researchers are also recognizing that pain management can be a critical determinant to exercise adherence. Some researchers believe that physicians should not hesitate to aggressively medicate pain if pain prevents regular exercise (Gremillion & Vollenhoven, 1998). Other researchers find that chronic pain in RA is exacerbated by stress, anxiety, and depression, and teaching patients relaxation techniques can be as important as medication therapy for pain management. Pain-management regimens that incorporate both types of interventions are considered desirable. Highly individualized pain-management programs that also take into consideration disease activity, level(s) of fatigue, and the need for rest periods are considered optimal (Allegrant, 1996; Newcombe & Jurisson, 1994).

As seen with OA, weight-management exercises are believed to be key components for the management of RA (Cooper et al., 1998). Excess body weight can interfere with the ability and the motivation to exercise regularly as well as exacerbate chronic RA pain conditions. Obesity is known to stress joints, exacerbate inflammation, and contribute to superimposed OA (Newcomber & Jurisson, 1994) As a result, regular inactivity and fatigue can lead to functional impairments (Komatireddy, Leitch, Cella, Browning, & Minor, 1997). In turn, functional impairments are known to worsen quality of life and mood (Allegrant, 1996).

Headache

Headache is one of the major public health concerns in all countries throughout the world. Headache drains a country's productivity, health system, individuals, families, and societies; and it is an enormous economic, psychosocial, and human burden. (Leonardi, Musico, & Nappi, 1998). In the United States, recurrent or chronic headache ranks seventh among the top 10 complaints for which people seek medical advice (American Medical Association [AMA], 1998). An estimated 50 million U.S. citizens suffer from chronic headache, and 70% of the families in the United States have at least one member plagued with this condition. Businesses in the United States lose one and half million workdays a year because of the severity of this problem (Hammill, Cook, & Rosecrance, 1996). Clearly, headache affects our society significantly; researchers and clinicians have yet to discover the best way to effectively treat and manage this chronic condition.

In 1988, the International Headache Society Classification Committee published diagnostic criteria for headache disorders (International Headache Society, 1988). Their criteria describe more than 100 headaches in detail, a scope that goes far beyond the focus of this chapter and tends to be controversial, particularly for the primary headache disorders. Furthermore, the aim of this chapter is to address early on the role of exercise in major chronic pain conditions. Therefore, some generally acceptable definitions and characteristics for the more common types of chronic headache, meaning tension, migraine, and cluster headaches, are outlined below.

A *tension headache* is the most common type of headache. It is characterized by pain that is best described for being mild-to-moderate, generalized, and bilateral, and is usually felt as a pressure or tightness around the head and neck. A tension headache is more common to women than men, and it can occur infrequently, episodically, or even on a daily basis. The major cause of a tension headache tends to be stress and the frustrations of everyday life. Other common causes include eye strain and poor posture, especially of the neck and shoulder regions. Recently, chronic muscular disorders of the head and neck regions have been found to possibly play a major role in the conversion of episodic tension headaches to chronic tension headaches. Such findings can begin to further clarify possible causes for chronic tension headaches, a clarification that can hopefully optimize treatment possibilities for this persistent condition (AMA, 1998; Jensen, Bendsten, Lars, & Olsen, 1998; Swain & Kaplan, 1997).

A *migraine headache* afflicts more than 26 million U. S. citizens per year. The AMA considers migraine headache to be a neurological disorder that occurs both with and without an aura and tends to be more common in women than men. A migraine headache usually lasts anywhere from 4 to 72 hours, and the frequency of occurrence tends to be affected by a variety of contributing factors discussed later in this chapter (Bic, Blix, Hopp, & Leslie, 1998). A migraine headache without an aura was formerly called the common migraine headache. This type of headache is characterized by pain that is often unilateral, pulsating, and moderate-to-severe in intensity, and it is associated with symptoms of nausea, vomiting, photophobia, and phonophobia (AMA, 1998; Swain & Kaplan, 1997). A migraine headache with an aura was formerly called the classic migraine headache. This type of headache shares all of the same characteristics as the migraine headache without an aura. However, a migraine headache with aura exhibits prodromal neurological symptoms such as homonymous visual disturbances, unilateral numbness or parasthesias, unilateral weakness, or speech difficulties. Prodromal symptoms can be differentiated from signs of a stroke because they manifest for a much shorter duration, meaning for usually less than 60 minutes. However, differentiating the prodromal symptoms from a transient ischemic attack is more difficult and requires acute clinical assessment (Swain & Kaplan, 1997).

The exact cause of migraine headache remains uncertain. Yet, dietary triggers (e.g., caffeine, chocolate, cheese), medications (aspartame, nitrates, nicotine, estrogens, progesterone), food preservatives (some nitrates, monosodium glutamate), sleep problems, stress, menstruation, alcohol, and head trauma are believed to contribute to or worsen a migraine headache. More recent research findings suggest that high levels of blood lipid and free fatty acids are additional significant underlying factors in the development of a migraine headache. Clearly, the causes of migraine headaches can be considered multifaceted (Bic et al., 1998).

A *cluster headache* is less common than a migraine headache, occurring in nearly 4% of the U.S. population. This type of headache occurs more frequently in men than women. There are basically two types of cluster headaches, namely chronic and episodic. Cluster headaches that tend to occur weekly and persist at this frequency for up to one year are called chronic. Cluster headaches that occur infrequently or have long periods of remission usually lasting months at a time are called episodic. In general, 10%–20% of cluster headache suffers have the chronic type. Cluster headaches themselves are characterized by severe, stabbing, unilateral pain in the supraorbital, orbital, or temporal areas of the head that usually persists for 20 to 30 minutes. Common symptoms that occur during a cluster headache include watery eyes, conjunctival injection, unilateral nasal congestion or rhinorrhea, forehead and facial sweating, constricted but reactive pupil, ptosis, and eyelid edema. Cluster-headache suffers are often unable to sit or lie prone due to the excruciating pain of this condition. Another type of episodic cluster headaches is one that occurs with concomitant migraine headache symptoms. This type of headache is called a cluster-migraine headache and can make proper diagnosis of a cluster headache difficult. Recent research findings indicate that diagnostic criteria for headaches do not consider the possibility of having two forms of headache persist together, as seen with the cluster-migraine headache. Apparently, diagnosing and therefore treating the cluster headache can be complicated (AMA, 1998).

Although less common, the sinus headache and the mixed headache are two chronic conditions that routinely require medical advice. The mixed headache commonly refers to headache symptoms that are usually a combination of tension headache and migraine headache complaints. The sinus headache is associated with chronic sinus problems and manifests as headache in the sinus areas. The symptoms of a sinus headache are often described as pulsing or throbbing sensations located in either the frontal sinus area or around the juncture of the temporal and parietal lobe regions. Even though this chapter will focus on the role of exercise in tension, migraine, and cluster headaches, it is useful to be familiar with other types of chronic headache conditions (AMA, 1998).

Exercise has the potential to be the most potent method for preventing and treating pain as well as promulgating health and fitness. Yet, the role of exercise in pain management has not received sufficient attention in the pain-management literature. In fact, a content analysis of the pain publications showed that only a few authors have mentioned the role of exercise in preventing or treating pain, and when they have, the discussions have been brief and generally lack robust research support (Fuchs & Zaichkowsky, 1997).

It has been well documented that chronic headache pain is pervasive and costly to treat (Stewart, Linet, Celentrano, & Reed, 1991).

Authors and researchers are now finally agreeing that a key to headache management is headache prevention. Empirical studies show that exercise is crucial because it is a healthy behavior and part of a lifestyle that reduces the occurrence of triggers or worsening of tension, migraine, and cluster headaches (Bic et al.,1998; de Bruijn-Kofman, van de Weil, Groenman, Sorbi, & Klip, 1997; Maizels, 1998). Furthermore, the AMA encourages healthy behavior and lifestyle changes for the management of chronic headache conditions and recommends moderate exercise as part of healthy lifestyle and behavioral changes (AMA, 1998). Not only is exercise being recommended as a first line of defense in the treatment and management of this chronic pain condition, but it also can improve the functional status of headache sufferers significantly.

Given that the more common causes of tension headache tend to be stress and frustrations of everyday life, moderate, regular exercise, preferably daily exercise, has been repeatedly shown to reduce a person's stress response and improve her overall physical and psychological well-being (Blanchard, 1980; Blanchard & Andrasik, 1982; Jensen et al., 1998). Brief or focused headache-treatment programs have demonstrated effectiveness in managing chronic tension headaches. Specifically, a 6-week treatment program studied the effectiveness of ergonomic and postural education, isotonic strengthening exercises for the cervical muscles, and massage and stretching for reducing symptoms of tension-type headaches. The findings reveal that the frequency of tension-type headaches was reduced significantly whereas the Sickness Impact Profile (SIP) scores improved significantly. Similarly, a 10-week mass-media behavioral program for the treatment of chronic headaches piloted their multimedia interventions and found highly significant reductions in headache activity, medication intake, and work absenteeism at the end of their program, as well as at the 4-month followup evaluation. The types of multimedia used included videotapes, audiocassettes, television, and workbook exercises (de Bruijun-Kofman et al., 1996; Hammill et al., 1996). Overall, the findings in both of these studies demonstrated a 40 to 60% improvement in the headache condition. Some limitations of these studies include a small sample size in the 6-week program and the pilot nature of the mass-media program. Yet, the mass-media study took research one step further and compared the effectiveness of the behavioral interventions for the treatment of tension headaches with the effectiveness of such interventions for treatment of migraine headaches. As a matter of fact, researchers found no significant differences between these two types of headache groups, nor was the interaction between diagnosis and treatment significant. This outcome is congruent with the results of other studies, which indicate that classification into tension and migraine types of headache might be of little value for the treatment of behavioral headache (de Bruijun-Kofman et. al., 1996).

As discussed, migraine headaches, both with and without an aura, tend to be brought on by a variety of factors such as diet, medications, hormonal changes, sleep problems, stress, alcohol, preservatives, and head trauma (Bic et al., 1998; Swain & Kaplan, 1997). Although the literature unanimously agrees that vigorous exercise is not recommended for the treatment of migraine headaches, moderate exercise has more recently been referred to as part of the "magic cure" for the treatment of this headache condition (Bic et al., 1998). The magic cure concept is part of a recent research finding that shows that elevated levels of blood lipids and free floating fatty acids are common denominators for the onset of migraine headaches. Hence, these researchers conclude that the magic cure for

migraine headaches may be to minimize the occurrence of factors that contribute to elevated levels of blood lipids and free floating fatty acids through lifestyle changes. In particular, they suggest the following interventions, including exercise, that are known to reduce blood lipids and free floating fatty acids:

1. Consume a low-fat diet.
2. Increase the intake of complex carbohydrates.
3. Get moderate, not vigorous, exercise.
4. Do not skip meals or experience prolonged hunger.
5. Quit smoking.
6. Decrease the consumption of alcohol and caffeine.
7. Decrease stress by using relaxation techniques.

These researchers go on to suggest that migraine headaches may be a warning signal of possible biochemical imbalances in the body that can lead to the development of chronic illnesses, like cardiovascular disease (Bic et al., 1998). These findings can possibly reshape how we conceptualize and deliver our care because they reflect the growing understanding that science has regarding the role that molecular biology can play in managing our health.

In general, the AMA endorses moderate exercise as a means to prevent the occurrence of migraine headache. The AMA, in accordance with other researchers (Swain & Kaplan, 1997), finds that once mild migraine headache symptoms have begun, any routine movement or physical activity can trigger a full-blown migraine headache attack. Clearly, exercise is not indicated once this type of event has occurred (AMA, 1998). Moreover, migraine headaches can be problematic for individuals who depend upon physical activity as part of their occupation as seen with professional athletes and other fitness experts. For these individuals, the ability to exercise is critical, and the occurrence of two or more migraine headache episodes per month can be problematic. Given this unique relationship, which applies for probably very limited cases that can be considered a professional risk, the prophylactic use of medications, not exercise, may be indicated. Medications like nonsteroidal anti-inflammatory drugs, tricyclic antidepressants, verapamil, or beta-blockers are commonly used as a first line of defense. Nonetheless, the use of prophylactic migraine-headache medication is not an option for many headache suffers because many of the recommended medications have potent side effects, and they can cause liver toxicity, addiction, or rebound headache (Bic et al., 1998; Swain & Kaplan).

Generally speaking, cluster headaches tend to be more difficult to treat and to manage. This is largely because they tend to occur episodically with no specific pattern and to be brief. Consequently, prevention is considered the key to managing this headache condition (AMA, 1998; Swain & Kaplan, 1997). Although the AMA recommends medications like ergotamine to treat acute cluster-headache attacks and lithium to prevent these headaches, they apparently do not recommend nonmedical interventions as a first line of defense for treatment of this sporadic headache condition. In reviewing the literature, we could not find sufficient data that explore the role of exercise in managing chronic cluster headaches. Therefore, we extrapolate from our clinical experiences, anecdotal research, and notes of some researchers that cluster headaches and migraine-headache symptoms occur concomitantly and ask, therefore, whether prevention of cluster headaches would not benefit from regular moderate exercise in the same way that migraine headaches can (D'Amico et al., 1997). Researchers who explored this question found that cluster and migraine headaches may co-exist, which supports a preconceived notion that migraine headaches transform into clus-

ter headaches (D'Amico et al., 1997). Rather than having one headache type precede or perhaps have a causal relationship to another, these findings indicate that cluster headaches often go undiagnosed because they can be difficult to assess and may have symptoms that are masked by migraine-headache phenomenon. Although this research has its limitations given the 10-patient sample size of the study, it is supportive of other researchers who criticize the International Headache Society (IHS), the AMA, and other organizations that do not consider the possibly of two headache types existing concurrently.

In summary, one can infer that concomitant headache disorders are either completely ignored or have yet to be "discovered." The role that exercise can have, particularly if headache disorder coexists, could be greater than imagined. At present, concluding that exercise needs to have an official role in the treatment of chronic headache conditions seems quite reasonable, but such a conclusion is not supported adequately by research. Still, to make the role of exercise effective, taking a thorough history and assessing for the possibility of concurrent headache conditions are necessary steps for building a comprehensive care plan for the chronic headache sufferer. These types of assessment tools provide both the headache sufferer and the health care provider a baseline of data from which all other office visits can build an understanding of the headache symptoms and pattern of occurrence, including the frequency, intensity, and duration of symptoms as well as recording possible headache triggers. From this type of ongoing assessment, integrating exercise can becomes a creative and rewarding intervention.

Fibromyalgia

Fibromyalgia (FM), primarily diagnosed in females, is a disorder characterized by musculoskeletal pain and stiffness. Complaints of weakness, swollen joints, and constant fatigue, neurovascular complaints of coldness, numbness, tingling, mottled skin, and a reticular skin pattern are common symptoms. Sleep disturbances, depression, and anxiety are other major components (Farrar, Locke, & Kantrowitz, 1995; Goldenberg, 1994).

Wolfe and his colleagues (1990) helped to establish, via the American College of Rheumatology, more robust criteria for classification of FM as a separate entity from other chronic fatigue syndromes. Their criteria emphasize a history of widespread pain, which is defined as bilateral bodily pain, both above and below the waist and axial skeletal pain. Verification of pain in 11 of 18 tender point sites on digital palpations is considered the major diagnostic tool (Wolfe et al., 1990). With an unknown etiology and no conclusive pathophysiology, the most common recommended symptomatic treatment consists usually of low doses of tricyclic antidepressants, Selective serotonin reuptake inhibitors (SSRIs), myofacial injections, low-grade aerobic exercise, and some form of psychological intervention (Baumstark & Buckelew, 1992; Feiffenberger & Amundson, 1996; Godfrey, 1996; Reveille, 1997; Wilke, 1995, 1996).

In examination of the supportive research literature for the use of exercise as an adjunct therapy for fibromyalgia (FM), it is clear that the presenting symptoms played initially a major role. Exercise seems a good way not only to try to combat the obvious musculoskeletal aching, stiffness, and soft-tissue tender points, but also to affect positively the symptoms of sleep disturbances, mild to moderate depression, and anxiety. These psychophysiological symptoms were demonstrated to be strongly amenable to exercise in various other populations (Fuchs & Zaichkowsky, 1997). However, the picture is more complex because it is quite established that some FM patients report aggravation of pain due to exercise, whereas others report pain relief. This mixed evaluation of exercise may also be present in the same patients at different times during the exercise regimen (Yunus, Masi, Calabro, Miller, & Feigenbaum, 1981).

The choice of selecting aerobic activity, as a preferred adjunct treatment modality for FM, originates in Moldofsky's early observation of a marathon runner who participated in a sleep study (Moldofsky & Scarisbrick, 1976). This study reports of great difficulties in inducing painful fibrositic tender points in this subject. Assuming that the runner's aerobic fitness and not his "Olympic spirit" may be the major attribute for this resistance, aerobic-training studies in FM patients (or as it was named then fibrositis/fibromyalgia) followed soon after. McCain, in two pioneering investigations, laid the preliminary foundation for such research by comparing a cardiovascular to a flexibility program. His findings of a moderate exercise program, lasting 20 weeks × three times weekly, showed a substantial increase in cardiovascular fitness and pain decreases in objective measurements and self-reports by the FM patients. However, the statistical analysis of these studies leaves much to be desired (McCain, 1986; McCain, Bell, Mai, & Halliday, 1988).

Since these initial cardiovascular investigations, most of the following treatment programs incorporated aerobic, anaerobic, and psychobehavioral conditions in their treatment regiment. Mengshole, Kømnaes, and Førre (1992) showed that a program of dynamic endurance work, of 60 minutes for 20 weeks twice weekly, did not exacerbate the pain in FM. However, only little functional improvement could be measured. Nichols and Glenn (1994) showed a trend of mainly psychological improvements and lower pain as a result of a 20-minute moderate-walk program that lasted 8 weeks, three times per week. Burckhardt, Mannerkorpi, Hedenberg, and Bjelle (1994) showed in an open-ended study, a decrease in pain of the tender points as well as an enhanced quality of life and self-efficacy in an FM group who received an educational program and walked moderately three times per week for 20 minutes or more at home. Similar results of decreased pain and higher self-efficacy associated with improved physical activities after a 6-week intervention of exercise and behavioral methods were documented by Buckelew, Murray, Hewett, Johnson, and Huyser (1995) and Buckelew et al. (1996). Regular self physical exercise, rather than drugs or specific physical therapies, were also correlated after a 2-year followup with improvement in pain, mood, and coping strategies (Granges, Zilko, & Littlejohn, 1994). From the short review of these preliminary investigations, it seems clear that FM patients who are involved in some regular aerobic-type activity program report fewer symptoms than sedentary patients do. However, the research designs of these studies, the construct validity and reliability of the outcome measurement tools, and the refinement of the other tests employed do not comply with basic research requirements (Bakker, van der Linden, van Santen Hoeufft, Bolwijn, & Hidding, 1995; Bakker, Rutten, et al., 1995; Hewett et al., 1995).

More vigorous, controlled exercise studies were published recently. Hørven Wigers, Stiles, and Vogel (1996) compared a 14-week treatment followed up by a 4-year testing period. Three groups with FM were studied. The first group exercised aerobically 20 to 45 minutes, three times weekly, up to 60 or 70% of their maximum heart rate. The second group was a stress-management group.

This group practiced cognitive behavioral stress-management techniques, which they maintained later at home. The third group was used as a control group and continued their regular therapies (e.g., medications, pool therapy). After 14 weeks, both experimental groups showed the expected psychosomatic gains. However, the most effective intervention seemed to be the aerobic exercise. At the followup, the groups seemed to lose their gains, probably due to noncompliance attributed to the lack of supervision.

Another relatively long-term group intervention combined 6 months once a week with lectures in behavioral modification, stress management, family support, and exercise instructions to be practiced at home (Bennet et al., 1996). In this study, the FM experimental group was followed for 2 years and was compared to a group of FM patients outside the program. Somatic and psychological improvements were evident in the experimental group after the active intervention, and improvements continued during the 2-year followup. Their pain and depression reductions were significantly better in comparison to those of the no-treatment group. Despite the impressive results, this study lacks adequate controls and blinded-outcome measurement procedures.

Martin et al. (1996) used 60 patients divided into two groups: exercise and relaxation. Each group met three times per week for 6 weeks for 1 hour of supervised treatment. The comprehensive exercise group practiced 20 minutes of walking at a pace sufficient to raise their heart rate to 60 or 70% of their individual maximal heart rate. The next 20 minutes were used for general flexibility exercises, and the remaining 20 minutes, for low-resistance weight training in a gym. The relaxation group divided its time among three relaxation techniques: visualization, mild yoga, and autogenic relaxation. At the end of the study, the exercise group showed a significant improvement in the number of tender points (TP) and myalgic scores in comparison to those of the relaxation groups. This study is important not only because it demonstrated positive effects of exercise on pain in FM patients, but also in demonstrating that these patients can be involved in a total fitness exercise program without adverse effects. This study, however, had no long-term followup that is crucial in such a variable condition as fibromyalgia.

Borenstein (1995) used a multidisciplinary program for only FM and FM/pain patients' groups, which included walking unsupervised at an increased pace, up to a maximum of 30 minutes per day for 12 months. He concluded that patients with primary fibromyalgia seem to benefit more than patients with secondary fibromyalgia with spinal pain. Finally, Goldenberg (1991) in one of his earlier studies, reports on 210 FM/Fibrositis patients who were instructed to exercise with a routine that seemed to have stretching elements for 15 minutes at least three times a week. He found that patients who entered the study with excessive joint hypermobility benefited more, when measuring symptoms of sleep disturbance and fatigue, than did patients with less joint hypermobility. His hypothesis was that the exercise regimen improved muscle support, muscle tone, and blood flow, which, in time, helped to improve the symptoms associated with "loose joints." This study, unfortunately, is a prime example of the lack of understanding of basic muscle physiology concepts, exercise regimens, and measurement methods by most physicians who were involved in the early stages of FM research. However, this study as well as the other earlier studies indicated strongly that FM patients can exercise in a variety of ways and benefit too, which seems to be a revolutionary concept at the time.

Some of the earlier and most of the recent studies on FM and exercise have not attempted to find the optimal exercise routine. Actually, these studies try to pinpoint the exact mechanism that is involved in the reduced physical performance of FM patients, except being sedentary. Furthermore, these studies try, usually via short but complex interventions, to expose the possible pathogenesis of FM. These studies seem to be solely interested in the underlying mechanisms that impair activity and induce pain in the muscles, especially at the cellular level. It is speculated that decreased maximal voluntary contractions (MVC) is one of the mechanical mechanisms in diminished muscle strength. The pain and fatigue may also be related to the inability to relax the muscle between contractions due to incomplete recuperation of electrical and/or metabolic muscle properties. Surface electromyography (EMG) and a variety of metabolic processes were investigated in order to try to decode the mystery during muscle rest, exercise, and exhaustion in FM patients. Jacobsen, Wildschiodtz, and Danneskiold-Samsoe (1991) found that electrical stimulation during isometric exercise produced more twitches in the quadriceps muscles of FM patients. Nørregaard, Bülow, and Danneskiold-Samsoe (1994) found no EMG differences in several myoelectric measurements when comparing FM patients to sedentary controls. Lindth, Johansson, Hedberg, and Grimsby (1994) and Mengshoel, Saugen, Førre, and Vøllestad (1995) found an increase in EMG during increased fatigue of the quadriceps muscle, but this can be a normal reaction of deconditioned muscles. Miller, Gabrielle, and Grandevia (1996) tested the biceps brachii hand muscle and found that neither reflex pain inhibition nor muscle contractile failure played a role in the pathogenesis of fatigue in FM patients. Also, no EMG abnormalities of the myoelectrical-metabolic relations during exercise and recovery in the leg's anterior tibialis muscle could be found by Vestergaard-Poulsen et al (1995). These findings should not be surprising because similar results of no gross abnormal electrical propagation, summation, or function of the pre-post synoptic area were already indicated in most of the early research literature (e.g., Bartels & Danneskiold-Samsoe, 1986; Bennett, 1989).

Naturally, EMG led to the combined investigation of metabolic processes inside the resting, working, and exhausted muscle in FM patients. Only some early findings by Yunus, Kalyan-Raman, Kalyan-Raman, and Masi (1986) and Bengtsson, Henriksson, and Larsson (1986) indicated pathological changes in the structure of the sarcomere, the energy production, and utilization of energy sources using biopsies of deconditioned muscles of FM patients. Nevertheless, most of the later more sophisticated studies failed to supply such evidence. Nørregaard, Bulow, Mehlson, and Danneskiold (1994) showed that potassium, lactate, creatine kinase, and myoglobin concentrations were not significantly different in FM patients than in deconditioned healthy controls who exercised on a bicycle ergometer. However, the patients reported significantly more pain for the same workload. Jacobsen, Jensen, Thomsen, Danneskiold-Samsoe, and Henriksen (1992), using 31 Phosphorous Nuclear Magnetic Resonance (31 PNMR) spectroscopy, showed no difference in inorganic phosphate and creatinine phosphate ratios (Pi/Pcr) during dynamic work and recovery in the calf muscle of FM patients as compared to the same muscle area/size in nonpatients. Yet, during anaerobic static exercise, these differences reached significance ($P < 0.003$). Vestergaard-Poulsen (1995) repeated a more comprehensive study where similar unremarkable metabolic differences emerged. Jubrias, Bennett, and Klug (1994) used the same method to study more exhaustive exercise in the forearms of FM patients versus nonpatients. They found that the Pi/Pcr ratios are similar during exercise, but higher metabolic activity (37% vs. 12%) was found in FM patients after the end of exercising. They concluded that the later differences were not related to the exercise regimen, but probably indicate some sarcolemmal abnormality, which should be further investigated. Finally, Simms et al. (1994) found no significant metabolic changes during exercise in the upper trapezius and no significant metabolic change in the tibialis anterior muscles during rest, exercise, and recovery. Their conclusion is also that FM patients demonstrate muscle-energy metabolism similar to that of sedentary controls and that phosphorous energy metabolism is probably not directly related to the etiology of FM.

Because all of the previously reviewed studies found no, or very small and usually insignificant, differences in FM patients' muscle metabolism, it is important to mention that only one controlled study showed major metabolic abnormalities in exercising FM patients, as compared to other pain patients and healthy controls (Eisinger, Plantamura, & Ayavou, 1994). This is a dissident study that definitely needs further serious investigation.

In conclusion, anaerobic exercise capacity, and especially aerobic exercise tolerance, were consistently shown to be lower in FM patients. However, it is almost certain that the lower VO2 max and exercise tolerance in FM patients is more a function of lower effort, due to increased pain, than a defined pathology (Mengshoel, Vøllestad, & Førre, 1995; Nørregaard, Bülow, Lykkegaard, Mehlsen, & Danneskiold-Samsoe, 1997; Sietsema, Cooper, Caro, Leibling, & Louie, 1993). This possibility is always mentioned in the researchers' conclusions but is poorly investigated. The pain and fatigue have probably little to do with peripheral electrical and metabolic mechanisms in the working muscles. We speculate that the perceived exertion, due to lower pain threshold, is mainly centrally mediated. It seems that a statement by Cafarelli, one of the outstanding investigators of healthy muscle threshold, fatigue, and pain, appears to be very adequate to conclude this section: "Muscle sensations arise from both peripheral feedback and central feed-forward, and that both are required for optimal control of the musculature" (Cafarelli, 1988, p.160). It is our impression that a distorted perception of pain, rather than gross cellular malfunction, is the main mechanism that differentiates FM patients from other sedentary healthy people. This different perception seems to greatly influence the irregular participation and poor adherence of FM patients in lifelong exercise regimens despite the clearly documented positive outcomes. However, we cannot absolutely exclude that some peripheral mechanisms may be involved in alteration of the distorted central pain perceptions in FM patients.

Conclusion

Musculoskeletal and neurovascular disorders, including low back, neck, shoulder upper and lower extremities pain, rheumatological diseases, headaches, and fibromyalgia, limit the physical and psychosocial function of people of all ages. These disorders have been estimated to affect about 10% of the U.S. population (Deuster, 1996), and their human, personal, and national costs are staggering. Physical exercise offers major benefits in many of these conditions and seems to have substantial effect on pain, which is a major complaint in the symptomology of all of these disorders.

Indeed, our conclusion based on the review of the relevant literature confirms that physical exercises are a potent remedy in the treatment, prevention, and progression of most of these conditions. Our extensive literature reviews strongly support, with some minor exceptions, the use of various physical exercise regimens as either a sole modality or major ingredient in a multidisciplinary pain-treatment approach. More specifically, the following conclusions can be drawn:

1. Active exercises are not recommended during the acute phase of chronic low back pain (the first 2 to 3 days). However, therapeutic passive exercises may be of some value.
2. Different exercise regimens are strongly recommended during subacute and especially chronic back pain. Actually, very high-intensity local and generalized fitness exercises, including working against increased intensity resistance (e.g., weights) and aerobics, are clearly indicated for treatment, maintenance, and prevention of CLBP.
3. Therapeutic and self-exercise regimens including range-of-motion (ROM) and strength exercises are necessary in the rehabilitation and reconditioning of neck, shoulder, and upper and lower extremities pain disorders.
4. Range-of-motion (ROM) exercises, stretching, and working against resistance (pool therapy, weights, etc.) are strongly recommended in all stages of osteoarthritis and rheumatoid arthritis.
5. Research in the area of headaches and exercise is in a very premature stage to draw robust conclusions. However, various exercise routines seem to benefit most types of headaches. It is clear that exercising during a headache, especially a migraine headache, is not recommended.
6. In fibromyalgia therapy, aerobic exercises are an integral part of the treatment, and that practice is substantiated strongly by our research findings. Anaerobic exercises also seem to have benefits, but need to be further investigated.

Overall, exercise can improve the clinical manifestations of chronic pain conditions.

Yet, it must be stressed that any exercise regimen is best started under the guidance of an exercise specialist and a physician. Following are some general guidelines meant to be used as an adjunct for practicing safe and effective exercise programs already prescribed by a medical professional:

1. Any exercise program should be started slowly. A gradual build-up of the amount of time spent doing a particular exercise task is best. This prevents stress and injury to the body.

2. The exercise program should be paced, and the exerciser should listen to the body. If the body feels tired, pushed or uncomfortable, the doctor should be consulted for advice on how to proceed with the exercise regimen while managing fatigue, pain, or distress.

3. When the body feels fatigued, easier exercise tasks should be substituted for more difficult ones. This keeps the body active and helps maintain this important daily habit.

4. Exercisers should learn proper body positioning for exercising. This can prevent fatigue and injury.

5. Wearing properly fitted exercise equipment, such as footwear, joint protectors, and hand or head gear, can prevent injury.

6. Exercise participants should learn to develop and use larger and stronger joints that can carry strength-training exercise loads.

7. Any exercise regimen should begin and end with adequate warm-up and cooldown periods. Up to 10 minutes of range-of-motion (ROM) exercises per warm-up and cooldown period is common.

8. Exercises should be varied to work different muscle groups. This style of conditioning is key for building strength, endurance, and flexibility.

9. Exercisers should realize that exercising is a lifelong activity that is essential for illness prevention and good health maintenance.

References

Accerro, P., & Braggs, W. J. (1993). Reflex sympathetic dystrophy: Challenges of diagnosis and management. *Journal of the American Academy of Physician Assistants, 16*, 24–31.

Allegrant, J. P. (1996). The role of adjunctive therapy in the management of chronic nonmalignant pain. *The American Journal of Medicine, 101*(Suppl. 1A), 35S–39S.

Altmaier, E. M., Lehmann, T. R., Russell, D. W., Weinstein, J. N., & Kao, C. F (1992). The effectiveness of psychological interventions for the rehabilitation of low back pain: A randomized controlled trial evaluation. *Pain, 49*, 329–335.

American Medical Association (1998). *Health Insight* [Online]. Available at: www.ama-assn.org/insight/spec-on/migraine/whatis/htm.

Arthritis Foundation. (1998). *Living well with arthritis* [Online]. Available at: www.arthritis.org/resource/tips/lwwo.shtml/

Bakker, C., Rutten, M., van Santen-Hoeufft, M., Bolwijn, P., van Doorslaer, E., Bennett, K., & van der Linden, S. (1995). Patient utilities in fibromyalgia and the association with other outcome measures. *Journal of Rheumatology, 22*, 1536–1543.

Bakker, C., van der Linden, S., van Santen Hoeufft, M., Bolwijn, P., & Hidding, A. (1995). Problem elicitation to assess patient priorities in ankylosing spondylitis and fibromyhalgia. *Journal of Rheumatology, 22*, 1304–1310.

Bartels, E. M., & Danneskiold-Samsoe, B. (1986). Histological abnormalities in muscle from patients with certain types of fibrositis. *Lancet, 1*, 755–757.

Baumstark, K. E., & Buckelew, S. P. (1992). Fibromyalgia: Clinical signs, research findings, treatment implications, and future directions. *Annals of Behavioral Medicine, 14*(4), 282–291.

Bengtsson, A., Henriksson, K. G., & Larsson, J. (1986) Reduced high-energy phosphate levels in the painful muscles of patients with primary fibromyalgia. *Arthritis and Rheumatism, 29*, 817–821.

Bennett, R. M. (1989) Physical fitness and muscle metabolism in the fibromyalgia syndrome: An overview. *Journal of Rheumatology, (Suppl.), 19*, 28–29.

Bennett, R. M., Burckhardt, C. S., Clark, S. R., O'Reilly, C. A., Wiens, A. N., & Campbell, S. M. (1996). Group treatment of fibromyalgia: A 6 month outpatient program. *Journal of Rheumatology, 23*, 521–528.

Bentsen, H., Lindgärde, F., & Manthorpe, R. (1997). The effect of dynamic strength back exercise and/or a home training program in 57-year old women with chronic low back pain: Results of prospective randomized study with a 3-year followup period. *Spine, 22*(13), 1494–1500.

Bic, Z., Blix, G., Hopp, H., & Leslie, M. (1998). In search of the ideal treatment for migraine headache. *Medical Hypotheses, 50*, 1–7.

Blake, C., & Garrett, M. (1997). Impact of litigation on quality of life outcomes in patients with chronic low back pain. *The Irish Journal of Medical Science, 166*(3), 124–126.

Blanchard, E. B. (1980). Migraine and tension headache: A meta-analytic review. *Behavior Therapy, 11*, 613–631.

Blanchard E. B., & Andrasik, F. (1982). Psychological assessment and treatment of headache: Recent developments and emerging issues. *Journal of Consulting and Clinical Psychology, 50*, 859–879.

Borenstein, D. (1995). Prevalence and treatment outcome of primary and secondary fibromyalgia in patients with spinal pain. *Spine, 20*(7), 796–800.

Bove, A. A. (1983). Exercise in the elderly. In A. A. Bove & D. T. Lowenthal (Eds.), *Exercise medicine: Physiological principles and clinical applications* (pp. 173–181). Orlando, FL. Academic Press Inc.

Bronfort, G., Goldsmith, C. H., Nelson, C. R., Boline, P. D., & Anderson, A. V. (1996). Trunk exercise combined with spinal manipulative or NSAID therapy for chronic low back pain: A randomized, observer-blinded clinical trial. *Journal of Manipulative Physiological Therapeutics, 19*(9), 570–582.

Buckelew, S. P., Huyser, B., Hewett, J. E., Parker, J. C., Johnson, J. C., Conway, R., & Kay, D. R. (1996). Self-efficacy predicting outcome among fibromyalgia subjects. *Arthritis Care and Research, 9*(2), 97–104.

Buckelew, S. P., Murray, S. E., Hewett, J. E., Johnson, J., & Huyser, B. (1995). Self-efficacy, pain and physical activity among fibromyalgia subjects. *Arthritis Care and Research, 8*(1), 43–50.

Burckhardt, C. S., Mannerkorpi, K., Hedenberg. L, & Bjelle, A. (1994). A randomized, controlled clinical trial of education and physical training for women with fibromyalgia. *Journal of Rheumatology, 21*(4), 714–720.

Buckwalter, J., & Lane, N. (1997). Athletics and osteoarthritis. *The American Journal of Sports Medicine, 25*, 873–881.

Burns, S. H., & Mierau, D. R. (1997). Chiropractic management of low back pain of mechanical origin. In L. G. F. Giles & K. P. Singer (Eds.), *Clinical anatomy and management of low back pain* (pp. 344–357). Oxford, UK: Butterworth-Honemann, Reed Educational and Professional Publishing, Ltd.

Cafarelli, E. (1988). Force sensation in fresh and fatigued human skeletal muscle. In K. B. Fandolf (Ed.), *Exercise and sport sciences reviews* (Vol. 16, pp. 139–168). New York: Macmillan Pub. Co.

Cailliet, R. (1995). *Low back pain syndrome* (5th ed.). Philadelphia: F. A. Davis Company.

Callahan, L. F., Rao, J., & Boutaugh, M. (1996). Arthritis and women's health: Prevalence, impact, and prevention. *American Journal of Preventive Medicine, 12*, 401–409.

Campello, M., Nordin, M., & Weiser, S. (1996). Physical exercise and low back pain. *Scandinavian Journal of Medicine and Science in Sport, 6*(2), 63–72.

Carey, T. S., Garrett, J., Jackman, A., McLaughlin, C., Fryer, J., Smucker, D. R., & The North Carolina Back Pain Project. (1995). The outcomes and costs of care for acute low back pain among patients seen by primary care practitioners, chiropractors, and orthopedic surgeons. *New England Journal of Medicine, 333*, 913–917.

Cherkin, D. C., Deyo, R. A., Street, J. H., Hunt, M., & Barlow, W. (1996). Pitfalls of patient education: Limited success of a program for back pain in primary care. *Spine, 21*, 345–355.

Cherkin, D. C., Deyo, R. A., Wheeler, K., & Ciol, M. A. (1995). Physician views about treating low back pain: The results of a national survey. *Spine, 20*, 1–20.

Clanton, T., & Solcher, B. (1994). Chronic leg pain in the athlete. *Clinical Sports Medicine, 13*, 743–759.

Cooper, C, Inskip, H., Croft, P., Campbell, L., Smith, G., McLaren, M., & Coggon, D. (1998). Individual risk factors for hip osteoarthritis: Obesity, hip, injury, and physical activity. *American Journal of Epidemiology, 147*, 516–522.

D'Amico, D., Centonze, V., Grazzi, L., Leone, M., Richetti, G., & Bussone, G. (1997). Co-existence of migraine and cluster headache: Report of 10 cases and possible pathogenetic implications. *Headache, 37*, 21–25.

Dabis M., Ettinger, W., & Neuhaus, J. (1990). Obesity and osteoarthritis of the knee: Evidence from the National Health and Nutrition Examination Survey (NHANES I). *Seminars in Arthritis and Rheumatology, 20*, 34–41.

Daniels, J. M. (1997). Treatment of occupationally acquired low back pain. *American Family Physician, 55*, 587–596.

de Brujin-Kofman, A. T., Van de Weil, H., Groenman, N. H., Sorbi, M. J., & Klip, E. (1997). Effects of a mass media behavioral treatment for chronic headache: A pilot study. *Headache, 37*, 415–420.

DeMichele, P. L., Pollock, M. L., Graves, J. E., Foster, D. N., Carpenter, D., Garzarella, L., Brechue, W., & Fulton, M. (1997). Isometric torso rotation strength: Effect of training frequency on its development. *Archives of Physical Medicine and Rehabilitation, 78*, 64–69.

Deuster, P. A., (1996). Exercise in the prevention and treatment of chronic disorders. *Women's Health Issues, 6*(6), 320–331.

Deyo, R. A. (1998, August). Low back pain. *Scientific American, 279*, 49–53.

Deyo, R. A., & Phillips, W. R. (1996). Low back pain: A primary challenge. *Spine, 21*, 2826–2832.

Dubbert, P. (1992). Exercise in behavioral medicine. *Journal of Consulting and Clinical Psychology, 60*, 613–618.

Eisenberg, D. M., Kessler, R. C., Foster, C., Norlock, R. E., Calkins, D. R., & Delbanco, T. L. (1993). Unconventional medicine in the United States: Prevalence, costs and patterns of use. *New England Journal of Medicine, 328*(4), 246–252.

Eisinger, J., Plantamura, A., & Ayavou, T. (1994). Glycolysis abnormalities in fibromyalgia. *Journal of the American College of Nutrition, 13*(2), 144–148.

Ettinger, W. H., Burns, R., Messier, S. P., Applegate, W.,

Rejeski, W. J., Morgan, T., Shumaker, S., Berry, M. J., O'Toole, M., Monu, J., & Craven, T. (1997). A randomized trial comparing aerobic exercise and resistance exercise with a health education program in older adults with knee osteoarthritis. *Journal of the American Medical Association, 277*, 25–31.

Faas, A. (1996). Exercises: Which ones are worth trying, for which patients, and when? *Spine, 21*(24), 2874–2878.

Faas, A., van Eijk, J. Th. M., Chavannes, A. W., & Gubbels, J. W. (1995). A randomized trial of exercise therapy in patients with acute low back pain: Efficacy on sickness absence. *Spine, 20*, 941–947.

Farrar, D. J., Locke, S. E., & Kantrowitz, F. G., (1995). Chronic fatigue syndrome I: Etiology and pathogenesis. *Behavioral Medicine, 21*, 5–16.

Felson D. T., Zhang, Y., Anthony, J. M., Naimark, A., & Anderson, J. J. (1992). Weight loss reduces the risk for symptomatic osteoarthritis in women: The Framingham Study. *Annals of Internal Medicine, 116*, 535–539.

Flavell, H. A., Carrafa, G. P., Thomas, C. H., & Disler, P. B. (1996). Managing chronic back pain: Impact of an interdisciplinary team approach. *Medical Journal of Australia, 165*(5), 253–255.

Foltz-Gray, D. (1997). In the swim. *Arthritis Today, 10*, 18–24.

Fordyce, W. (1976). *Behavioral methods for chronic pain and illness.* St. Louis: Mosby.

Fox, E. L. (1979). *Sports physiology.* Philadelphia: W. B. Saunders Company.

Fuchs, Z., & Zaichkowsky, L. (1997). Exercise in aging and pain control. In D. I. Mostofsky, D. & J. Lomranz (Eds.), *Handbook of pain and aging* (pp. 347–364). New York: Plenum Press.

Gatchel, R. J., & Turk, D. C. (1996). *Psychological approaches to pain management, A practitioner's guidebook.* New York: Guilford Press.

George, E., Creamer, P., & Dieppe, P. (1994). Clinical subsets of osteoarthritis. *The Journal of Musculoskeletal Medicine, 11*, 14–29.

Godfrey, R. G. (1996). A guide to the understanding and use of tricyclic antidepressants in the overall management of fibromyalgia and other chronic pain syndromes. *Archives of Internal Medicine, 156*, 1047–1052.

Goldenberg, D. L. (1994). Fibromyalgia, chronic fatigue syndrome and myofascial pain syndrome. *Current Opinions in Rheumatology, 6*, 223–233.

Gotlieb, H., Strite, L. C., Koller, R., Madorsky, A., Hockersmith, V., Kleeman, M., & Wagner, J. (1977). Comprehensive rehabilitation of patients having chronic low back pain. *Archives of Physical Medicine and Rehabilitation, 58*, 101–108.

Granges, G., Zilko, P., & Littlejohn, G. O. (1994). Fibromyalgia syndrome: Assessment of the severity of the condition 2 years after diagnosis. *Journal of Rheumatology, 21*(3), 523–529.

Gremillion, R. B., & Vollenhoven, R. F. (1998).

Rheumatoid arthritis: Designing and implementing a treatment plan. *POSTGRADUATE Medicine, 103*, 103–123.

Hakkinen, A., Malkia, E., Hakkinen, K., Jappinen, I., Laitinen, L., & Hannonen, P. (1997). Effects of detraining subsequent to strength training on neuromuscular function in patients with inflammatory arthritis. *British Journal of Rheumatology, 36*, 1075–1081.

Hall, H. (1989). The Back School. In C. D. Tollison & M. L. Kriegel (Eds.), *Interdisciplinary rehabilitation of low back pain* (pp. 291–304). Baltimore, MD: Williams and Wilkins.

Hammill, J., Cook, T., & Rosecrance, J. (1996). Effectiveness of a physical therapy regime in the treatment of tension-type headache. *Headache, 36*, 149–153.

Hartigan, C., Miller, L., & Liewehr, S. C. (1996). Rehabilitation of acute and subacute low back and neck pain in the work-injured patient. *Orthopedic Clinics of North America, 27*(4), 841–860.

Haskell, W. L. (1994). Health consequences of physical activity: Understanding and challenges regarding dose-response. *The Official Journal of the American College of Sports Medicine, 26*, 649–660.

Heller, A. (1994). Carpal tunnel syndrome—an industrial epidemic. *Clinical Review, 7/8*, 61–74.

Hewett, J. E., Buckelew, S. P., Johnson, J. C., Shaw, S. E., Huyser, B., & Zheng Fu, N. G. (1995). Selection of measures suitable for evaluating change in fibromyalgia clinical trials. *Journal of Rheumatology, 22*, 2307–2312.

Hides, J. A., Richardson, C. A., & Jull, G. A. (1996). Multifidus muscle recovery is not automatic after resolution of acute, first episode low back pain. *Spine, 21*(23), 2763–2769.

Hørven Wigers, S., Stiles, T. C., & Vogel, P. A. (1996). Effects of aerobic exercise versus stress management treatment in fibromyalgia. *Scandinavian Journal of Rheumatology, 25*, 77–86.

Hupli, M., Hurri, H., Luoto, S., Risteli, L., Vanharanta, H., & Risteli, J. (1997). Low synthesis rate of type I procollagen is normalized during active back rehabilitation. *Spine, 22*(8), 850–854.

Hutchinson, M., & Ireland, M. (1994). Common compartment syndromes in athletes. *Sports Medicine, 17*, 200–208.

Huyser, B., Buckeley, S. P., Hewett, J. E., & Johnson, J. C. (1997). Factors affecting adherence in rehabilitation interventions for individuals with fibromyalgia. *Rehabilitation Psychology, 42*(2), 75–91.

International Headache Society. (1988). Classification and diagnostic criteria for headache disorders, cranial neuralgias and facial pain. *Cephalalgia, 8* (Suppl. 7), 1–96.

Jacobsen, S., Jensen, K. E., Thomsen, C., Danneskiold-Samsoe, B., & Henriksen, O. (1992). 31P Magnetic resonance spectroscopy of skeletal muscle in patients with fibromyalgia. *Journal of Rheumatology, 19*(10), 1600–1603.

Jacobsen, S., Wildeschiodtz, G., & Danneskiold-Samsoe, B. (1991) Isokinetic and isometric muscle strength combined with transcutaneous electrical muscle stimulation in primary fibromyalgia syndrome. *Journal of Rheumatology, 18*, 1390–1393.

Jensen, R., Bendsten, L., & Olsen, J. (1998). Muscular factors are of importance in tension-type headache. *Headache, 38*, 10–17.

Jordan, A., & Ostergaard, K. (1996). Rehabilitation of neck and shoulder pain in primary health care clinics. *Journal of Manipulative Physiological Therapies, 19*, 32–36.

Jubrias, S. A., Bennett, R. M., & Klug, G. A. (1994). Increased incidence of a resonance in the phosphodiester region of 31P nuclear magnetic resonance spectra in the skeletal muscle of fibromyalgia patients. *Arthritis and Rheumatism*, 37(6), 801–807.

Karas, B. E., Cohn, S., & Conrad, K. M., (1996). Back injury prevention interventions in the workplace: An integrative review. *American Association of Occupational Health Nurses Journal, 44*(4), 189–196.

Katz, R. T. (1994). Carpal tunnel syndrome: A practical review. *American Family Physician, 49*, 1371–1379.

Koes, B. W., Bouter, L. M., Beckerman, H., van der Heizden, G. J., & Knipschild, P. G., (1991). Physiotherapy exercises and back pain: A blinded review. *British Medical Journal, 302*, 1572–1574.

Koes, B. W., Bouter, L. M., & van der Heizden, G. J. (1995). Methodological quality of randomized clinical trials on treatment efficacy in low back pain. *Spine, 20*(2), 228–235.

Komatireddy, G. C., Leitch, R. W., Cella, K., Browning, G., & Minor, M. (1997). Efficacy of low load resistive muscle training in patients with rheumatoid arthritis Functional Class II and II. *Journal of Rheumatology, 24*, 1531–1539.

La Croix, A. Z., Newton, K. M., Leville, S. G., & Wallace, J. (1997). Healthy aging: A women's issue. *Western Journal of Medicine, 167*, 220–232.

Lahad, A., Malter, A. D., Berg, A. O., & Deyo, R. A. (1994). The effectiveness of four interventions for the prevention of low back pain. *Journal of the American Medical Association, 272*(16), 1286–1291.

Lane, N. E., & Thompson, J. M. (1997). Management of osteoarthritis in the primary care setting: An evidence-based approach to treatment. *American Journal of Medicine, 103* (Suppl. 6A), 25S–30S.

Leonardi, M., Musico, M., & Nappi, G. (1998). Headache as a major public health problem: Current status. *Cephalalgia, 18* (Suppl. 21), 66–69.

Linchitz, R. M. (1987). *Life without pain.* Reading, MA: Addison-Wesley Publication Co.

Lindh, M. H., Johansson, L. G., Hedberg, M., & Grimsby, G. L. (1994). Studies on maximal voluntary muscle contraction in patients with fibromyalgia. *Archives of Physical Medicine and Rehabilitation, 75*, 1217–1222.

Ljunggren, A. E., Weber, H., Kogstad, O., Thom, E., & Kirkesola, G., (1997). Effect of exercise on sick leave due to low back pain: A randomized, comparative, long-term study. *Spine, 22*(14), 1610–1617.

Lobstein, D. D., Rasmussen, C. L., Dunphy, G. E., & Dunphy, M. J. (1989). Beta-endorphin and components of depression as a powerful discriminators between joggers and sedentary middle-aged men. *Journal of Psychosomatic Research, 33*(3), 293–305.

MacIntyre, D. L., Reid, W. D., & McKenzie, D. C. (1995). Delayed muscle soreness: The inflammatory response to muscle injury and its clinical implications. *Sports Medicine, 20*(1), 24–40.

Maizels, M. (1998). Topic in primary care medicine: The clinician's approach to the management of headache. *Western Journal of Medicine, 168*, 203–212.

Mälkiä, E., & Kannus, B. (1996). Editorial: Low back pain B to exercise or not to exercise? *Scandinavian Journal of Medicine and Science in Sport, 6*, 61–62.

Mälkiä, E., & Ljunggren, A. E. (1996). Exercise programs for subjects with low back disorders. *Scandinavian Journal of Medicine and Science in Sport, 6*, 73–81.

Malmivaara, A., Häkkinen, U., Aro, T., Heinrichs, M. J., Koskenniemi, L., Kuosma, E., Lappi, S., Paloheimo, R., Servo, C., Vaaranen, V., & Hernbrg, S. (1995). The treatment of acute low back pain: Bed rest, exercises, or ordinary activity? *New England Journal of Medicine, 332*(6), 351–355.

Manniche, C. (1995). Assessment and exercise in low back pain. With special reference to the management of pain and disability following first time lumbar disc surgery. *Danish Medical Bulletin, 42*(4), 301–313.

Manniche, C. (1996). Clinical benefit of intensive dynamic exercises for low back pain. *Scandinavian Journal of Medicine and Science in Sport, 6*(2), 82–87.

Manniche, C., Hesselsøe, G., Bentzen, L., Christensen, I., & Lundberg, E. (1988). Clinical trial of intensive muscle training for chronic low back pain. *Lancet*, ii *24/31.* 1473–1476.

Manniche, C., Lundberg, E., Christensen, I., Bentzen, L., & Hesselsøe, G. (1991). Intensive dynamic back exercises for chronic low back pain: A clinical trial. *Pain, 47*(1).

Marlowe, S. M. (1994). It's time to stop treating arthritis generically. *Advance PA, 1,* 15–16.

Martin, L., Nutting, A., Macintosh, B. R., Edworthy, S. M., Butterwick, D., & Cook, J. (1996). An exercise program in the treatment of fibromyalgia. *Journal of Rheumatology, 23*, 1050–1053.

McCain, G. A. (1986). Role of physical fitness training in the fibrositis/fibromyalgia syndrome. *The American Journal of Medicine, 81* (Suppl. 3A), 73–77.

McCain, G. A., Bell, D. A., Mai, F. M., & Halliday, P. D. (1988). A controlled study of the effects of a supervised cardiovascular fitness training program on the manifestation of primary fibromyalgia. *Arthritis and Rheumatism, 31*(9), 1135 B1141.

McCracken, L. M., Zayfert, C., & Gross, R. T. (1992). The pain anxiety symptoms scale: Development and validation of a scale to measure fear of pain. *Pain, 50*, 67–73.

McGill, S. M. (1997). Distribution of tissue loads in the

low back during a variety of daily and rehabilitation tasks. *Journal of Rehabilitation Research and Development, 34*(4), 448–458.

Mengshoel, A. M., Saugen, E., Førre, Ø., & Vøllestad, N. K. (1995). Muscle fatigue in early fibromyalgia. *Journal of Rheumatology, 22,* 143–150.

Mengshoel, A. M., Vøllestad, N. K., & Førre, Ø. (1995). Pain and fatigue induced by exercise in fibromyalgia patients and sedentary healthy subjects. *Clinical and Experimental Rheumatology, 13,* 477–482.

Miller, T. A., Gabrielle, M. A., & Gandevia, S. C. (1996) Muscle force, perceived effort, and voluntary activation of the elbow flexors assessed with sensitive twitch interpolation and fibromyalgia. *Journal of Rheumatology, 23,* 1621–1627.

Moldofsky, H., & Scarlsbrick, P. (1976). Induction of neurasthenic musculoskeletal pain syndrome by selective sleep stage deprivation. *Psychosomatic Medicine, 38,* 35–44.

Murphy, D., Lindsay, S., & Williams, A. C. (1997). Chronic low back pain: Predictions of pain and relationship to anxiety and avoidance. *Behavioral Research and Therapy, 35*(3), 231–238.

Nasim, A. (1997). Surgical decompression of thoracic outlet syndrome; Is it a worthwhile procedure? *The Royal College of Surgeons of Edinborough, 42,* 319–323.

National Institutes of Health: Consensus Development Conference Statement. (1986). *The Integrated Approach to the Management of Pain.* (3). Bethesda, MD: U.S. Department of Health and Human Services.

National Institute of Neurological Disorders and Stroke. (1996). *Thoracic outlet syndrome* [Online]. Available at www.ninds.nih.gov/healinfo/disorder/thoracic/thoracic/htm.

Nelson, B. W., O'Reilly, E., Miller M., Hogan, M., Wegner, J. A., & Kelly, C. (1995). The clinical effects of intensive, specific exercise on chronic low back pain: A controlled study of 895 consecutive patients with 1-year followup. *Orthopedics, 18*(10), 971–981.

Neuberger, G. B., Press A. N., Lindsley H. B., Hinton R., Cagle P. E., Carlson K., Scott S., Dahl J., & Kramer B. (1997). Effects of exercise on fatigue, aerobic fitness, and disease activity measures in persons with rheumatoid arthritis. *Research in Nursing and Health, 20,* 95–204.

Newcomber, K., & Jurisson, M. I. (1994). Rheumatoid arthritis: The role of physical therapy. *The Journal of Musculoskeletal Medicine, 11,* 14–26.

Nicholas, M. K., Wilson, P. H., & Goyen, J. (1992). Comparison of cognitive-behavioral group treatment and an alternative nonpsychological treatment for chronic low back pain. *Pain, 48,* 339–347.

Nichols, D. S., & Glenn, T. M. (1994). The effects of aerobic exercise on pain perception, affect, and level of disability in individuals with fibromyalgia. *Physical Therapy, 74,* 327–332.

NIH Technology Assessment Panel. (1996). Special communication: Integration of behavioral and relaxation approaches into the treatment of chronic pain and insomnia. *Journal of the American Medical Association, 276,* 313–318.

Nordin, M. (1995). Back pain: Lessons from patient education [Patient Education 2000 Congress, 1994, Geneva, Switzerland]. *Patient Education & Counseling, 26*(1–3), 67–70.

Nørregaard, J., Bülow, P. M., & Danneskiold-Samsoe, B. (1994). Muscle strength, voluntary activation, twitch properties and endurance in patients with fibromyalgia. *Journal of Neurology, Neurosurgery, and Psychiatry, 57,* 1106–1111.

Nørregaard, J., Bülow, P. M., Lykkegaard, J. J., Mehlsen, J., & Danneskiold-Samsoe, B. (1997). Muscle strength, working capacity and effort in patients with fibromyalgia. *Scandinavian Journal of Rehabilitation Medicine, 29,* 97–102.

Nørregaard, J., Bülow, P. M., Mehlsan, J., & Danneskiold-Samsoe, B. (1994) Biochemical changes in relation to a maximal exercise test in patients with fibromyalgia. *Clinical Physiology, 14*(2), 159–167.

Pate, R., Pratt, M, Blair, S. N., Haskell, W. L., Macera, C. A., Bouchard, C., Buchner, D., Ettinger, W., Heath, G. W., King, A. C., Kriska, A., Leon, A. S., Marcus, B. H., Morris, J., Paffenbarger Jr., R. S., Patrick K., Polloc, M. L., Rippe, J. J., Sallis, J., & Wilmore, J. H. (1995). Physical activity and public health: A recommendation from the Centers for Disease Control and Prevention and the American College of Sports Medicine. *Journal of the American Medical Association, 273*(5), 402–407.

Physical Therapy Corner. (1998). *Thoracic outlet syndrome: More than just a pain in the neck* [Online]. Available at www.nismat.org/ptcor/thoracic_outlet/index.html.

Rainville, J., Sobel, J., Hartigan, C., Monlux, G., & Bean, J., (1997). Decreasing disability in chronic back pain through aggressive spine rehabilitation. *Journal of Rehabilitation Research and Development, 34*(4), 383–393.

Rall, L. C., Meydani, S. N., Kehayias, J., J., Dawson-Huges, B., & Roubenoff, R. (1996). The effects of progressive resistance training in rheumatoid arthritis. *Arthritis and Rheumatism, 39,* 415–426.

Reflex Sympathetic Dystrophy Association. (1998). *Hope* [Online]. Available at: www.rsdshope.org/medical/medical/html.

Reflex Sympathetic Dystrophy Syndrome Association of America. (1998). *Reflex sympathetic dystrophy syndrome* [Online]. Available at: www.rsdsd.org/#What.

Repetitive Motion Injuries. (1998). *Repetitive motion disorders* [Online]. Available at: www.dogpile.com/repetitive motion disorders/ IM-airport.com/html.

Reveille, J. D. (1997). Soft-tissue rheumatism: Diagnosis and treatment [Review]. *American Journal of Medicine, 102*(1A), 23S B29S.

Revel, M. (1995). Rehabilitation of low back pain patients: A review. *Revue de Rhumatisme English Edition, 62,* 35–44.

Ross, C. (1997). A comparison of osteoarthritis and rheumatoid arthritis: Diagnosis and treatment. *Nurse Practitioner, 22,* 20–28.

Saal, J. A. (1996). Natural history and nonoperative

treatment of lumbar disc herniation. *Spine, 21*(24 Suppl), 2S–9S.

Sarno, J. E. (1998). *The mindbody prescription: Healing the body, healing the pain.* New York: Warner Books.

Scheer, S. J., Radack, K. L., & O'Brien, D. R., Jr. (1995). Randomized controlled trials in industrial low back pain relating to return to work. Part 1. Acute interventions. *Archives of Physical Medicine and Rehabilitation, 76,* 966–973.

Scheer, S. J., Watanabe, T. K., & Radack, K. L. (1997). Randomized controlled trials in industrial low back pain. Part 3. Subacute/chronic pain interventions. *Archives of Physical Medicine and Rehabilitation, 78,* 414–423.

Schepsis, A. A., & Lynch, G. (1996). Exertional compartment syndromes of the lower extremity. *Current Opinion in Rheumatology, 8,* 143–147.

Schlike, J., Johnson, G., Housh, T., & O'Dell, J. (1996). Effects of muscle-strength training on the functional status of patients with osteoarthritis of the knee joint. *Nursing Research, 45,* 68–72.

Shekelle, P. G., Adams, A. H., Chassin, M. R., Hurwitz, E. L., & Brook, R. H. (1992). Spinal manipulation for low back pain. *Annals of Internal Medicine, 117,* 590–598.

Shekelle, P. G., Markovich, M., & Louie, R. (1995). Comparing the costs between provider types of episodes of back pain care. *Spine, 20,* 221–227.

Shepard R. J., & Shek, P. N. (1997). Rheumatoid disorders, physical activity, and training with particular reference to rheumatoid arthritis. *Exercise, Immunology, Review, 3,* 53–67.

Shields, R. K., & Givens Heiss, D., (1997). An electromyographic comparison of abdominal muscle synergies during curl and double straight leg lowering exercises with control of the pelvic position. *Spine, 22*(16), 1871–1879.

Sietsema, K. E., Cooper, D. M., Caro, X., Leibling, M. R., & Louie, J. S. (1993). Oxygen uptake during exercise in patients with primary fibromyalgia syndrome. *Journal of Rheumatology, 20*(5), 860–865.

Simms, R. W., Roy, S. H., Hrovat, M., Anderson, J. J., Skrinar, G., LePocle, S. R., Zerbini, C. A., de Luca, C., & Jolesz, F. (1994), Lack of association between fibromyalgia syndrome and abnormalities in muscle energy metabolism. *Arthritis and Rheumatism, 37*(6), 791–800.

Smidt, G. L., Blanpied, P. R., & White, W. R. (1989). Exploration of mechanical and electromyographic responses of trunk muscles to high-intensity resistive exercise. *Spine, 14*(8), 815–830.

Sobel, D., & Klein, A. C. (1994). *Backache: When exercises work.* New York: St. Martin's Press.

Sollner, W., & Doering, S. (1997). Psychologishe therapieverfahren bei chronischen nicht-radikularen ruckenschmerzenk. *Orthopade, 26*(6), 535–543.

Soric, R. (1989). Role of physical medicine modalities, In C. D. Tollisson & M. L. Kriegel (Eds.), *Interdisciplinary rehabilitation of low back pain* (pp. 101–105). Baltimore, MD: William and Wilkins.

Stenstrom, C. H., Arge, B., & Sundbom, A. (1997). Home exercise and compliance in inflammatory rheumatic disease: A prospective clinical trial. *The Journal of Rheumatology, 24,* 470–480.

Stewart, W. F., Linet, M. S., Celentrano, D. D., & Reed, M. L. (1991). Prevalence of migraine headache in the United States. Relation to age, income, race, and other sociodemiographic factors. *American Journal of Epidemiology, 134,* 1111–1120.

Sullivan, M. S., Kues, J. M., & Mayhew, T. P. (1996). Treatment categories for low back pain: A methodological approach. *Journal of Orthopedic and Sport Physical Therapy, 24*(6), 359–364.

Swain, R., & Kaplan, B. (1997). Diagnosis, prophylaxis and treatment of headache in the athlete. *Southern Medical Journal, 90,* 878–888.

Szabo, R., & Madison, M. (1992). Carpal tunnel syndrome. *Orthopedic Clinics of North America, 23,* 103–108.

Teasell, R. W., & Harth, M. (1996). Functional restoration: Returning patients with chronic low back pain to work: Revolution or fad? *Spine, 21*(7), 844–847.

Thorén, P., Floras, J. S., Hoffmann, P., & Seals, D. R. (1990). Endorphins and exercise: Physiological mechanisms and clinical applications. *Medicine and Science in Sports and Exercise, 22*(4), 417–428.

Turner, J. A., Clancy, S., McQuade, K. J., & Cardenas, D. D. (1990). Effectiveness of behavioral therapy for chronic low back pain: A component analysis. *Journal of Consulting and Clinical Psychology, 58*(5), 573–579.

Twomey, L., & Taylor, J. (1995). Exercise and spinal manipulation in the treatment of low back pain. *Spine, 20*(5), 615–619.

Exercise and arthritis: the importance of a regular program. [University of California at Berkeley Wellness Letter]. (1994). Berkeley: University of California at Berkeley Publishers.

Van Tulder, M. W., Koes, B. W., & Bouter, L. M., (1997). Conservative treatment of acute and chronic nonspecific low back pain: A systematic review of randomized controlled trials of the most common interventions. *Spine, 22*(18), 2128–2156.

Vestergaard-Poulsen, P., Thomsen, C., Nørregaard, J., Bülow, P., Sinkjaer, T., & Henriksen, O. (1995). P NMR spectroscopy and electromyography during exercise and recovery in patients with fibromyalgia. *Journal of Rheumatology, 22,* 1544–1551.

Webster's new collegiate dictionary (2nd ed.). (1981). Springfield: G. & C. Merriam Company.

Wheeler, A. H. (1995). Diagnosis and management of low back pain and sciatica. *American Family Physician, 52*(5), 1333–1341.

Wheeler, A. H., & Hanley, E. N., Jr. (1995). Nonoperative treatment for low back pain: Rest to restoration. *Spine, 20*(3), 375–378.

Wilke, W. S. (1995). Treatment of "resistant" fibromyalgia [Review]. *Rheumatic Diseases Clinics of North America*, *21*(1), 247–260.

Wilke, W. S. (1996). Fibromyalgia: Recognizing and addressing the multiple interrelated factors. *Postgraduate Medicine*, *100*(1), 153–170.

Wolfe, F., Smythe, H. A., Yunus, M. B., Bennett, R. M., Bombardier, C., Goldenberg, D., Tugwell I., Campbell, P., Abeles, S. M., Clark, P., Fam, A. G., Farber, S. J., Fiechtner, J. J., Franklin, C. M., Gatter, R. A., Hamaty, D., Lessard, J., Lichtbroun, A. S., Masi, A. T., McCain, G. A., Reynolds, W. J., Romano, T. J., Russel, I. J., & Sheon, R. P. (1990). The American College of Rheumatology 1990 criteria for the classification of fibromyalgia. *Arthritis and Rheumatism, 33*(2), 160–172.

Yamamoto, S. (1997). A new trend in the study of low back pain in workplaces. *Industrial Health*, *35*, 173–185.

Yunus, M. B., Kalyan-Raman, U. P., Kalyan-Raman, K., & Masi, A. T. (1986). Pathologic changes in muscle in primary fibromyalgia syndrome. *American Journal of Medicine*, (Suppl. 3A), *81*, 38–42.

Yunus, M. B., Masi, A. T., Calabro, J. J., Miller, K. A., & Feigenbaum, S. L. (1981). Primary fibromyalgia (fibrositis): Clinical study of 50 patients with matched normal controls. *Seminars in Arthritis and Rheumatism, 11*, 151–171.

14
Sleep Problems

Glenn S. Brassington

The purpose of this chapter is to provide current knowledge about the relationship between sleep problems and exercise behavior and to offer practical guidelines for prescribing exercise to patients with sleep problems. This chapter consists of five parts:

- First, the importance of continuing to study sleep and to develop effective and non-pharmacological methods for treating sleep problems is discussed.
- Second, typically studied sleep parameters are presented so that the reader can gain an understanding of how sleep variables have been assessed in the scientific literature.
- Third, research on exercise as a treatment for sleep problems is presented with an emphasis on synthesizing the results from review articles, meta analyses, and true experiments.
- Fourth, mechanisms that have been proposed to explain how exercise may improve sleep are outlined.
- Finally, future directions for research into the medical application of exercise in the treatment of sleep problems are proposed.

Before beginning to discuss the material outlined above, it is important for the reader to be aware that very little literature is available about the impact of exercise on specific sleep disorders (e.g., obstructive sleep apnea), but, rather, investigations conducted on the relationship between sleep and exercise have been concerned with physiological variables, sleep quality, or symptoms of what is called insomnia rather than a particular sleep disorder. For this reason, the term sleep *problems* will be used when talking about sleep rather than the term sleep *disorders*.

The Importance of Studying Sleep Problems

Sleep problems pervade our society. In the 1993 *Wake Up America: A National Sleep Alert Report of the National Commission on Sleep Disorders Research* presented to Congress, researchers stated that approximately 70 million Americans have a problem sleeping, with 60% of this group having a chronic sleep disorder (National Commission on Sleep Disorders Research, 1993). The authors of the report stated that sleep problems affect men and women of every age, race, and socioeconomic class. Further, it was estimated that if the population of the U.S. increases according to the Bureau of Census projections, and the incidence and prevalence of sleep problems remain unchanged, by the year 2010, approximately 79 million Americans will have difficulty falling asleep, and approximately 40 million Americans will experience debilitating levels of daytime sleepiness. Interestingly, sleep problems are not limited to Americans. In a recent study of 2,398 Italian community-dwelling adults aged 65 years or older, researchers reported the prevalence of insomnia as 36% in men and 54% in women (Maggi et al., 1998). In terms of major sleep disorders, it is estimated that obstructive sleep apnea affects 5 to 10 million Americans, whereas narcolepsy affects 250,000 to 375,000 Americans (National Commission on Sleep Disorders Research).

Disturbed sleep can have a profound effect on the quality of life of patients. Patients report a great deal of frustration and anxiety about not being able to fall asleep at night knowing that they will in all likelihood perform poorly the next day while trying to meet their occupational and family responsibilities. However, beyond the level of frustration associated with having trouble falling asleep at night is the effect that poor sleep can have on the level of one's daytime functioning. Poor sleep has been shown to be associated with depressed mood and reduced motivation. Poor sleep is not only associated with symptoms of depression, but it is also associated with reduced mental acuity (i.e., concentration, memory, cognitive processing) and poor physical performance.

Sleep problems can sap the enjoyment from a person's life and diminish motivation to such an extent that the individual cannot function. Although many people make the connection between poor sleep and feeling a bit "blue," they often do not believe that their physical performance is hindered by a lack of quality sleep. Unfortunately, this belief is misguided and has often been promoted outside the sleep research community in introductory textbooks (e.g., Weiten, 1995). There

exists a great deal of data connecting inadequate amounts of quality sleep with poor work performance as well as occupational, automotive, and other physical injuries. In a recent meta-analysis of 19 original research studies, researchers reported that sleep deprivation strongly impaired human functioning (Pilcher & Huffcutt, 1996). The results of the meta-analysis concluded that sleep-deprived subjects performed at a level 1.37 standard deviations lower than that of the nonsleep-deprived subjects. Another way of representing the findings was that a person at the 50th percentile in the deprived group performed roughly equivalent to a person at the 9th percentile in the nondeprived group. Mood was found to be even more strongly affected by sleep deprivation. (For a more thorough discussion of the effect of sleep deprivation and sleepiness on performance, see Monk, 1991.)

In addition to the prevalence of sleep problems and the impact they have on an individual's happiness and performance, sleep problems contribute to health care costs. It has been reported that habitual short sleepers are at risk of increased morbidity and mortality. A 9-year followup study found that individuals sleeping fewer than 6 hours each night had a 70% higher mortality rate as compared to those who slept 7 or 8 hours per night (National Commission of Sleep Disorders Research, 1993). This relationship remained significant even after controlling for age, gender, race, smoking history, physical inactivity, alcohol consumption, social support, and physical health (National Commission of Sleep Disorders Research). Further, shift workers have been observed to have greater mortality and morbidity as well as a higher incidence of illnesses such as gastrointestinal and cardiovascular disorders than do nonshift workers. Health care costs attributable to sleep problems were estimated to be $46 billion a year by an economist working for the National Commission on Sleep Disorders Research (National Commission of Sleep Disorders Research).

Another consequence of poor sleep that has received a great deal of attention is motor vehicle accidents. Driver sleepiness has been estimated to be a causative factor in 1% to 3% of all motor vehicle accidents (Lyznicki, Doege, Davis, & Williams, 1998; Webb, 1995). The National Highway Traffic Safety Administration (NHTSA) claims that 100,000 police-reported automobile accidents each year have sleepiness as a causative factor. In addition, the NHTSA claims that 4% of all fatal motor vehicle accidents or greater than 1,500 deaths can be attributed to driver sleepinesss. Finally, even the medical treatment of sleep problems can have adverse effects. For example, prescription and over-the-counter hypnotics may have adverse effects on individuals, especially older adults, that may include daytime sleepiness, fall, confusion, and harmful interactions with other medications (Morin & Azrin, 1988). Therefore, in terms of patient quality of life, lost productivity, health care costs, and accidents, the impact of sleep problems in American society is staggering.

Measuring Sleep

Sleep includes two distinct states called non-rapid eye movement (non-REM) and rapid eye movement (REM) sleep. These two states of sleep are very different from one another, as different as the sleeping and waking states. These two states of sleep are defined and described by continuous electroencephalographic (EEG), electro-oculographic (EOG), and electromyographic (EMG) measurements. Non-REM consists of a relatively inactive physiological state. Non-REM sleep generally occurs first in the transition from wakefulness to sleep and occupies 75–80% of sleep. Non-REM sleep is divided into four states (i.e., stages 1, 2, 3, and 4) that roughly

correspond to the depth of sleep. Stage 1 is a transitional phase from waking to sleep, whereas stage 2 is usually considered the onset of sleep. During stages 3 and 4, sleep gradually becomes deeper. These two stages of sleep are collectively know as slow-wave sleep (SWS). SWS consists of high-amplitude and low-frequency waves on the EEG. During SWS, body oxygen consumption is lowest, and awakening a person is more difficult than at the earlier stages (Chokroverty, 1999). There are internationally accepted standards for staging sleep that were documented in 1968 (Rechtschaffen & Kales, 1968). However, recently computer-facilitated staging of sleep coupled with sophisticated statistical techniques (e.g., spectral analysis) have been used to more accurately quantify sleep physiology (Dijk, Hayes, & Czeisler, 1993; Geering, Achermann, Eggimann, 1993). Unlike the stages of non-REM sleep, REM sleep is characterized by rapid eye movements, higher levels of brain activity, increases in blood flow, elevated heart rate, loss of temperature regulation, and paralysis of some muscles, including those of the chin. Non-REM sleep alternates cyclically with REM sleep approximately every 90–100 minutes throughout the night. Non-REM sleep usually occurs first and accounts for approximately 75–80% of sleep, whereas REM sleep accounts for 20–25% of each night's sleep (National Commission of Sleep Disorders Research, 1993).

Although most studies that have examined the relationship between exercise and sleep have operationalized sleep using polysomnography, some researchers have employed self-report measures of sleep. Self-report measures used in the literature to date have either been retrospective questionnaires that ask subjects to recall characteristics of their sleep over a certain period of time (e.g., 30 days) or prospective sleep diaries. An example of one of the more popular retrospective measures is the Pittsburgh Sleep Quality Index (Buysee, Reynolds, Monk, Berman, & Kupfer, 1989). The PSQI is a self-rated questionnaire that assesses sleep quality and disturbances over a 30-day period. Seven 3-point component scores are derived from 19 individual items (e.g., subjective sleep quality, sleep latency, sleep duration, habitual sleep efficiency, sleep disturbances, use of sleep medication, and daytime dysfunction). These component scores are totaled to yield a global score.

Researchers employing prospective recordings of sleep typically have asked subjects to complete a 14-day sleep diary, making entries each morning upon awakening and each evening upon retiring to bed. Subjects are asked to record the time they went to bed, the approximate time they fell asleep, the number of times they awoke during the night and for approximately how long, the time they awoke in the morning, the total time they slept, the number of daytime naps, and the length of each nap (Brassington & Hicks, 1995). Other information (e.g., medication use) may be collected for subjects completing sleep diaries (King, Oman, Brassington, Bliwise, & Haskell, 1997). Although self-report measures do not capture as precisely some of sleep as polysomnography (e.g., sleep onset latency, sleep duration), self-report measures provide information about a subject's perception of his or her sleep, which, in terms of patient distress, is important information. Also, it may be the case for some subjects that they experience their sleep as restless whereas the architecture of their sleep appears normal based on polysomnographic measurements.

In addition to directly assessing nighttime sleep, many researchers have looked to levels of daytime alertness or sleepiness as a means of assessing the quality of a person's sleep. It has been demonstrated that daytime sleepiness results from inadequate nighttime sleep rather than external conditions such as attending a boring lecture or engaging in a tedious work assignment (Monk, 1991). The gold standard for assessing daytime sleepiness is the Multiple Sleep Latency Test (MSLT; Carskadon, Dement, & Mitler, 1986). During the MSLT, subjects are asked to lie down in a dark, quiet, distraction-free room and to try to fall asleep. Continuous EEG, EMG, and EOG readings are gathered, and the number of minutes it takes the subject to fall asleep is recorded. It takes a subject who has had adequate amount of sleep about 20 minutes to fall asleep whereas it can take subjects with sleep problems less than 5 minutes to fall asleep (Carskadon, 1994; Dement, 1992). As with the assessment of nighttime sleep, there are self-report measures of daytime sleepiness. One example of this type of measure is the Epworth Sleepiness Scale (ESS; Johns, 1991). The ESS asks subjects to rate the likelihood that they would doze off or fall asleep—on a scale ranging from *never doze* to *high chance of dozing*— during a number of frequently occurring daily activities (e.g., sitting and reading, watching TV). The ESS has been shown to distinguish normal subjects from subjects in a number of diagnostic groups, including obstructive sleep apnea syndrome, narcolepsy, and idiopathic hypersomnia (Johns).

Exercise as a Treatment for Sleep Problems

Studies of the relationship between sleep and exercise can generally be categorized as epidemiological, experimental, or quasi-experimental in design. Epidemiological studies have focused on exploring the relationship between current levels of habitual physical activity and sleep in large community samples. For example, a recent epidemiological study of sleep was conducted with participants from the Tucson Epidemiological Study of Obstructive Airway Disease (Sherrill, Kotchou, & Quan, 1998). Subjects were 722 eligible individuals from a larger random-stratified sample of 3,805 individuals in 1,655 households. The authors concluded that higher levels of habitual physical activity are associated with greater sleep quality. Quasi-experimental or cross-sectional study designs have generally compared the sleep of groups of fit versus unfit individuals or habitual exercisers versus sedentary individuals. One of the main limitations of epidemiological studies and quasi-experimental/cross-sectional study designs is that the direction of the relationship between exercise and sleep cannot be determined. Although these types of studies shed light on the relationship between exercise and sleep, they do not tell one whether engaging in exercise/physical activity increased sleep quality or whether individuals who sleep better felt more like engaging in a variety of health-promoting behaviors, including exercise. Conversely, true-experimental studies are those in which levels of exercise have been manipulated, a control group was included in the design, and attempts were made to control potentially confounding variables. The strength of this type of design is that it permits researchers to speak about exercise as a cause of changes in sleep.

Over the past 15 years, a number of reviews and meta-analyses have been conducted on the relationship between exercise and sleep (Driver & Taylor, 1996; Horne, 1981; Kubitz, Landers, Petruzzello, & Han, 1996; O'Connor & Youngstedt, 1995; Shapiro, 1981; Shapiro & Drivers, 1988; Torsvall, 1981; Trinder, Montgomery, & Paxton, 1988; Youngstedt, O'Connor, & Dishman, 1997). This part of the chapter will attempt to summarize and integrate the findings of these reviews to give the reader a good sense of what was known about sleep and exercise up until the last few years.

Then, examples of well-conducted experimental studies not included in past reviews will be presented.

Three narrative review articles examining the relationship between exercise and sleep were published in 1981 and included approximately 30 studies (Horne, 1981; Shapiro, 1981; Torsvall, 1981). The authors of these three reviews concurred that exercise increased slow wave sleep (SWS; stages 3 and 4) in physically fit subjects. In addition, Torsvall and colleagues reported that exercise was related to increased reported nighttime tiredness, increased sleep duration, and decreased sleep onset latency.

Two more narrative reviews of the sleep and exercise literature were published in 1988 and included approximately 50 studies (Shapiro & Drivers, 1988; Trinder et al., 1988). Although Shaprio and Driver came to almost the same conclusions as those of the authors of the 1981 reviews, Trinder and colleagues found less support for the notion that exercise affects sleep. Trinder and colleagues argued that only three of the studies reviewed in 1981 showed an unequivocal increase in SWS and 6 showed no effect of exercise on SWS or either of its components (i.e., stages 3 or 4). Further, Trinder et al. argued that 9 of the other studies reviewed in 1981 had equivocal results. Hence, Trinder and colleagues claimed that the generally positive conclusions made by earlier reviewers were a misinterpretation of the results of these studies, especially in terms of the impact of acute exercise (i.e., a single bout of exercise) on sleep. Nevertheless, Trinder and colleagues did conclude that there was evidence for the effect of habitual endurance training on sleep parameters, specifically SWS and total nighttime sleep. The impact of exercise on these sleep parameters was evident regardless of the level of physical fitness of the subjects studied. A common criticism made by all reviews was that the majority of studies included in these reviews suffered from a number of methodological limitations (e.g., small number of subjects, poor measurements of exercise).

Between 1995 and 1997, four more reviews of the sleep and exercise literature were conducted (Driver & Taylor, 1996; Kubitz et al., 1996; O'Connor & Youngstedt, 1995; Youngstedt et al., 1997). O'Connor and Youngstedt, in a comprehensive narrative review, divided all of the studies conducted until 1994 into six categories (i.e., epidemiological, cross-sectional comparisons, longitudinal investigations, acute exercise experiments, experiments with rigorous control over the environment). O'Connor and Youngstedt concluded that the small amount of epidemiological evidence suggested that subjects perceive exercise to be beneficial in promoting sleep. However, the authors cautioned that the direction of the relationship could not be determined by this type of epidemiological data. In terms of the cross-sectional comparisons, O'Connor and Youngstedt cited a substantial amount of research by Trinder and colleagues demonstrating that groups with greater physical activity histories slept better (i.e., greater SWS, less sleep onset latency) than did sedentary groups of subjects. Interesting to note, in one of the studies by Trinder and colleagues, subjects involved in aerobic exercise had less sleep onset latency and a greater amount of SWS than did a weight-lifting group and controls (Trinder, Paxton, Montgomery, & Fraser, 1985). Hence, the data from this study suggest that the type of exercise one engages in may influence both sleep onset latency and SWS.

In terms of longitudinal studies, O'Connor and Youngstedt (1995) reported that well-controlled experimental studies were rare. Further, the intervention studies available for O'Connor and Youngstedt's review examined subjects who frequently had no sleep problem upon entering the study, a condition that precluded the possibility of improving

subjective sleep quality. In the few available studies, O'Connor and Youngstedt reported that the results concerning the impact of exercise on sleep were mixed.

Employing a new statistical technique called meta-analysis, Kubitz and colleagues (1996) examined the effect of acute and chronic exercise on sleep. Meta-analysis is a statistical technique designed to quantitatively synthesize the results of a group of studies. Many researchers believe that this is an improvement over traditional narrative reviews because it minimizes the influence of a researcher's subjective opinion biasing the conclusions drawn from the review. Kubitz and colleagues found 32 studies that examined the effect of acute exercise on sleep. They were able to calculate 828 effect sizes. Significant mean effect sizes were found for stage 3, stage 4, overall SWS, REM sleep, sleep onset latency, total sleep time, and REM latency. The largest effect size was for stage 4 ($ES = 0.75$), and the smallest was for REM sleep ($ES = -.014$). Correspondingly, these researchers reported that habitual exercise was related to positive effect sizes for SWS and total sleep time as well as negative effect sizes for observed REM sleep, sleep onset latency, and awake time during the night.

Unlike the meta-analysis by Kubitz and colleagues (1996), which included studies that measured sleep by self-report as well as by polysomnography, Youngstedt and colleagues (1997), in a review of acute exercise and sleep, included only studies that measured sleep using polysomnography. Youngstedt and colleagues' review reported significant but smaller effect sizes than those reported by the Kubitz study. They reported moderate effect sizes for SWS, REM, REM-Latency, and total sleep time. Both meta-analytic reviews stated that the major limitation of all of the studies reviewed was that none of the studies assessed the impact of acute exercise on poor sleepers. All of the participants in these studies had *no* sleep problems, which in all likelihood limited the amount of variability one would expect to see in their sleep.

In summary, more recent meta-analytic reviews support the notion that both acute and chronic exercises have a moderate effect on various aspects of sleep (i.e., SWS, sleep onset latency, nighttime awakenings, REM sleep, and total sleep time). Unfortunately, few studies include a control group and effectively manipulate exercise levels. Further, it is equally rare to see a study that includes subjects with sleep problems in its design. Finally, few studies solicited subjective ratings of sleep; instead, they generally relied on polysomnographic measurements. Unfortunately, the design characteristics of these study limit the inferences one can draw about the impact of exercise on sleep.

A recent study designed to address these issues was conducted by King and colleagues (King et al., 1997) at the Stanford Center for Research in Disease Prevention and will be described here both to provide evidence of the effectiveness of exercise in promoting sleep quality as well as to describe the type of study needed to advance our knowledge about the relationship between sleep and exercise. This study was a randomized controlled experiment designed to test the effect of 16 weeks of exercise training on self-reported sleep quality. Subjects were a volunteer sample of 29 women and 14 men aged 50 to 76 years who were sedentary (i.e., no participation in a regular program of physical activity two or more times per week for at least 30 minutes per session or in a sport at least twice per week during the preceding 6 months) and free of cardiovascular disease, and who reported moderate sleep complaints. Moderate sleep complaints were defined as ratings of 3 or higher on a 5-point scale on 2 out of 3 sleep items drawn from the Sleep Questionnaire and Assessment of

Wakefulness (Miles, 1982). Subjects were randomized to either a wait-list control group in which they were asked to maintain their current level of activity and lifestyle or a 16-week exercise-training program. Subjects in the exercise-training program were given an exercise prescription based on a symptom-limited treadmill exercise test. A 12-lead electrocardiogram was recorded, and oxygen uptake was determined during testing. Exercise intensity was gradually increased over the first 6 weeks of the study to 60 to 75% of heart-rate reserve based on the peak heart rate achieved during treadmill testing. Subjects were asked to engage in four 60-minute exercise sessions per week over the 16-week training period. Two exercise periods per week were conducted at a local YMCA and were supervised by study staff and included a minimum of 30 minutes of low-impact aerobic exercise. For the other two sessions each week, subjects were asked to exercise at home and to complete their exercise before dinner. The home-based exercise consisted of brisk walking or stationary cycling sessions. Small to moderate changes in cardiovascular functional capacity were observed at the end of the 16-week training period. This is in all likelihood due to the moderate intensity of the exercise prescription and the brief time period being studied.

Sleep quality was assessed by the Pittsburgh Sleep Quality Index (PSQI; Buysee et al., 1989) and a 14-day sleep diary. Baseline scores on the PSQI placed subjects in the moderate range for sleep problems. Significant changes were seen for the exercise group on the global scale of the PSQI as well as on several of the PSQI subscales (i.e., rated sleep quality, sleep-onset latency, sleep duration). Table 1 illustrates these mean differences.

Results obtained from the PSQI were further supported by the 14-day sleep diary data. Subjects in the exercise group reported improvements in overall sleep quality, sleep

Table 1. Mean sleep scores for the exercise and control groups

	Exercise Group		Control Group	
	Baseline	Posttest	Baseline	Posttest
Sleep Onset Latency (min.)	28.4	14.6	26.1	23.8
Sleep Duration (hrs.)	6.0	6.8	5.8	6.0

onset latency, and degree of restedness upon awakening in the morning as compared to the sleep reported by the control group. Interestingly, improvements in sleep were not noted when subjects were tested 8 weeks into the study. Hence, it may be the case that to achieve improvement in sleep, one must engage in exercise for a period longer than 8 weeks. Although not statistically significant, a small reduction in sleep medication use was observed in the exercise group. These data provide support for the notion that participation in a moderate-intensity exercise program, regardless of increases in fitness, can have a positive impact on self-rated sleep quality.

In another well-designed randomized controlled study conducted at the Harvard Medical School (Singh, Clements, & Fiatarone, 1997), researchers examined the impact of high-intensity progressive resistance training of large muscle groups (i.e., weight training) on the sleep of depressed patients. Subjects were either randomized to a health-education attention control program or a 3-day-per-week exercise machine-based strength-training program for 10 weeks. The exercise resistance was set at 80% of the one repetition maximum. Each exercise session lasted 60 minutes, and resistance was increased to the degree that each subject could tolerate. Ninety percent of the sessions were supervised by the primary investigator of the study. Researchers reported a 93% compliance with the exercise group prescription. Subjective sleep quality

was assessed by the PSQI and two Likert-type scales created by the investigators. Results showed that overall subjective-sleep quality was improved in the exercise group as compared to that of the attention control group as were levels of depression, whereas (nonexercise) activity was unchanged in both the exercise and control groups. Not only does this well-controlled study contribute to our knowledge about the effect of a virtually unstudied type of exercise (i.e., strength training), but it also suggests a possible mechanism by which this type of exercise may affect sleep (i.e., by reducing symptoms of depression).

In summary, a synthesis of past reviews and current randomized controlled studies suggests that exercise, both acute and chronic, endurance and resistance, may play a role in improving both physiological as well as self-report dimensions of sleep. Nevertheless, the study of exercise and sleep is in its relative infancy in terms of well-controlled studies and understanding the mechanisms by which exercise may improve sleep. Hence, the final sections of this chapter propose possible mechanisms that may explain the relationship between exercise and sleep as well as point the way for future research in this area.

Mechanisms by Which Exercise May Affect Sleep

Almost nothing is known empirically about the mechanisms by which exercise may influence sleep. The most cited mechanisms in the literature are

1. The body heating hypothesis and
2. The restorative hypothesis.

The *temperature hypothesis* suggests that increases in body temperature that occur during exercise have a positive effect on sleep architecture (Horne & Staff, 1983). However, this hypothesis was not supported by either of the two recent meta-analyses (Kubitz et al., 1996; Youngstedt et al., 1997). This does not necessarily mean that the heating effect of exercise has absolutely no effect on sleep. It has been suggested by some researchers that heating may affect sleep by altering circadian temperature rhythms (Trinder et al., 1988). The *restorative hypothesis* suggests that sleep is deeper following exercise because the body needs to restore itself and recover from the strain of exercise. This notion is said to be supported by studies that show increased SWS (i.e., the deeper stages of sleep) in association with increased exercise.

Unfortunately, given that most studies of exercise have not included measures of possible mediating variables such as cognition, other behavior, and environmental factors, little is known empirically at the present time about how exercise may be affecting sleep. Hence, proposing a general structure

for how exercise may affect sleep may broaden the discussion of mechanisms and suggest some new avenues of research. It may be helpful to think about exercise as having both a direct influence on sleep (e.g., body heating, restorative, circadian pacemaker resetting) as well as an indirect effect on sleep in which exercise improves sleep by modifying other variables that may be related to sleep problems (e.g., depression, anxiety). Figure 1 shows categories of variables that exercise has been shown to influence and that have often been implicated in sleep problems.

As can be seen from Figure 1, each of the five categories of variables listed above has been shown to influence sleep. Cognitions and moods associated with depression and anxiety disorders are related to poor sleep as are behaviors such as caffeine consumption, poor diet, and alcohol use. Further, physical reactions such as increased arousal and panic have been shown to disrupt sleep. Finally, environmental factors such as exposure to sunlight have been implicated in the development and maintenance of poor sleep. Importantly, all of these variables may be positively influenced by exercise. Exercise has been shown to elevate mood, reduce arousal and anxiety, encourage the adoption of other health behaviors, and, if done during

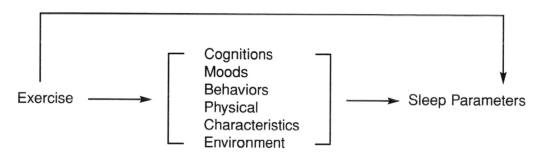

Figure 1
Categories of variables that have been shown to influence, and have been implicated in sleep problems.

the day, may increase one's exposure to sunlight. These are only some of the variables that may mediate the effect of exercise on sleep.

At least one study has attempted to tease out the unique effect of exercise on sleep as opposed to the effect of exercise on sleep mediated by psychological variables such as depression, anxiety, stress, and physical symptoms. Brassington and Hicks (1995) compared the sleep quality (measured by the PSQI) of older adult regular exercisers with that of a sedentary group and found that the groups differed on the global sleep index, sleep quality, sleep onset latency, and daytime dysfunction. However, when an analysis of covariance was conducted controlling for anxiety, depression, stress, and physical symptoms, the global sleep score, onset latency, and daytime dysfunction means only approached significance. These results suggest that exercise may have a limited effect on overall ratings of sleep quality that is not dependent on the modulation of psychological variables, but that this direct effect is small.

Conclusion and Future Directions for Research

Clearly, the study of exercise as a treatment of sleep problems is an important area of research that could benefit millions of people. It is equally clear that we have a long way to go before we can say that we have a good understanding of this relationship. Nevertheless, it is reasonable to conclude that the evidence looks promising that exercise has a positive effect on both physiological as well as self-report measures of sleep quality. Exercise appears to increase physiological parameters of sleep such as SWS that are associated with a deeper, more restful sleep. Exercise of both endurance and resistance types appear to reduce the time it takes one

to fall asleep at night and the number of nighttime awakenings and to increase the restfulness of sleep.

Although the evidence to date is promising, a number of methodological components must be included in future designs to further our understanding of this important relationship. First, more randomized controlled experiments need to be conducted in which exercise and sleep are rigorously measured. This would increase our knowledge about the dose-response relationship between exercise and sleep (i.e., the optimal frequency, duration, and intensity). Second, polysomnographic and self-report measures need to be included together in studies. This type of information would help researchers determine the relationship between physiological measures of sleep and subjective appraisals of sleep quality. The meaning of some physiological measurements of sleep are not well understood as they relate to sleep quality. Correspondingly, with the advent of new technologies for quantifying EEG activities, many new physiological measures of sleep may become available without a good understanding of how these measures relate to an individual's experience of nighttime sleep or daytime functioning. Third, studies need to be conducted in which the time of day of exercise is controlled so as to determine the optimal time of day to exercise to promote sleep quality. Fourth, the above studies need to be conducted with subjects who have at least a moderate amount of difficulty with their sleep or a diagnosed sleep disorder. Including subjects like these will make it possible to observe changes in sleep over time as well as to begin to determine the impact of exercise on specific sleep disorders. Finally, measures of mediating variables need to be included in all future studies of exercise and sleep in order to begin to understand the mechanism by which exercise improves sleep.

References

Brassington, G. S., & Hicks, R. A. (1995). Aerobic exercise and self-reported sleep quality in elderly individuals. *Journal of Aging and Physical Activity, 3,* 120–134.

Buysee, D. J., Reynolds, C. F. I., Monk, T. H., Berman, S. R., & Kupfer, D. J. (1989). The Pittsburgh Sleep Quality Index: A new instrument for psychiatric practice and research. *Psychiatry Research, 28,* 193–213.

Carskadon, M. A. (1994). Measuring daytime sleepiness. In M. H. Kryger, T. Roth, & W. C. Dement (Eds.), *Principles and practice of sleep medicine* (2nd ed., pp. 961–966). Philadelphia: W. B. Saunders Company.

Carskadon, M. A., Dement, W. C., & Mitler, M. M. (1986). Guidelines for the Multiple Sleep Latency Test (MSLT): A standard measure of sleepiness. *Sleep, 9,* 519–524.

Chokroverty, S. (Ed.). (1999). *Sleep disorders medicine: Basic science, technical considerations, and clinical aspects* (2nd ed.). Boston: Butterworth-Heinemann.

Dement, W. C. (1992). *The sleepwatchers.* Stanford, CA: Stanford Alumni Association.

Dijk, D. J., Hayes, B., & Czeisler, C. A. (1993). Analysis of spindle activity by transient pattern recognition software and power spectral analysis. *Sleep Research, 22,* 426.

Driver, S., & Taylor, S. R. (1996). Sleep disturbances and exercise. *Sports Medicine, 21*(1), 1–6.

Geering, B. A., Achermann, P., & Eggimann, F. (1993). Period-amplitude analysis and power spectral analyis: A comparison based on all night EEG recordings. *Journal of Sleep Research, 2,* 121–129.

Horne, J. A. (1981). The effects of exercise upon sleep: A critical review. *Biological Psychology, 12*(4), 241–290.

Horne, J. A., & Staff, L. H. (1983). Exercise and sleep: Body-heating effects. *Sleep, 6*(1), 36–46.

Johns, M. W. (1991). A new method for measuring daytime sleepiness: The Epworth Sleepiness Scale. *Sleep, 14*(6), 540–545.

King, A. C., Oman, R. F., Brassington, G. S., Bliwise, D. L., & Haskell, W. L. (1997). Moderate-intensity exercise and self-rated quality of sleep in older adults: A randomized controlled trial. *Journal of the American Medical Association, 277*(1), 32–37.

Kubitz, K. A., Landers, D. M., Petruzzello, S. J., & Han, M. (1996). The effects of acute and chronic exercise on sleep. A meta-analytic review. *Sports Medicine, 21*(4), 277–291.

Lyznicki, J. M., Doege, T. C., Davis, R. M., & Williams, M. A. (1998). Sleepiness, driving, and motor vehicle crashes. *Journal of the American Medical Association, 279*(23), 1908–1913.

Maggi, S., Langolis, J. A., Minicuci, N., Grigoletto, F., Pavan, M., Foley, D. J., & Enzi, G. (1998). Sleep complaints in community-dwelling older persons. *Journal of the American Geriatic Society, 46,* 161–168.

Miles, L. E. (1982). A sleep questionnaire. In C. Guilleminault (Ed.), *Sleeping and waking disorders: Indications and techniques* (pp. 383–413). Menlo Park, CA: Addison-Wesley.

Monk, T. H. (1991). *Sleep, sleepiness, and performance.* New York: John Wiley & Sons.

Morin, C. M., & Azrin, N. H. (1988). Behavioral and cognitive treatments of geriatric insomnia. *Journal of Consulting and Clinical Psychology, 56,* 748–753.

National Commission on Sleep Disorders Research. (1993). *Wake up America: National sleep alert.* Rockville, MD: U.S. Department of Health and Human Services.

O'Connor, P. J., & Youngstedt, S. D. (1995). Influence of exercise on human sleep. *Exercise & Sport Sciences Reviews, 23,* 105–134.

Pilcher, J. J., & Huffcutt, A. I. (1996). Effects of sleep deprivation on performance: A meta analysis. *Sleep, 19*(4), 318–326.

Rechtschaffen, A., & Kales, A. (1968). *A manual of standardized terminology: Techniques and scoring system for sleep stages of human subjects.* Los Angeles: UCLA Brain Information Service/Brain Research Institute.

Shapiro, C. M. (1981). Sleep and the athlete. *British Journal of Sports Medicine, 15*(1), 51–55.

Shapiro, C. M., & Drivers, H. S. (1988). *Exercise and sleep—A review. NATO Colloquium.* New York: Plenum Press.

Sherrill, D. L., Kotchou, K., & Quan, S. F. (1998). Association of physical activity and human sleep disorders. *Archives of Internal Medicine, 158*(17), 1894–1898.

Singh, N. A., Clements, K. M., & Fiatarone, M. A. (1997). A randomized controlled trial of the effect of exercise on sleep. *Sleep, 20*(2), 95–101.

Torsvall, L. (1981). Sleep after exercise: A literature review. *Journal of Sports Medicine & Physical Fitness, 21*(3), 218–225.

Trinder, J., Montgomery, I., & Paxton, S. J. (1988). The effect of exercise on sleep: The negative view. *Acta Physiologica Scandinavica. Supplementum, 574,* 14–20.

Trinder, J., Paxton, S. J., Montgomery, I., & Fraser, G. (1985). Endurance as opposed to power training: Their effect on sleep. *Psychophysiology, 22*(6), 668–673.

Webb, W. (1995). The cost of sleep-related accidents: A reanalysis. *Sleep, 18,* 276–280.

Weiten, W. (1995). *Psychology themes and variations.* New York: Brooks/Cole Publishing Co.

Youngstedt, S. D., O'Connor, P. J., & Dishman, R. K. (1997). The effects of acute exercise on sleep: A quantitative synthesis. *Sleep, 20*(3), 203–214.

15
The Role of Exercise in the Management of Depression

Egil W. Martinsen

Until the last two decades, most physicians have paid little attention to the lifestyles adopted by their patients. For many years, the most common advice to patients was to take it easy, and rest was considered the best way of preserving good health. Although exercise has not been taken seriously among health professionals, many people intuitively have known the beneficial effects of physical activity on mental health. This is well illustrated by the following quotations:

Above all, do not lose the desire to walk. Every day I walk myself to my daily well-being and from every disease. I have walked myself to my best thoughts, and know no thought so heavy, that one cannot walk away from it.
—Søren Kierkegaard, Danish Philosopher
1813–1847 (Kierkegaard [1991])

I have always believed that exercise is a key not only to physical health but to peace of mind. Many times in the old days I unleashed my anger and frustration on a punchbag rather than taking it out on a comrade or even a policeman. Exercise dissipated tension, and tension is the enemy of serenity. I found that I worked better and thought

more clearly when I was in good physical condition, so training became one of the inflexible disciplines of my life.
—Nelson Mandela,
President of South Africa, 1995

Depression is a major health problem. The lifetime prevalence risk for major depressive disorder in the community is estimated to be 17%: 13% among males and 21% among females. The lifetime prevalence of dysthymic disorder is 6%–5% among females and 8% among males (Kessler et al., 1994). Only one half of subjects suffering from depression seek treatment, and out of these only one half get a correct diagnosis.

The standard forms of therapy are antidepressant medication and various forms of psychotherapy and, in severe cases, electroconvulsive therapy. Psychotherapy is expensive, and the capacity for treatment is far less than the need. The new generations of antidepressant drugs are also expensive, and medication may have troublesome side effects. Neither psychotherapy nor antidepressant medication is always effective. The number of patients responding to initial antidepressant medication is no more than 50% among all patients beginning treatment, if dropouts are accounted for (Nelson, 1998).

There is overwhelming evidence that individuals with depression are being seriously undertreated (Hirshfield et al., 1997). The health care system can probably never meet the need for treatment for this large group of patients. If a simple and inexpensive approach like exercise might be helpful in the treatment or prevention of depression, this might be important for public health.

Population studies have shown clear correlations between physical activity level and mental health at a given point of time (Stephens, 1988). Depressed patients have reduced physical work capacity as compared with the general population (Martinsen, Strand, Paulsson, & Kaggestad, 1989; Morgan, 1969). This kind of correlational evidence, however, leaves open the question of causality: Are patients depressed because they are unfit and inactive, are they unfit because they are depressed, or is there some third factor, like social class or genetics, that is connected to both reduced fitness and depression?

Longitudinal population studies indicate that subjects who are depressed and sedentary at baseline are much more likely to be depressed at followup compared to those who are depressed and physically active (Farmer et al., 1988). Even such studies do not give causal evidence, however, due to the problem of self-selection. Experimental intervention studies are necessary to answer these questions, and this chapter will focus on the antidepressant effects of exercise with clinically depressed individuals.

Assessment of Depression

Modern criteria-based diagnostic systems have greatly increased diagnostic reliability in psychiatry. Research diagnostic criteria (RDC; Spitzer, Endicott, & Robins, 1978), the *Diagnostic and Statistical Manual of Mental Disorders* (DSM-III; American Psychiatric Association, 1980), and DSM-IV (American Psychiatric Association, 1994) are commonly used. These diagnostic systems make it easier to compare results across studies.

Several instruments have been developed to measure the level of depression. The Beck Depression Inventory (BDI; Beck, Ward, Mendelsohn, Mock, & Erbaugh, 1961), and the Self-Rating Depression Scale (SDS; Zung, 1965) are well validated self-report instruments. The Hamilton Depression Rating Scale (Hamilton, 1960), the Comprehensive Psychopathological Rating Scale (CPRS) depression subscale (Åsberg, Perris, Schalling, and Sedvall, 1978) and the Montgomery Åsberg Depression Rating Scale (MADRS; Montgomery & Åsberg, 1979) are commonly used therapist-assisted ratings.

In some of the scales, like BDI and SDS, normal ranges of the item scores are given. These instruments may be used to identify cases or patients. In some exercise-intervention studies, the scores on such scales are used as the only means of classification of a given patient, and no formal diagnoses are made. This is not optimal. There are several conditions in addition to clinical depression—grief reactions as well as various somatic and psychiatric disorders—that are associated with elevated depression scores. Studies where elevated depression scores are the only means of classification, therefore, have limited value because it is difficult to generalize the results to other populations.

Clinical Exercise-Intervention Studies

During the last few years, quasi-experimental as well as experimental exercise-intervention studies on clinically depressed subjects have started to emerge. In some of the studies, various forms of exercise are compared.

Sime (1987) used a multiple-baseline single-case design in a study of 15 subjects with moderately elevated scores on the BDI.

Depression scores were not significantly changed during a screening phase and a 2-week pre-exercise period, but dropped significantly during a 10-week exercise period. Doyne, Chambless, and Beutler (1983) used the same design in a study of four women with RDC major depressive disorder. Significant reductions in depression scores were obtained during a 6-week exercise period, and these reductions were significantly larger than what occurred in the pre-exercise screening phase.

The first experimental study was performed by Greist et al. (1979). Running was compared with two forms of individual psychotherapy in 28 outpatients with RDC minor depression. No significant differences were found in treatment outcome among the various conditions after 12 weeks: Significant reductions in depression scores were found in all groups.

Eighteen subjects with elevated BDI scores, without formal diagnoses, were studied by Rueter, Mutrie, and Harris (1982). These were randomly assigned to counseling alone or supervised running in addition to counseling. The reductions in BDI scores were significantly larger in the combined running-and-counseling group than in the counseling-alone group.

Another study, by Klein et al. (1985), had 74 patients with RDC major or minor depression who were randomly assigned to running, meditation-relaxation or group psychotherapy. After 12 weeks, significant reductions in depression scores were obtained in each treatment group, but there were no significant differences among the groups. The followup results indicated a better outcome for the exercise and the meditation groups.

McCann and Holmes (1984) studied 41 women with elevated BDI scores, without formal diagnoses, who were randomly assigned to either aerobic exercise, relaxation training, or a waiting-list control condition. After 10 weeks, there were significant reductions in depression scores in each treatment group, but the reduction in the aerobic exercise group was significantly larger than in the two other groups.

Again, persons with elevated BDI scores, without formal diagnosis, were studied. Freemont and Craighead (1987) randomly assigned 49 people to cognitive therapy, aerobic exercise, or the combination of the two. Significant reductions in depression scores were obtained in all treatment groups after 10 weeks, but there were no significant differences among the groups.

The study by Martinsen, Medhus, and Sandvik (1985) had 49 inpatients of both sexes, mean age 40, with DSM-III major depression. They were randomly assigned to aerobic exercise or a control condition. Patients in the training group exercised aerobically, most commonly brisk walks and jogging, for one hour three times a week for 6 to 9 weeks, whereas those in the control group attended occupational therapy. Patients in both groups received psychotherapy, individually as well as in groups, and milieu therapy. The increase in aerobic capacity and reduction in depression scores, CPRS as well as BDI, were significantly larger in the training group, indicating that aerobic exercise and increased fitness were associated with an antidepressive effect in these patients.

An additional finding in this study was that the antidepressive effect seemed to depend on increase in aerobic fitness. Patients in the training group with less than 15% increase in maximum oxygen uptake had an antidepressive effect similar to that in the control group, whereas those with moderate (15%–30%) and large (>30%) increases had similar and larger reductions in depression scores. A further analysis of these data showed that this relation seemed to be particularly important in males (Martinsen, 1987).

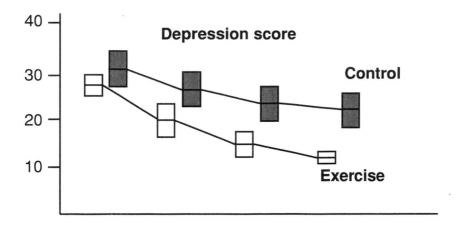

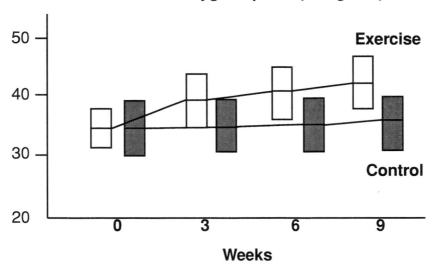

Figure 1

Mean depression scores (Beck Depression Inventory) and maximum oxygen uptake, with 95% confidence intervals. Printed with permission from British Medical Journal *1985; 291:109).*

The correlation between increase in aerobic capacity and reduction in BDI scores was .40 in males ($p<.05$) and -.13 ($p>.05$) in females, using the Spearman rank order correlation.

Aerobic Versus Other Forms of Exercise

To study these interesting findings further, Martinsen and coworkers performed another study, in which they compared aerobic and nonaerobic forms of exercise (Martinsen, Hoffart, and Solberg, 1989). This study included 99 inpatients of both sexes (mean age 41) with DSM-III-R major depression, dysthymic disorder, or depressive disorder not otherwise specified. Patients were randomly assigned to aerobic (brisk walks or jogging) and nonaerobic exercise (training of muscular strength and endurance, relaxation, and flexibility) for one hour three times a week for 8 weeks.

Patients in the aerobic group achieved significant increase in aerobic capacity, whereas those in the nonaerobic group were unchanged. In both groups, there were significant reductions in depression scores, MADRS as well as BDI, but the differences between the groups were small and not statistically significant. Patients with substantial increases in aerobic capacity (>15%) had reductions in depression scores almost similar to those of patients with little or no increase. The correlations between increased aerobic capacity and reduced BDI scores were .26 for males and .13 for females. None of these values reached statistical significance ($p > .01$ for both) although the value for males is not far from being significant. Thus, the authors were not able to replicate the findings from their first study. In this larger study, they found no significant correlation between increase in fitness and reduction in depression, for neither males nor females.

Other investigators have followed the same line of research, comparing aerobic exercise with other forms.

Mutrie (1988) studied 24 subjects with elevated BDI scores, without formal diagnoses, who were randomly assigned to aerobic and nonaerobic (stretching and strengthening exercises) and a waiting-list control condition. Subjects trained alone three times a week and met with a physical educator every 2 weeks for instructions and physical tests. After 4 weeks, subjects in both training groups had larger reductions in BDI scores than those of the waiting-list control condition, with superior results in the aerobic group. Only the difference between the aerobic and the control group reached statistical significance. This is probably due to the small number of subjects in each group.

Doyne et al. (1987) compared running (aerobic) with weight lifting (nonaerobic training) in 40 outpatients with RDC minor or major depression. In both exercise groups, the reductions in depression scores were larger than in a waiting-list control group. The differences between the two forms of exercise were minimal and not statistically significant.

Sexton, Mære, and Dahl (1989) studied 25 inpatients with DSM-III unipolar depression, randomly assigned to running and walking. In both groups, there were significant reductions in depression scores, but the differences between the groups were small and not statistically significant.

Discussion of Exercise-Intervention Studies

The results in these studies all point in the same direction: Aerobic exercise is more effective than no treatment, and not significantly different from other forms of treatment, including various forms of psychotherapy. These conclusions are supported by meta-analyses (North, McCullagh & Tran, 1990; Stich, 1998) and review articles (Ernst, Rand, & Stevinson, 1998). Increase in aerobic fitness does not seem to be important; patients without physiological gains have psychological effects similar to the effects of those with improved fitness.

The studies comprise outpatients and inpatients, males and females, and age-groups from 17 to 60 years old. Exercise settings vary from home-based exercise alone to exercise in outpatient and inpatient clinical settings. The same trend is seen in all studies, indicating that the antidepressant effect associated with exercise is general.

These results are limited to unipolar depressive disorders without melancholic and/or psychotic features, commonly called mild to moderate forms of depression. In the official American classification system, DSM-IV, this includes mild and moderate forms of major depression, dysthymic disorder, and depressive disorder not otherwise specified.

Whether these results may be generalized to major depressive episodes in patients with bipolar disorder is an open question. Similarly, there are no good studies addressing the value of exercise intervention in the most severe forms of major depression. Clinical experience, however, indicates that exercise has limited value (Greist, 1987). Severe depression usually requires medication, electroconvulsive therapy, and/or psychotherapy, with exercise as an adjunct.

No study has yet addressed whether systematic exercise may prevent relapse in bipolar disorder. The author has personally followed three male patients with this disorder. They were between 20 and 40 years of age and enthusiastic runners. All were lithium responders, but wanted to taper lithium and see if daily running could replace it. Within one year, all had relapsed and had to start again with lithium. In the author's opinion, exercise may have many beneficial effects for patients with bipolar disorder, by giving feelings of well-being and mastery, and increase in self-esteem, but it is probably not effective in prevention of manic or depressive episodes.

A few studies have compared exercise with psychotherapy and counseling in the treatment of depression and have found them to be about equally effective (Freemont & Craighead, 1987; Greist et al., 1979; Klein et al., 1985). There has been a rapid development within the field of psychotherapy research the last years. These studies do not meet modern methodological demands of psychotherapy research, but they do open up interesting perspectives and should be followed by new, better designed studies.

The number of studies still is relatively small, and many have methodological shortcomings: Some have used BDI score as the only way of classification; the intensity, frequency, form and duration of exercise are not always precisely described; and some have not included measures of fitness. There is, therefore, still a need for more methodologically sound studies.

Prevention

An interesting question is whether exercise may prevent the occurrence of depression in vulnerable individuals and prevent relapse for those who have recovered from a depressive episode. Gøtestam and Stiles (1990) studied Norwegian soldiers exposed for a stressful life situation. Soldiers who were actively engaged in sports were significantly less depressed 12 weeks after exposure to the stressful life situation, compared with the physically sedentary ones.

Martinsen, Sandvik, and Kolbjørnsrud (1989) found that previous adult experience with exercise and sports predicted less chance of relapse in nonpsychotic patients one year after discharge from hospital and that continuous exercise at followup was associated with lower symptom scores. Population studies indicate that subjects who are sedentary and not depressed at baseline are more likely to be depressed at followup than are those who are more physically active (Camacho, Roberts, Lazarus, Kaplan, & Cohen, 1991; Farmer et al., 1988).

Exercise may have a prophylactic effect, but more evidence is needed before safe conclusions can be drawn.

Patients' Evaluation

At a one year followup of their 1985-study, Martinsen and Medhus (1989) asked patients to evaluate the usefulness of physical fitness training, as compared to other forms of therapy, during a hospital stay. Patients ranked physical fitness training as the therapeutic element that had helped them most, prior to individual psychotherapy. The same trend was seen in another study of 92 inpatients with various nonpsychotic mental disorders (Martinsen, Sandvik, et al., 1989)

Sexton et al. (1989) reported the same trend from their study. Many patients reported that physical fitness training had helped them more than traditional forms of therapy, including psychotherapy and medication.

These studies, of course, give no proof for the efficacy of exercise treatment, but the findings are interesting.

Practical Management

Several components in the depressive syndrome may make it difficult to exercise. Fatigue, lassitude, low self-esteem, and psychomotor retardation are common symptoms. For those receiving antidepressant medication, side effects like dryness of mouth, drowsiness, and increased heart rate may cause additional problems. This was especially true for the older generation of antidepressants.

Because of these factors, many patients will need encouragement and support when starting to exercise. It is important that the intensity of exercise be no higher than the patients can master because most patients are unfit. The aim is to arrange exercise in such a way that every session will be a mastery experience for the patients. During the last year, the author has observed some 100 patients taking part in hospital exercise programs. The experience is that it is possible to help a large proportion of depressed patients to start with regular exercise.

Exercise and Medication

Patients taking the tricyclic antidepressant agents (TCA) should be informed about the possibility of experiencing hypotension both when standing up and during exercise. These patients may have higher risk of fainting or falling during exercise. Studies of the effect of these drugs during maximal exercise have not been performed (Powles, 1981). Orthostatic hypotension is also a common side effect from the monoamine oxidase inhibitors (MAOI), which is the other large group of antidepressants. During the last decade, new classes of antidepressants have been developed. The selective serotonin reuptake inhibitors (SSRI), in general, have fewer side effects and interfere less with exercise (Martinsen & Stanghelle, 1997). The author has personally followed several hundred patients who have taken part in various forms of exercise programs. No serious side effects of the combination of exercise and medication have been observed.

Two studies have addressed whether exercise and medication can potentiate each other. In the first study, Martinsen (1987) found no synergistic effect of the combination of exercise and TCA, compared to exercise alone, in a study involving 43 subjects with DSM-III major depression. In a second study, involving 99 patients with DSM-III-R unipolar depressive disorders, there was a nonsignificant trend toward a larger reduction in depression scores in patients who received TCAs in addition to exercise, compared to those who only exercised (Martinsen, Hoffart, et al., 1989). For the moment, we do not know whether exercise may potentiate the effects of antidepressant medication or vice versa.

Hypotheses About Mechanisms

Several hypotheses have been forwarded to explain how the psychological effects associated with exercise are mediated. For most of them, empirical evidence is to a large degree lacking. In the following, the most important of them will be shortly reviewed.

Anthropological hypothesis. For thousands

of years, humans have been gatherers and hunters. Only in the last decades it has been possible for large population groups to survive without hard physical work. Inactivity has detrimental effects on physical health, and it may not be good for mental health either (Åstrand & Rodahl, 1985).

Biological hypotheses. During physical activity, the deep body temperature is elevated. It has been postulated that this transient warming may explain the psychological effects of exercise, the thermogenic hypothesis. Efforts to test the thermogenic hypothesis by blocking customary rise in core temperature associated with vigorous physical activity have failed to yield consistent findings. For the moment, it seems reasonable to conclude that the temperature hypothesis still remains tenable (Koltyn, 1997).

Endorphine hypothesis. Both animal and experimental data indicate that prolonged aerobic exercise will lead to a release of endogenous opioids in the central nervous system. Whether this may explain the psychological effects associated with exercise is an open question (Hoffmann, 1997).

Monoamine hypothesis. Central serotonergic and noradrenergic systems are the targets for numerous antidepressant agents. Data derived from animal and human studies favor the hypothesis that central serotonergic systems are modified by physical activity, but it remains to be shown whether such a contribution is significant in exercising subjects (Chauloff, 1997). It is also possible that chronic exercise affects the brain's noradrenergic system in ways qualitatively similar to the effects of pharmacological interventions (Dishman, 1997).

Psychological hypotheses. Several psychological hypotheses have been forwarded. Bahrke and Morgan (1978) have proposed that the psychological benefits associated with exercise may be due to mere distraction from stressful stimuli. They based their hypothesis on a study in which they found acute exercise to be associated with reduction in state anxiety. Later they found that the same anxiolytic effect might be achieved by mere resting in a sound-filtered room. Some have postulated that regular, monotonous exercise may be looked upon as a kind of meditation or self-hypnosis, inducing an altered state of consciousness. Others claim that the important thing about exercise is the development of a positive addiction (Glasser, 1976). The concepts of competence and mastery (White, 1959) may easily fit into exercise psychology. From social learning theory, Bandura (1977) has presented a self-efficacy theory, saying that a treatment will be effective if it restores a sense of self-efficacy by arranging self-mastery experiences.

Different hypotheses are available, but the empirical evidence supporting them is limited. Probably there is not only one mechanism mediating the psychological effects of exercise. Different mechanisms may work for different people, and biological, psychological, and social mechanisms may interplay in concert.

Summary

In clinically depressed patients, aerobic exercise seems to be more effective than no treatment and not significantly different from other interventions, including various forms of psychotherapy. Aerobic and nonaerobic forms of exercise seem to be equally effective. The results are restricted to mild to moderate forms of unipolar depression; DSM-IV mild to moderate forms of major depression, dysthymic disorder, and depressive disorder not otherwise specified. Patients appreciate exercise and find it to be a useful form of therapy. Physical exercise may be an alternative or adjunct to traditional forms of treatment in mild to moderate forms of unipolar depression.

References

American Psychiatric Association. (1980). *Diagnostic and statistical manual of mental disorders* (3rd ed.). Washington, DC: Author.

American Psychiatric Association. (1994). *Diagnostic and statistical manual of mental disorders* (4th ed.). Washington, DC: Author.

Åsberg, M., Perris, C., Schalling, D., & Sedvall, G. (1978). The CPRS: Development and applications of a psychiatric rating scale. *Acta Psychiatrica Scandinavica* (Suppl. 271), 1–27.

Åstrand, P. O., & Rodahl, K. (1985). *Textbook in work physiology.* New York: McGraw-Hill.

Bahrke, M. S., & Morgan, W. P. (1978). Anxiety reduction following exercise and meditation. *Cognitive Therapy and Research, 4,* 323–333.

Bandura, A. (1977). Self-efficacy: Toward a unifying theory of behavioral change. *Psychological Review, 84,* 191–215.

Beck, A. T., Ward, C. H., Mendelson, M., Mock, J., & Erbaugh, H. (1961). An inventory for measuring depression. *Archives of General Psychiatry, 4,* 561–571.

Camacho, T. C., Roberts, R. E., Lazarus, N. B., Kaplan, G. A., & Cohen, R. D. (1991). Physical activity and depression: Evidence from the Alameda County Study. *American Journal of Epidemiology, 134,* 220–231.

Chauloff, F. (1997). The serotonin hypothesis. In W. P. Morgan (Ed.), *Physical activity and mental health* (pp. 179–198). Washington, DC: Taylor & Francis.

Dishman, R. (1997). The norepinephrine hypothesis. In W. P. Morgan (Ed.), *Physical activity and mental health.* Washington, DC: Taylor & Francis.

Doyne, E. J., Chambless, D. L., & Beutler, L. E. (1983). Aerobic exercise as a treatment for depression in women. *Behavioral Therapy, 14,* 434–440.

Doyne, E. J., Ossip-Klein, D. J., Bowman, E. D., Osborn, K. M., McDougall-Wilson, I. B., & Neimeyer, R. A. (1987). Running versus weight-lifting in the treatment of depression. *Journal of Consulting and Clinical Psychology, 55,* 748–754.

Ernst E., Rand J. I., & Stevinson C. (1998) Complementary therapies for depression. *Archives of General Psychiatry, 55,* 1026–1032.

Farmer, M. E., Locker, B. Z., Moscicki, E. K., Dannenberg, A. L., Larson, D. B., & Radloff, L. S. (1988). Physical activity and depressive symptoms: The NHANESI epidemiologic followup study. *American Journal of Epidemiology, 128,* 1340–1351.

Freemont, J., & Craighead, L. W. (1987). Aerobic exercise and cognitive therapy in the treatment of dysphoric moods. *Cognitive Therapy and Research, 2,* 241–251.

Glasser, W. (1976). *Positive addiction.* New York: Harper & Row.

Gøtestam, K. G., & Stiles, T. C. (1990). *Physical exercise and cognitive vulnerability: A longitudinal study.* Paper presented at the Annual Meeting for the Association for the Advancement of Behavior Therapy, San Francisco.

Greist, J. H. (1987). Exercise intervention with depressed outpatients. In W. P. Morgan & S. E. Goldston (Eds.). *Exercise and mental health* (pp. 117–121). Washington, DC: Hemisphere.

Greist, J. H., Klein, M. H., Eischens, R. R., Faris, J., Gurman, A. S., & Morgan, W. P. (1979). Running as treatment for depression. *Comprehensive Psychiatry, 20,* 41–54.

Hamilton, M. (1960). A rating scale for measuring depression. *Journal of Neurology, Neurosurgery and Psychiatry, 23,* 56–62.

Hirshfield, R. M. A., Keller, M. B., Panico, S., Arons, B. S., Barlow, D., Davidoff, F., Endicott, J., Froom, J., Goldstein, M., Gorman, J. M., Gutrie, D., Marek, R. G., Maurer, T. A., Meyer, R., Phillips, K., Ross, J., Schwenk, T. L., Sharfstein, S. S., Thase, M. E., & Wyatt, R. J. (1997). The national depressive and manic-depressive association consensus statement on the undertreatment of depression. *Journal of the American Medical Association, 277*(4), 333–340.

Hoffman, P. (1997). The endorphin hypothesis. In W. P. Morgan (Ed.), *Physical activity and mental health* (pp. 163–177). Washington, DC: Taylor & Francis.

Kessler, R. C., McGonagle, K. A., Zhao, S., Nelson, C. B., Hughes, M., Eshleman, S., Wittchen, H.-U., & Kendler, K. (1994). Lifetime and 12-months prevalence of DSM-III-R psychiatric disorders in the United States. *Archives of General Psychiatry, 51,* 8–19.

Kierkegaard, S. (1991). *Collected works.* Copenhagen: Gyldendal.

Klein, M. H., Greist, J. H., Gurman, A. S., Neimeyer, R. A., Lesser, D. P., Bushnell, N. J., & Smith, R. E. A. (1985). A comparative outcome study of group psychotherapy vs exercise treatments for depression. *International Journal of Mental Health, 13,* 148–177.

Koltyn, K. (1997). The thermogenic hypothesis. In W. P. Morgan (Ed.), *Physical activity and mental health* (pp. 213–226). Washington, DC: Taylor & Francis.

Mandela, N. (1995). *Long walk to freedom.* London: Abacus.

Martinsen, E. W. (1987). The role of aerobic exercise in the treatment of depression. *Stress Medicine, 3,* 93–100.

Martinsen, E. W., Hoffart, A., & Solberg, Ø. (1989). Comparing aerobic and nonaerobic forms of exercise in the treatment of clinical depression: A randomized trial. *Comprehensive Psychiatry, 30,* 324–331.

Martinsen, E. W., & Medhus, A. (1989). Exercise adherence and patients' evaluation of exercise in a comprehensive treatment programme for depression. *Nordic Journal of Psychiatry, 43,* 521–529.

Martinsen, E. W., Medhus, A., & Sandvik, L. (1985). Effects of aerobic exercise on depression: A controlled study. *British Medical Journal, 291,* 109.

Martinsen, E. W., Sandvik, L., & Kolbjørnsrud, O. B. (1989). Aerobic exercise in the treatment of nonpsychotic mental disorders. *Nordic Journal of Psychiatry, 43,* 411–415.

Martinsen, E. W., & Stanghelle, J. K. (1997). Drug

therapy and physical activity. In W. P. Morgan (Ed.), *Physical activity and mental health* (pp. 81–90). Washington, DC: Taylor & Francis.

Martinsen, E. W., Strand, J., Paulsson, G., & Kaggestad, J. (1989). Physical fitness in patients with anxiety and depressive disorders. *International Journal of Sports Medicine, 10*, 58–61.

McCann, I. L., & Holmes, D. S. (1984). Influence of aerobic exercise on depression. *Journal of Personality and Social Psychology, 46*, 1142–1147.

Montgomery, S. A., & Åsberg, M. (1979). A new depression scale designed to be sensitive to change. *British Journal of Psychiatry, 134*, 382–389.

Morgan, W. P. (1969). A pilot investigation of physical work capacity in depressed and nondepressed psychiatric males. *Research Quarterly, 39*(4), 1037–1043.

Mutrie, N. (1988). Exercise as a treatment for moderate depression in the UK health service. In *Sport, health, psychology and exercise symposium* [Proceedings]. S. Biddle (Ed.) Bisham Abbey National Sports Centre, Buckinghamshire.

Nelson, J. C. (1998). Overcoming treatment resistance in depression. *Journal of Clinical Psychiatry, 59*(Suppl. 16), 13–19.

North, T. C., McCullagh, P., & Tran, Z. V. (1990). Effects of exercise on depression. *Exercise and Sport Science Reviews, 18*, 379–415.

Powles, A. C. P. (1981). The effects of drugs on the cardiovascular response to exercise. *Medicine and Science in Sports and Exercise, 13*, 252–258.

Rueter, M., & Mutrie, N., & Harris, D. (1982). *Running as an adjunct to counseling in the treatment of depression.* Unpublished manuscript, The Pennsylvania State University.

Sexton, H., Mære, Å., & Dahl, N. H. (1989). Exercise intensity and reduction in neurotic symptoms. *Acta Psychiatrica Scandinavica, 80*, 231–235.

Sime, W. E. (1987). Exercise in the treatment and prevention of depression. In W. P. Morgan & S. E. Goldston (Eds.), *Exercise and mental health* (pp. 145–152). Washington, DC: Hemisphere.

Spitzer, R. L., Endicott, J., & Robins, E. (1978). Research diagnostic criteria: Rationale and reliability. *Archives of General Psychiatry, 35*, 773–782.

Stephens, T. (1988). Physical activity and mental health in the United States and Canada: Evidence from four population surveys. *Preventive Medicine, 17*, 35–47.

Stich, F. A. (1998). *A meta-analysis of physical exercise as a treatment for symptoms of anxiety and depression.* Unpublished doctoral dissertation, University of Wisconsin-Madison.

White, R. W. (1959). Motivation reconsidered: The concept of competence. *Psychological Review, 66*, 297–333.

Zung, W. W. K. (1965). Self-Rating Depression Scale. *Archives of General Psychiatry, 12*, 63–70.

16
Diabetes in Sport and Exercise

Tony Morris

Michael is 11 years old. He loves sport, especially soccer. During an intense soccer match, Michael passes out. Michael is diabetic. He self-administers insulin injections daily to ensure his blood sugar level does not rise to dangerous levels. Michael took his medication, but the intensive physical activity of the match depleted the artificially lowered blood sugar to a level where Michael did not have sufficient energy to continue the match. For Michael, involvement in sport is part of a balancing act he must conduct every day of his life, trying to keep his blood sugar in that narrow region between hyperglycemia and hypoglycemia.

Ellen is 57 years of age. She is 15 kilos overweight and leads a very sedentary life. Ellen visits her doctor because she has been experiencing dizziness, hot flushes, intense thirst by day, and multiple visits to the bathroom during the night. Blood tests indicate that Ellen has diabetes. Her doctor prescribes a change of diet and a regular exercise program. Ellen does not know how she will cope. All the foods she likes the most are prohibited. Worst of all, she hates physical activity. It is often painful and always feels unpleasant to the point of being noxious. Ellen is not confident that she can meet the lifestyle challenges that face her.

From the cases of Michael and Ellen, it can be seen that diabetes is a life-threatening condition that has a major impact on peo-

ple's lives. It is also evident that it is complex. Diabetes can be diagnosed in apparently active, normal children or only appear much later in life, typically in obese, inactive people. In some cases, physical activity must be approached with caution; in others, it is a central element in treatment. Our understanding of diabetes has increased greatly in recent times, but this has raised many questions. It is now known that there are several different types of diabetes. Michael has one, insulin-dependent diabetes, and Ellen has another, non-insulin-dependent diabetes.

Diabetes is a group of conditions that affect people everywhere, but it is more prevalent in Western societies than in developing countries. This relates to the link between diabetes, diet, and exercise (e.g., Wing, 1989) and the association between diabetes and stress (e.g., Halford, Cuddihy, & Mortimer, 1990). It is particularly prevalent in indigenous groups in such societies. For example, Native Americans are 11 times more likely to develop diabetes than are white Americans (e.g., Harris, 1985). As the Western lifestyle, especially diet, inactivity, and stress, permeates many areas of the world, the incidence of diabetes could be expected to rise in developing countries too.

Diabetes is a major health concern. For example, the American Diabetes Association (1993) estimated there are more than 13 million diabetics in the United States. This is more than 5% of the American population. The incidence of diabetes in the United States is increasing by 6% each year. Thus, diabetes is considered to be the third most prevalent chronic illness in the United States, accounting for in excess of 160,000 deaths per year, either directly or through the complications that arise from diabetes. Similar statistics apply to other Western societies, such as Canada (Derksen & Rorke, 1996) and Australia (M. W. Simmons & Owen, 1992).

Diabetic conditions arise from the failure of the pancreas to produce insulin, or from the inability of the body to use the insulin effectively. Insulin is intimately involved in the transfer of glucose from the blood to the cells. If diabetes is not treated, glucose builds up in the blood, leading to hyperglycemia, which can induce coma and, ultimately, death (Taylor, 1995). Exercise can facilitate the transfer of glucose from the blood to the cells, especially when insulin is present, but not functioning. Thus, exercise is prescribed in the treatment of non-insulin-dependent diabetes. Conversely, when diabetes is being treated by medication, especially insulin injection, glucose transfer to the cells is artificially controlled, to maintain blood glucose at a normal level. Excessive physical activity, especially soon after the diabetic has taken medication, can lead to the level of glucose in the blood dropping too low, hypoglycemia. Thus, in some situations, sport and exercise generally can be dangerous for diabetics, whereas in other circumstances, physical activity is a critical component of the treatment of diabetes.

This chapter examines the relationship between diabetes and sport and exercise. It focuses primarily on the psychological aspects of this relationship. To provide an understanding of the illness, the nature of diabetes is, first, briefly discussed. This discussion is restricted, as there are adequate reviews of the pathophysiology and epidemiology of

diabetes (e.g., Kaplan, Sallis, & Patterson, 1993; Taylor, 1995). The chapter then focuses on involvement in sport and exercise activities for those with diabetes, emphasizing the impact of diabetes on life, especially for children and adolescents. Greatest attention in this chapter is given to self-management of diabetes treatment because it has the potential to make the largest impact. Adherence to regimens of physical activity is central to self-care. Prevention of diabetes is then briefly considered, and the chapter concludes with discussion of important areas for research.

What Is Diabetes?

The term diabetes mellitus covers a number of conditions that involve dysfunction of the energy systems of the body. Insulin plays a key role in the transfer of glucose from the blood to the cells. Glucose, extracted from the food we eat, is a major source of energy. When glucose is not metabolized efficiently, the energy systems of the body do not function effectively. Excess glucose circulating in the blood causes damage to major organs, including the heart, kidneys, and eyes, as well as the lower limbs, over a period of time. The two types of diabetes that are most common are insulin-dependent diabetes mellitus and non-insulin-dependent mellitus.

Insulin-Dependent Diabetes Mellitus (IDDM)

IDDM, also called Type I diabetes mellitus, early-onset diabetes mellitus, and juvenile-onset diabetes mellitus, is the most serious form of the illness. It accounts for about 10% of diabetes (Kaplan, Sallis, et al., 1993). Diagnosis is usually made in childhood, between 5 and 6, or in adolescence, from 10 to 13. Timings do vary, for example with sex, girls typically developing IDDM earlier than boys. Common symptoms are weight loss, but a strong craving for food, especially sweets; excessive thirst; frequent urination, especially at night; weakness and fatigue; dizziness and fainting (Taylor, 1995).

IDDM develops when the pancreas stops producing insulin. Evidence exists for a role for genetics in IDDM (e.g., Harris, 1985), predisposing the individual, rather than causing IDDM per se (Taylor, 1995). Development of the condition has also been linked to viral infections (e.g., Rossini, Mordeis, & Handlar, 1989) that, again, play a role, but do not constitute the cause of IDDM. Currently, a favored view is that IDDM is an autoimmune disorder, brought on by an infection, like measles and mumps, that interacts with a genetic predisposition. IDDM is a life-threatening illness and it must be treated with daily injections of insulin (American Diabetes Association, 1986).

Non-Insulin-Dependent Diabetes Mellitus (NIDDM)

Estimates of the incidence of NIDDM, also called Type II, late-onset, or adult-onset diabetes mellitus, have increased substantially in recent times. It is now believed to account for approximately 90% of all diabetes. The development of NIDDM is gradual. It is typically diagnosed in people over 40 years old. Most of those who have NIDDM are overweight or obese, although estimates vary between 60% and 90% (Herman, Teutsch, & Geiss, 1987). Symptoms include dryness of mouth and thirst; frequent urination, especially at night; pain or cramps in legs, feet, or fingers; frequent gum, skin, or urinary infections; slow healing of cuts and bruises; and drowsiness. People at high risk for NIDDM often lead sedentary lives. Because of its slow onset, NIDDM is much harder to diagnose than IDDM. It is estimated that about as many NIDDM sufferers remain undiagnosed, as have been identified, in a country like Australia (M. W. Simmons & Owen, 1992).

In NIDDM, insulin no longer facilitates the transfer of glucose from the blood to the cells, a state termed insulin resistance. Thus, a surfeit of glucose remains in the blood. The specific mechanism has not been identified. NIDDM can be treated by a combination of diet, exercise, and blood glucose monitoring. Together, these can improve glycemic control, to keep blood glucose within a normal range (Kaplan et al., 1993). There is evidence that weight loss, through diet and exercise, can enhance glycemic control (Wing, 1989). Unfortunately, people do not comply very well with lifestyle changes, such as adopting a diabetic diet and maintaining a regular exercise program. Thus, many NIDDM sufferers progress to the prescription of oral medication, to supplement diet and exercise.

The two main types of diabetes, IDDM and NIDDM, have different relationships with physical activity. In the case of NIDDM, physical activity is considered a central aspect of treatment. For IDDM sufferers, exercise can be a major component of treatment, but it can also be contraindicated. Research shows that exercise does not reduce blood glucose in people with IDDM, but it is valuable to reduce the incidence of complications, such as coronary artery disease (Albright, 1997). When blood glucose control is poor, exercise can lead to an increase in the level of sugar in the blood. When blood glucose control is good, the primary concern is to ensure that physical activity does not induce hypoglycemia.

Participating in Physical Activity With Diabetes

When diabetics undertake any systematic regimen of physical activity, they must monitor their diabetic status. The following discussion of issues relating to physical activity for people with diabetes focuses on involvement in competitive sport because this is the most complex context. Most of the principles and practices discussed apply also to participation in exercise activities.

Consideration of diabetes in competitive sport leads to a focus on IDDM because competitive sport performers tend to be children, adolescents, and young adults. NIDDM is usually recognized later in life. In Western societies, the leading sports performers are media idols, shaping the dreams of the generations to follow. Parents and schools frequently encourage sport participation for its health, social, and skill development benefits. Children are also attracted to sport because their friends participate. Children diagnosed with diabetes in early childhood could be denied sport participation, which might make them feel different from their friends. They could be excluded from other peer-based social activities. For diabetics diagnosed during adolescence, a successful junior sport career could already be in progress. Even during late adolescence and adulthood, there is potential for lack of understanding on the part of sports organizations. The chairman of the board of trustees of the British Diabetic Association wrote in the *British Journal of Sports Medicine* that people with diabetes are sometimes treated by sports bodies as if they were disabled (Hall, 1997). Hall cited cases of athletes banned from competition because they were diabetic. At the same time, he referred to leading professional athletes, competing in many sports, who were diabetic. Hall emphasized that, with careful monitoring of blood glucose and adjustments to insulin intake and food eaten, people with diabetes can participate in most physical activities, including high-level sports.

Participation in sport and exercise has a number of benefits for people with IDDM. It can reduce the risk of cardiovascular disease, the major cause of death in diabetics (Bell, 1992). Physical activity has also been associated with decreases in cholesterol and triglyceride levels, reduction of high blood pressure, and increase of insulin sensitivity (Horton, 1988). Fahey, Stallkamp, and Kwatra (1996) argued that exercise also enhances self-esteem and body image in diabetics. Participation in physical activity does involve risks for people with IDDM. These include hyperglycemia, during periods of poor glycemic control; hypoglycemia, during and after activity; foot damage, for those with neuropathy; and ocular complications, which might arise for IDDM patients with retinopathy, especially in activities where blood pressure is increased substantially, such as weight lifting.

Careful monitoring and control of blood glucose levels are essential, before, during, and after activity. In general, tight glycemic control reduces the risk of diabetic retinopathy, neuropathy, and nephropathy by 35 to 70% (Diabetes Control and Complications Trial Research Group, 1993). Importantly, such monitoring and control reduce the risk of hypoglycemia, which frequently occurs when an IDDM person in good glycemic control indulges in a substantial period of physical activity without any adjustment to allow for the effects of the exercise. It is often necessary for the individual to modify insulin intake and calories consumed before and after participation (Puffer, 1996). The recommended forms of insulin treatment for people who are physically active are three or more daily insulin injections or use of an external insulin pump (Fahey et al.). This is because insulin dosage can be fine-tuned to a greater extent when there are many small doses than when there are few large ones. The risk of hyperglycemia typically arises when diabetic athletes are in periods of poor glycemic control. This is because when blood glucose is above 250 mg/dl, rather than reducing the level of glucose, exercise increases the level further (Berg, 1996). It is strongly recommended that diabetics be in good glycemic control before they play competitive sport or participate in exercise activities (Fahey et al.).

Once a program has commenced, glucose should be monitored before, during, and after activity. Because each individual has a unique pattern of response to diet, medication, and exercise, it is important for a number of other factors to be monitored. These include type and amount of insulin and time it is given; insulin injection site; types and amounts of food consumed and times of meals; and duration and intensity of the activity. By examining the effects of all these factors on blood glucose in relation to training and to competition, patterns can be observed that will lead to the development of an individualized regimen. The insulin dose administered before activity often needs to be reduced by as much as 30 to 50% (Kemmer, 1992; Shiffrin & Parikh, 1985) to prevent hypoglycemia, even for moderate intensity and duration exercise sessions. Fahey et al. (1996) indicated that the optimal site for insulin injection before physical activity is debatable, but others have concluded that major muscle groups involved in the exercise should not be used (e.g., Berg, 1996; Thompson, 1996). Bantle, Neal, and Frankamp (1993) found that the abdomen is an efficient site. This suits many sports because the legs and arms are often heavily used, so insulin injected into a limb is absorbed into the blood faster than normal, leading to a rapid drop in blood glucose level and increased risk of hypoglycemia.

It is important to monitor glycemic level into the night following sport or exercise participation (Fahey et al.). Exercise increases insulin sensitivity, as well as metabolism. These increases are prolonged into the evening. When activity occurs in the evening, the effects are maintained during the night. This can result in nocturnal hypoglycemia.

Depending on the levels of blood glucose identified by regular monitoring, the bedtime insulin dose might need to be reduced.

Studies have indicated that overall blood-glucose control does not improve as a result of regular exercise in people with IDDM because they tend to overeat in anticipation of the exercise (Zinman, Zuniga-Guajardo, & Kelly, 1984). Diet should consist of 70% carbohydrates and monounsaturated fats, around 20% proteins, and less than 10% saturated fats. As one guide, Fahey et al. reported suggestions that diabetic athletes should eat a meal comprising 85 to 200 g of carbohydrates between 2 and 6 hours before performance in an endurance activity lasting more than one hour. When people with diabetes participate in spontaneous physical activity, they can only manage their blood glucose level by eating carbohydrates before and during the activity. Berg suggested that in prolonged activity or athletic tournaments that last all day, diabetic athletes should consume carbohydrates every half-hour. Fluid intake also needs to be monitored during exercise. For events lasting less than one hour, water is the best drink. Carbohydrate solutions can be useful sources of fluid and carbohydrates in long duration events or all-day tournaments.

It is clear from the discussion in this section that involvement in physical activity, including competitive sports, for people with IDDM, requires substantial extra preparation before performance, especially during training, and the need to monitor blood glucose during the event. This is all extremely demanding and could be considered a distraction to performers in competitive sport. Support from the coach and teammates is important to ensure that the diabetic athlete plays safely. The likelihood of diabetic precautions lapsing during competition is perhaps greatest in children, especially once they are engrossed in an activity they enjoy.

Here, parents play a vital role. In general, it seems that a critical aspect is to make the activity and the diabetic practices that surround it as regular and systematic as possible. Once a balance has been found for that individual, control will be easier if those levels of activity, medication, and diet are maintained. Under these conditions, as Hall (1997) stated, people with diabetes can participate at international and professional levels in many sports.

Treating Diabetes: The Role of Physical Activity

Today, exercise is recommended as an integral part of the treatment of NIDDM, whereas its involvement in IDDM, although less clear-cut, is generally supported. Perhaps surprisingly, physicians have recommended exercise as a treatment for diabetes for at least 200 years (e.g., Allen, Stillman, & Fitz, 1919; Rollo, 1798; Trousseau, 1882) although some doctors suggested that, in severe cases, patients be confined to bed (Rollo). The study of IDDM has revealed the role of exercise to be complex, including the paradoxical effect of exercise when glycemic control is not good (blood glucose level greater than 250 mg/dL). Here, exercise leads to an increase in glucose level. It is only during the last 20 years that research has been conducted in earnest on exercise and NIDDM. Results of the research indicate that regular physical activity reduces blood glucose level (e.g., Blair et al., 1996; Vranic, Wasserman, & Bukowiecki, 1990), but there are still many unanswered questions. NIDDM is associated with insulin resistance; that is, insulin is produced and transported in the blood, but the cells are resistant to it. The reason that the cells become resistant is not yet understood although there are a number of hypotheses (Vranic et al.). Further, the influence of exercise depends on many factors, including whether the person is obese and whether the treatment involves diet, oral medication, or insulin injection. Vranic et al. reported that, in the attempt to maintain homeostasis, metabolic and circulatory changes occur in the body during exercise. The extent of the changes in blood glucose level, during and after acute bouts of exercise, depends on a number of factors, including the type, intensity, and duration of the activity; the physical condition of the exerciser; the person's nutritional state; and the muscles used in the exercise. The regular performance of intense or moderate physical activity leads to long-term adaptations in people with NIDDM that include increased glucose tolerance and enhanced insulin sensitivity (Vranic et al.). The importance of long-term, regular exercise is that these changes are evident at rest, as well as during and immediately after exercise, and they are maintained for some time after the exercise regimen is terminated (Vranic et al.). Hasson (1994), however, reported little ongoing effect of exercise programs of fewer than 20 to 25 weeks. For more extensive discussions of the physiological effects of acute and long-term physical activity in diabetics, see Vranic et al., Hasson, or Blair et al.

Although researchers such as Vranic et al. (1990) have emphasized the need for more extensive research on both acute exercise and physical conditioning effects in NIDDM, the work done to date does clearly support the central role exercise plays in managing the metabolic processes of diabetics. Research also indicates that people with NIDDM are not very good at maintaining treatment regimens. They are worst at managing the lifestyle changes (diet and exercise) that they must make (M. W. Simmons & Owen, 1992; Wing, 1992). This chapter now addresses the difficulties of maintaining physical activity in a diabetes management regimen.

Management of Physical Activity in Diabetes

Physical activity is an important element of the typical diabetes treatment regimen. The term *physical activity* is preferred here to exercise, as it encompasses competitive sport, organized exercise programs, and lifestyle changes to enhance the extent of daily activity. Although researchers are currently seeking to understand the mechanisms underlying the effects of physical activity on diabetic metabolism, it is widely accepted that sport and exercise are associated with increased glucose metabolism and enhanced insulin sensitivity in NIDDM individuals and protection against cardiovascular disease and hypertension in people with IDDM. For both groups, exercise can alleviate stress, which affects glucose metabolism. Physical activity is usually prescribed as part of a complex, multicomponent treatment regimen, including adherence to a specific diet and regular monitoring of blood glucose, and often requiring oral medication or insulin injection. Because diabetes is a chronic illness, these behaviors must be sustained for life. Management of the components of diabetes treatment affects the length and quality of life. The issue of management of the elements of the diabetic regimen is, thus, critical to the long-term care of individuals with diabetes. This section considers the critical issue of the management of physical activity in the treatment regimen of individuals with IDDM and NIDDM.

Management of IDDM

Insulin-dependent diabetes mellitus is typically identified during childhood or early adolescence. Its management places great demands on patients and their families. Children with IDDM must understand the nature of the illness, appreciate the risks, recognize symptoms of hyperglycemia and hypogly-cemia, remember all the elements of the treatment regimen, and understand how to modify them under specific conditions, such as when they expect to participate in extended physical activity. Although parents can help when children are younger, IDDM children, like their friends, must develop independence. Consequently, sooner or later, control of their diabetes must become an issue of self-management.

Research on the self-management of IDDM in children is complicated by factors including memory and understanding, which can undermine the reliability of self-reports. Johnson, Silverstein, and their colleagues have studied IDDM management in children and adolescents, using 24-hour recall interviews originally developed to study dietary behavior, but extended by Johnson's group to all areas of diabetes management (Johnson, Silverstein, Rosenbloom, Carter, & Cunningham, 1986). They have shown that children and adolescents can produce accurate self-reports, which are corroborated by parents (Johnson et al., 1986) and objective observers (Reynolds, Johnson, & Silverstein, 1990). It was found that younger children did not produce such accurate reports, but with multiple interviews, their recall increased (Freund, Johnson, Silverstein, & Thomas, 1991). It was also found that younger children tended to underestimate the amount of time spent exercising and the strenuousness of the activity more than older children did (Freund, et al.; Johnson et al., 1986; Reynolds, et al.). It is important that Johnson, Silverstein, and their colleagues have shown satisfactory reliability and validity for use of the 24-hour recall technique with children, based on a variety of methods.

The Johnson–Silverstein group examined the relationship between adherence, measured by 24-hour recall, and health status, reflected in blood glucose control. Earlier work typically combined all aspects of the diabetes regimen to produce a composite score. Results of this research were equivocal. Several studies found no significant relationship between adherence and diabetic control (Cox, Taylor, Nowacek, Holley-Wilcox, & Pohl, 1984; Hanson, Henggeler, & Burghen, 1987a; Simonds, Goldstein, Walker, & Rawlings, 1981), whereas low, statistically significant correlations were found by others (Brownlee-Duffeck et al., 1987; Hanson, Henggeler, & Burghen, 1987b). A strong correlation was found by Kaplan, Chadwick, and Schimmel (1985), but they also found a significant correlation between glycosylated hemoglobin levels and score on a lie scale, so some doubt must be cast on the validity of the self-reported adherence data (Johnson, Tomer, Cunningham, & Henretta, 1990). Johnson et al. (1990) argued that evidence suggests that diabetes regimen behaviors are relatively independent (e.g., Glasgow, McCaul, & Schafer, 1987; Johnson et al., 1990). Glasgow et al. (1987) found no consistent relationship between patients' adherence to their regimen and their diabetic control. This contradicted an earlier study by Glasgow's group (Schafer, Glasgow, McCaul, & Dreher, 1983), but was consistent with another study, involving a larger sample (Schafer, McCaul, & Glasgow, 1986).

Johnson et al. (1990) followed Glasgow in using 13 measures of adherence, including indicators of exercise frequency, duration, and type. Adding further methodological sophistication, Johnson et al. (1990) acquired 24-hour recall reports from the primary caretaker, as well as from the patient. They also assessed the multiple-regimen adherence measures nine times over the same period for which the diabetes control measure was taken. (Glycosylated hemoglobin, the usual measure of diabetic control, reflects average control over the past 3 months, whereas recall, which is usually measured at about the same time that blood is drawn, assesses adherence over the past 24 hours. Thus, Johnson et al., 1990, obtained three 24-hour recall tests for the first, middle, and final 2-week periods of the 3 months covered by the diabetic control measure.) There were few differences based on demographic characteristics, but boys exercised significantly more than girls did. Also, comparison of four age-groups (6–9, 10–12, 13–15, 16–19) indicated that adherence to exercise regimen decreased with age. Exercise-regimen adherence contributed no unique variance to a hierarchical multiple regression, examining demographic characteristics and adherence measures as predictors of diabetic control. Johnson et al. (1990) also measured triglyceride levels because IDDM sufferers are likely to die of atherosclerotic heart disease in adulthood (Barrett-Connor & Orchard, 1985). Exercise did contribute to the regression in this case, in interaction with glycosylated hemoglobin at the start of the study. Thus, greater adherence to exercise schedule (more exercise in this case) was associated with lower triglycerides, but only in participants who had poor glycemic control. Exercise was also a stronger predictor variable for girls. Johnson et al. (1990) concluded that adherence behavior was different for patients in good versus fair or poor diabetic control. Johnson et al. (1992) tested a longitudinal causal model that was analyzed using structural equation modeling (LISREL). Despite the strengths of structural equation modeling in testing for causal links, few were found, and none involved exercise. Again, adherence and diabetic control declined with age, and the adherence measures for different aspects of the regimen showed little intercorrelation.

Bond, Aiken, and Somerville (1992) tested the health belief model (HBM) in a cross-sectional study of 56 adolescents with IDDM, aged 10 to 19. For health beliefs, susceptibility and severity were collapsed into a threats measure, costs and benefits were combined, and cues to action remained independent. The multiple indicators of compliance to diabetes regimen were based on the measures developed by Johnson et al. (1990) and by McCaul, Glasgow, and Schafer (1987). In hierarchical multiple regression, older adolescents were found to be less compliant. Nor did compliance generally, or exercise compliance specifically, relate to metabolic control, as measured by glycosylated hemoglobin. Bond et al. stated that health professionals should guard against making assumptions about compliance, based on measures of metabolic control. The best compliance occurred when threat was low and benefits were high. Bond et al. noted an implication that health professionals should avoid the use of threat as a motivator for compliance. Metabolic control was best when threat was low and cues were high. Because this study was cross-sectional, no inferences should be made about the directions of relationships. Bond et al. also reported that 70% of parents were unable to report reliably on their child's activities.

The research on IDDM suggests that greater attention needs to be paid to exercise adherence in adolescents than in children. This could reflect effects of a number of factors, including increasing influence of peers during this period and decreasing guidance and monitoring by parents. Surprisingly, reasons underlying this pattern do not seem to have been examined systematically. The absence of relationships between adherence to different aspects of the diabetic regimen is also a consistent finding that has not been adequately explained. There is little work that has investigated the reasons for this lack of consistency within each individual. Finally, the absence of any strong relationship between adherence and diabetic control has been established by the recent, methodolog-

ically more sophisticated studies. This clearly has practical implications for the motivation of child or adolescent IDDM patients, who fastidiously follow the required regimen only to be told by their physician that their 3-monthly glycosylated hemoglobin test shows poor diabetic control. Perhaps, after several years of this sort of experience, adolescents become disillusioned with their treatment. Thus, health professionals might inadvertently contribute to lack of adherence. Further research is needed on these matters.

Management of NIDDM

Non-insulin-dependent diabetes mellitus, which typically accounts for around 90% of diabetes, generally affects people who are older (over 40), overweight, especially obese, and sedentary. Population statistics indicate that older people will form a larger part of society in future. The incidence of NIDDM and the personal, social, and economic demands it imposes will increase, unless substantial lifestyle change occurs. Thus, the attention of health policy-makers and researchers has focused more on NIDDM during the last 15 years. This section considers a number of research perspectives on the management of NIDDM, including characteristics related to effective management; application of behavioral methods; relationships among knowledge, practice, and health status; and identification of barriers and problem-solving skills.

Characteristics that influence management. In a 6-year project, Anderson et al. (1995) examined the association of a number of variables with diabetes management in Canadian women of European and Chinese descent. Based on the findings of an ethnographic study, Anderson et al. studied the effects of perception of professional care, reported level of social support, self-reported biomedical knowledge, fluency in English, and ethnicity on the standard areas of self-management measured by a section of the same interview. Anderson et al. found that no variable related to all areas of diabetes management. Exercise management was only related to one variable, satisfaction with social support from family and friends, whereas medication management was associated with perceived quality of professional care. The most striking finding was that not one of the 196 women met the criteria for effective exercise management, based on the recommendations of the Canadian Diabetes Association. Anderson et al. concluded that diabetes management is a complex, multifaceted process.

Much research has examined adherence of NIDDM patients to their existing regimen. Some studies have investigated involvement in specific diabetes programs. Wierenga and Wuethrich (1995) considered the attrition of African Americans and white Americans from a diabetes program. Attrition of African Americans from diabetes education programs had previously been shown to be nearly double that of whites (Brownlee-Duffeck et al., 1987). The sample of 171 NIDDM patients comprised 80 African Americans and 91 white Americans, who were between 20 and 50% overweight. Wierenga and Wuethrich found that compared with white Americans, African Americans perceived that they experienced more social support for diet, taking medication, and exercise, and more barriers for diet and exercise, but fewer for taking medication. Thirty-three percent of the African American group dropped out of the program, whereas only 10% of the white Americans left. Those who stayed reported, at the start of the study, more difficulty in living with diabetes, a greater expectation of change in their health behavior as a result of participation, and less previous success in losing weight, but fewer barriers to diet. These results suggest that it is important to tailor education programs to suit different cultural groups.

Wierenga (1994) examined the relationship between a number of lifestyle variables and health status of diabetics. Meta-analyses have indicated that diabetes education programs increase knowledge about diabetes (Brown, 1988, 1990), but this is not necessarily sufficient to produce lifestyle changes in diet and exercise needed for diabetes management (Bernal, 1986). Zimmerman and Connor (1989) found social support influenced exercise behavior more than other aspects of diabetes management. Using multiple regression, Wierenga found that knowledge and social support influenced health practices and that health practices explained the largest amount of variance (18%) in health status. A reservation concerning this study, as with the study by Anderson et al. (1995), is that all the measures, including measures of adherence, were self-reported.

Behavioral approaches to diabetes management. Wierenga (1994) administered a behavioral modification program to promote weight loss as this is considered to be "the cornerstone of therapy" (Wierenga, p. 33). Based on Prochaska and DiClemente's (1983) stages-of-change model and Marlatt and Gordon's (1980) relapse-prevention model, the intervention aimed to modify life-long exercise and eating patterns gradually. It comprised five weekly 90-minute group sessions, focused on the selection of one behavior for modification, identifying barriers and situations where there was a high risk of relapse, and finding sources of social support. Changes were examined at 4-month followup. Analyses revealed that self-reported health practices in the treatment group changed significantly more than did those in the control group. The lifestyle program did not enhance social support or health status, nor was there any benefit in terms of weight loss. Wierenga noted that the initial high scores on the health status questionnaire probably produced a ceiling effect. She agreed with the recommendation of Beeny and Dunn (1990) that diabetes education programs go beyond increasing knowledge to changing behavior.

Wing and her colleagues (Wing, 1992) argued that the treatment of choice for NIDDM individuals is weight loss. In a major American survey, the relative risk of diabetes for overweight people aged 20 to 79 was 2.9 times the risk for people of comparable age who were not overweight (VanItallie, 1985). Prospective studies have shown a nonlinear relationship between obesity and diabetes; that is, there is only a modest relationship across most of the weight range, but a substantial increase in diabetes in the most obese people (Jarret, 1989). Between 60 and 90% of people with NIDDM are obese (Wing, Nowalk, & Guare, 1988). Obesity also increases the likelihood of diabetic complications. For example, increased retinopathy and nephropathy were found by Pirart (1979) and by Ballard et al. (1986), but others have failed to find this pattern (Wing, 1992). Manson et al. (1990) found increased risk of coronary heart disease (CHD) in an 8-year prospective study of 115,886 women aged 30 to 55. The risk of CHD in nonobese diabetics was twice that of nonobese nondiabetics, whereas the risk for obese women increased 12 times. Wing (1992) reported that studies of the short-term effects of weight loss; that is, effects observed soon after the weight is reduced suggest rapid improvements in glycemic control. There is evidence for both increased insulin secretion and reduced peripheral insulin resistance. Followup after more than a year showed much smaller improvements, compared to pre-weight loss-levels (Wing, 1985), but this is largely accounted for by the difficulty experienced in maintaining the initial weight loss. Thus, it appears that programs that can help obese

(that is, most) diabetics to achieve weight loss are likely to be of great benefit to their diabetic control, reduce the probability of complications, and enhance their quality of life, especially if such programs lead to the weight loss being maintained in the long term.

Wing and Jeffery (1979) found that behavior modification improved long term weight loss in nondiabetics. Wing, Epstein, Nowalk, Koeske, and Hagg (1985) found that a behavioral condition led to significantly greater weight losses at the end of the 16 week program than nutrition education, but there were no differences at 1-year followup. In terms of metabolic control, results did not favor the behavioral treatment. To improve the effectiveness of behavioral programs, especially in the longer term, Wing and her colleagues have examined the components of the programs more closely (e.g., Wing, Epstein, Paternostro-Bayles et al., 1988). Few studies have examined the effect of exercise as an adjunct to diet in diabetes although there is evidence that exercise improves weight loss compared with diet alone (Wing, 1992). Bogardus et al. (1984) found no significant difference in weight loss, over 12 weeks, for a very low calorie diet (VLCD) alone and a VLCD plus exercise, but the diet produced a 9.9 kg loss (as opposed to 11.1 kg for diet plus exercise), so it might have been that maximum results were achieved with the diet alone in this study. Wing, Epstein, Paternostro-Bayles et al. (1988) found that a diet-plus-exercise group showed significantly greater weight loss at 10 weeks, 20 weeks, and at 1 year followup, than a diet-alone group. Improvements in glycemic control were significant for both groups at 10 weeks and 1 year (no results given for 20 weeks), but with no differences between the two groups. These results were achieved by the exercise group with a greater reduction in medication. Hartwell, Kaplan, and Wallace (1986) also found a long-term advantage in glycemic control for diet plus exercise over diet alone even though weight reductions at the end of the program were modest. In further studies by Wing and her colleagues, with NIDDM samples, VLCDs and behavior modification produced significantly greater short- and long-term weight loss and glycemic control than did behavior modification alone (Wing, Marcus, Salata, et al., 1991). Improvements in mood, measured by the Beck Depression Inventory and the State Anxiety subscale of the State-Trait Anxiety Inventory were also found (Wing, Marcus, Blair, & Burton, 1991), but careful self-monitoring of blood glucose had no effect (Wing, Epstein, Nowalk, & Scott, 1988; Wing et al., 1986). Wing (1992) concluded that long-term weight losses reported in the research are typically modest, but cited support for their positive physical and psychological effects (e.g., Bauman, Schwartz, Rose, Eisenstein, & Johnson, 1988; Wing et al., 1987).

Barriers, problem solving, and self-care. Perhaps the most substantial body of work related to understanding diabetes self-management, including the role of exercise as a major component, is the research by Glasgow and his colleagues. Glasgow (1994) has adopted a social learning approach, including cognitive and behavioral concepts. It is not possible to review all of Glasgow's work here. Instead, three major aspects will be introduced, namely research on levels of self-care, barriers to self-care, and problem solving to enhance self-care.

Toobert and Glasgow (1994) explained that the term *levels of specific self-care* (behaviors) evolved from concern about the words *compliance* and *adherence*, which were felt to imply "one person bending their will to another" (p. 352) or "the patient doing what the doctor orders" (p. 352). Shillitoe and Christie (1990) also argued for avoid-

ance of the term *compliance*. Toobert and Glasgow preferred the term *levels of diabetes self-care* to refer to the absolute frequency or consistency of regimen behaviors, reserving *adherence* specifically for comparison of the behavior of individuals with the advice of medical or other health professionals.

Glasgow and colleagues developed the Summary of Diabetes Self-Care Activities (SDSCA) questionnaire to measure self-care behavior (e.g., Glasgow, McCaul, & Schafer, 1987; Schafer et al., 1983; Toobert & Glasgow, 1994). It was first used by Schafer et al. (1983) and then by Glasgow et al. (1987). The SDSCA has been refined, so that the form presented by Toobert and Glasgow (1994) consisted of 12 items. Self-care was measured for diet, exercise, medication administration, and glucose testing. The three items for exercise asked on how many of the past 7 days the individual had participated in 20 minutes or more of physical exercise (an absolute self-care measure), what percentage of the time (last 7 days) the person exercised the amount suggested by their doctor (an adherence measure), and how many times the diabetic participated in a specific exercise session, aside from work or household activities (a more specific absolute measure of structured exercise). Three studies were undertaken to validate the SDSCA. Together, they showed acceptable test-retest reliability, internal consistency, factor structure, and concurrent validity (Glasgow et al., 1992; Glasgow, Toobert, Mitchell, Donnelly, & Calder, 1989; Glasgow, Toobert, Riddle, et al., 1989). Predictive validity was not so convincing, with no SDSCA subscale correlating with glycosylated hemoglobin or fasting blood glucose and exercise only showing a significant correlation with desired weight in two studies. Glasgow (1994) noted that metabolic control might be influenced by a range of factors other than self-care. These include appropriateness of regimen, type and duration of diabetes, individual differences in response to stress, social support, and heredity. Thus, the repeated finding of no link between self-care and metabolic control is not so surprising although it is problematic for the long-term maintenance of treatment, as previously noted.

Glasgow (1994) described barriers to self-care as factors, such as cost, time, social pressures, competing demands, and thoughts associated with aspects of the regimen, that affect attempts to follow the regimen closely. Because diabetes regimens are multifaceted, each component of the regimen can have its own set of barriers. A separate barriers subscale was developed for each element of self-care. The 31-item Barriers to Self-Care Scale was based on an earlier 15-item scale developed for IDDM (Glasgow, McCaul, & Schafer, 1986). The revised scale for general use included seven items in the exercise barriers subscale, asking how often each happens for the individual. Examples of items are "The weather is bad when I would like to exercise" and "I think about how much time it takes to exercise." Responses are made on a Likert scale from 1 (*Very rarely or never*) to 7 (*Daily*), with 0 (*Does not apply to me*). The scale was tested in the first two studies that also tested the SDSCA (Glasgow, Toobert, Mitchell, et al., 1989; Glasgow, Toobert, Riddle, et al., 1989). In both studies, barriers to dietary self-care were most frequently reported, followed by exercise barriers, with testing and medication taking less problematic. Internal consistency, stability over 3 and 6 months, and construct validity, both concurrent and predictive, were supportive, the only nonsignificant correlation for exercise emerging for a 6-month prospective self-monitoring measure. Irvine, Saunders, Blank, and Carter (1990) also developed a barriers scale, the 60-item Environmental Barriers to Adherence Scale (EBAS). Glasgow noted that there appears to

be an assumption in the EBAS that if something does not prevent adherence, then it is not a barrier, whereas diabetics might exert considerable effort to overcome a barrier. For example, for many overweight, sedentary people, exercise is a noxious experience, but many still perform exercise as prescribed by their regimen. Exploration of these sorts of thoughts and feelings represents an important direction for future research.

Glasgow and colleagues have shown that barriers, such as those related to exercise, do affect self-care in the predicted direction (e.g., Glasgow et al., 1989a, 1989b). Long-term management of chronic illnesses, like diabetes, requires the development of self-regulation skills in individuals with the illness, so that they take responsibility for their own regimen. Thus, Glasgow has focused attention on problem-solving skills to cope with the barriers to self-care and adherence that people with diabetes meet, whether those barriers are personal, social, or environmental in origin. Toobert and Glasgow (1991) suggested that diabetes education should benefit from the identification of specific problem-solving skills associated with successful coping with the complex diabetes regimen. Further, it will be valuable to be able to identify those diabetic individuals who need training in such problem-solving skills.

Previous paper-and-pencil measures of problem solving, typically developed with IDDM samples, had not revealed significant relationships with self-care or adherence (Johnson et al., 1982; McCaul et al., 1987), so Toobert and Glasgow (1991) chose to develop a structured interview instrument. The Diabetes Problem Solving Interview (DPSI) invites people with diabetes to describe how they cope with 13 situations that can interfere with diabetes self-care. There are five sections, relating to the five main areas of care. Each section starts with a hypothetical situation that is described to diabetic people, who then explain how they would cope. Then the diabetics are asked to describe a problematic situation in that domain that they have actually experienced and to recount how they coped. Finally, they are asked to report how they generally cope with problems in that domain. Toobert and Glasgow (1991) found that exercise did not produce as large a range of strategies as diet, but a greater number of strategies were suggested for exercise problem solving than for glucose testing. Hierarchical multiple regression revealed that exercise problem-solving variables were stronger predictors of self-care than were patient characteristics. Cognitive strategies were most strongly related to exercise regimen observance. No significant relationships were found between problem-solving skills and glycemic control. Toobert and Glasgow (1991) concluded that behavioral problem-solving skills are probably more important in the diet domain, as coping here involves "an almost continuous flow of interpersonal interactions" (p. 82), so the diabetic person must adopt many behaviors to avoid eating inappropriate food. Exercise, on the other hand, probably requires the person to develop a range of motivational strategies for adherence and self-care to be effective in the long-term. Toobert and Glasgow (1991) considered that the problem-solving approach held promise and deserved further elaboration.

The progress made by Glasgow's group in identifying critical variables in the self-management of diabetes by physical activity, demonstrating their involvement in regimen observance, is noteworthy. Glasgow's work has also identified several central principles of diabetes management. Preeminent here is the observation that self-care is not unitary. The intuition that some people will be good at maintaining all aspects of the diabetes regimen, whereas others are poor in all domains, has been refuted. Determining why this is the case would seem to be a fruitful re-

search direction. The practical implication, at this stage, seems to be that health professionals should work with each diabetic they treat individually in terms of self-management and, further, should consider each regimen area separately for each individual. In particular, experts whose role is to engender a long-term exercise regimen should not rely on behavior in other areas of diabetes self-care although they would be wise to ensure their picture of each individual is complete. Another essential result of the work of Glasgow's group and others has been to allay the misapprehension that good self-care or adherence leads to good metabolic control. Toobert and Glasgow (1994) listed many factors that can influence diabetic control, but that are unrelated to adherence. A model in which self-care is predicted by barriers and problem-solving strategies to cope with them has promise, although, again, an exercise-specific version needs to be developed. Not only is the modeling approach an exciting direction for research, but its implications for treatment also are immediate and compelling. Identification of exercise barriers and training in problem-solving skills to overcome them should help many diabetics to better manage physical activity, which has proved especially difficult for the older, largely obese, and sedentary NIDDM population.

Exercise Therapy

Recent papers on exercise therapy for diabetes have focused on the important role of exercise in the treatment of diabetes, often presenting relatively brief sections on the actual development of programs (Albright, 1997; Iverson, 1996; Staten, 1991). Albright, in her chapter in the American College of Sports Medicine's text on exercise management for persons with chronic diseases and disabilities, listed the main effects of exercise on diabetic individuals. She noted that nearly everyone with diabetes can benefit from exercise "although not all benefits will necessarily be realized by each person with diabetes" (p. 96). Artal (1996) reported that exercise can be undertaken by women with gestational diabetes, as well as by NIDDM women with diabetes, who become pregnant. Artal described a home-based program and a hospital-based program, each involving regular laboratory checks of mother and fetus. In both cases, women showed no ill effects. Having written substantially about the reasons for exercise in diabetes, Albright stated the recommendations for exercise testing in a section no longer than half a column. She advised that protocols used for populations at risk of coronary artery disease should be employed for most diabetic individuals. Albright then noted the main reasons for performing exercise tests. These are to identify the presence and extent of coronary artery disease and to determine the appropriate intensity range for aerobic-exercise training for that individual. The final section of Albright's chapter, entitled "Recommendations for Exercise Programs for People With Diabetes," briefly noted that programs must be individualized according to medication, diabetic complications, and goals of the program. Following contra-indications, a list of precautions was given. These include having a source of rapidly acting carbohydrate available during exercise; consuming adequate fluids before, during, and after exercise; practicing good foot care; wearing proper shoes; and carrying medical identification. On this point, the paper, rather abruptly, ends. A paper on diabetes in a seminal text on "exercise management" should include some information about programs for exercise management in diabetic people, including advice on techniques to enhance adherence.

Although other papers on exercise therapy do give more guidance on developing programs, none that were found substantively addressed the major issue of achieving long-term lifestyle change. Staten (1991) focused on managing diabetes, from an exercise perspective, in older adults. She pointed to the considerations for starting exercise, such as determining an appropriate type of exercise, as well as duration and intensity, and deciding how rapidly the exercise regimen should progress. She recommended that an exercise stress test be carried out to determine a safe target heart rate. Because peripheral or autonomic neuropathy can lead to loss of sensation in feet and hands, Staten advised that, in addition to wearing supportive shoes, exercisers check feet for redness before and after exercise and change footwear and that the form of exercise be terminated if redness persists. Staten suggested that the first step in managing exercise in an older person is to appreciate the relationship of the exercise to insulin, nutrition, and glucose. Then fears about cardiovascular events might need to be addressed by visiting an exercise physiologist. Other fears about falls, exercising in unsafe neighborhoods, or walking alone need to be dealt with sympathetically, according to Staten. She proposed mall walking or aerobics classes designed for older adults in these cases. She also noted that checking blood glucose before and after exercising can be motivating, as a decrease is often seen. Staten recommended support from family members, who, by taking an interest or actually participating in the exercise with the diabetic person, can enhance and sustain motivation. Staten proposed that the healthy, independent person with diabetes should gradually increase duration to between 20 and 60 minutes per session, for 3 to 5 sessions per week. Intensity should be within 60 to 90% of maximal heart rate. Staten emphasized that the most important principle is to make the first exercise regimen easy, so the person has a positive experience. Finally, Staten advised that it is important to stress the health benefits of exercise and make sure that it is enjoyable.

Iversen (1996) made some additional suggestions for people with NIDDM. Recognizing likely lower achievable maximal oxygen uptake and endurance than those of nondiabetics, she advised that exercise intensity be maintained in the lower range, monitored by perceived exertion. Low-impact aerobic activities are preferred because of the potential foot problems, so swimming and cycling are better than running or step aerobics, for example. Only one brief comment was made by Iverson about motivation, in which it was acknowledged that motivation is a problem, so "exercise programs for NIDDMs should incorporate variety, individual incentives and social support" (p. 27).

The literature on exercise therapy appears to be strongly oriented to the physical and physiological aspects of exercise in people with diabetes. Although these are important to know for health professionals who are associated with promoting exercise in diabetic populations, there seems to be a great need for papers that present accessible guidance on psychological factors that are likely to affect long-term adherence to exercise programs.

Programs for the Prevention of Diabetes

Despite the focus of this chapter being physical activity, it would be remiss not to comment on the critical role of physical activity in the prevention of diabetes. As discussed in the earlier sections of the chapter, although heredity and other biological factors play a role, NIDDM is largely associated with obesity and physical inactivity. Thus, it has been proposed that lifestyle changes that improve diet and increase exercise can lead to the primary prevention of this form of diabetes (Stern, 1991, Zimmet, 1988). Herman et al. (1987) suggested that up to 50% of NIDDM cases could be prevented by lifestyle changes.

Studies including exercise as an intervention have shown that NIDDM can be prevented or delayed in those with impaired glucose tolerance, especially if the intervention produces weight loss (D. Simmons, Fleming, Cameron, & Leakehe, 1996). Although the practical problems of obtaining sustained lifestyle change are substantial (Cox & Gonder-Frederick, 1992), it can be done, even with high-risk, cultural groups. For example, Heath, Leonard, Wilson, Kendrick, and Powell (1987) employed a successful intervention that was culturally tailored to encourage weight reduction and exercise habits in Zuni Indians, and Foreyt, Ramirez, and Cousins (1991) achieved a similar effect with Mexican Americans.

In a recent study, D. Simmons et al. (1996) presented a culturally appropriate diabetes education and lifestyle intervention to a multi-ethnic hospital ancillary workforce in Auckland, New Zealand. Many of the participants were Maori and Pacific Islanders, who have a high prevalence of NIDDM (D. Simmons, Gatland, Leakehe, & Fleming, 1995). The sample also comprised mainly women, who were unfit and obese, but who had not been diagnosed as diabetic, at the time. The intervention group attended small group diabetes education sessions run by diabetes educators of the same ethnicity, viewed a 17-minute diabetes awareness video *Let's Stop Diabetes Now*, and participated in low-impact exercise classes led by a physiotherapist. The control group completed baseline testing and was monitored during the intervention period. D. Simmons et al. (1996) reported that exercise was well attended and that knowledge increased, as a result of the intervention. Examination of the data indicated that increases, though significant, were small. Thus, at 6 months, total knowledge score was 35% for the intervention group and 26% for the control group, about a quarter to a third of the score possible on the test.

A month after termination of the program, there was a 2% increase in those reporting regular physical activity in the intervention group, compared to a 9% decrease in the control group. D. Simmons et al. (1996) concluded that diabetes knowledge and exercise can be increased in unfit participants by the combination of a culturally tailored exercise program and diabetes education. An interesting aspect of this study was that the ethnically matched diabetes educators were unemployed and unqualified individuals, trained for a community project.

Although community-based programs like the D. Simmons et al. (1996) project are important, there is wide agreement that changing established lifestyle in adults and older people is difficult. It is likely that lifestyle changes specific to the prevention of diabetes will be most effective if children in school are targeted. Although no studies of diabetes-specific lifestyle-education programs were found in the literature, Derksen and Rorke (1996) proposed a model program that could form the basis of such research. The program was designed to meet lifestyle and education needs in Canada, but seems to have general applicability. Deksen and Rorke argued that obesity should be addressed, for reasons canvassed in this chapter. They noted that stress has been shown to play a role in the incidence of NIDDM (Herd, 1990), so stress management was included. Derksen and Rorke adopted a framework developed for business employee health promotion (Association for Fitness in Business, 1992). This approach has four phases: initial planning, conceptual definition, implementation, and evaluation. Derksen and Rorke presented details of underlying processes in each phase and a specific program of activities in the form of figures, which they did not discuss in the text. They argued for a top-down approach, as education and health officials must provide support, but at the same time there is a need for teachers and students to take responsibility for ownership. They emphasized the need for environmental change to be consistent with the diabetes education. For example, school catering facilities should offer appropriate nutritional choice; school sport and exercise facilities should be widely accessible to all students and staff; and teaching and evaluation processes should be structured to reduce stress.

The development of diabetes-specific prevention programs in the community, at work, and at school seems to be in its infancy. Perhaps general health-education programs are thought to achieve the same goals. Certainly, the clear association of diet and exercise with NIDDM and the likely effect of NIDDM on length and quality of life give diabetes education the potential for powerful impact, whether as part of a more general program or as diabetes-specific education. Research is needed on the form of such education and the support that should be provided to achieve lifestyle change, following the provision of knowledge. Prevention research and programs must be a priority.

Conclusion

This chapter has considered the role of physical activity in the management of diabetes. Noting that physical activity has long been accepted as a part of diabetes treatment, only being contraindicated in a small proportion of cases, the author described the pathophysiology of insulin-dependent (IDDM) and non-insulin-dependent diabetes mellitus (NIDDM). Today, medical and physiological researchers continue to seek the underlying mechanisms. The difficulties of managing these illnesses were discussed. For IDDM in children, these difficulties involve the risk of participating in too much or too intense physical activity, leading to hypoglycemia, if blood glucose is under good control prior to the activity, or to hyperglycemia, if glycemic control is poor before exercise. Diabetics who are involved in sport must take precautions against both of these possibilities.

The major concern for IDDM and, especially, for NIDDM individuals is that exercise is an important component of the complex diabetes-management regimen. Research has indicated that, along with diet, the other lifestyle factor, the physical activity regimen, is hardest to maintain in the long term. The chapter, thus, focused on research on the management of the diabetes regimen, with particular reference to physical activity. A number of consistent findings were identified. First, increasing diabetes knowledge does not lead to changes in regimen behavior. Also, self-care in different components of the diabetes regimen is independent, so each element needs to be considered in different ways. Further, adherence to the diabetes regimen, including exercise, is not strongly associated with good metabolic control. This is especially frustrating for diabetics, as the ultimate goal of physicians is usually for the person to maintain normal blood-glucose control. This chapter reviewed the work of three prominent groups, in particular. Johnson's group highlighted the concern with worsening physical activity self-management in adolescent IDDM individuals. Wing focused on the combination of behavior modification, very low calorie diets, and exercise to reduce the weight of obese NIDDM individuals. Glasgow and colleagues examined barriers to self-care and ways of overcoming them through problem solving.

At this time, no panacea exists for managing the diabetic lifestyle. Refining the approach taken by Wierenga (1994), the combination of a number of techniques and perspectives might be promising. These could include social cognitive theory (Bandura, 1986); problem solving of barriers; cognitive and behavior modification techniques, based on the Health Belief Model (Becker &

Maiman, 1975); relapse prevention (Marlatt & Gordon, 1980); and the stages-of-change or transtheoretical model (Prochaska & DiClemente, 1983). It seems surprising that the approach of Prochaska has not received more attention in diabetes research, considering its success in other areas of exercise (see Prochaska & Marcus, 1994, for a discussion).

Based on the current research, a number of implications for health professionals involved in the management of diabetes were proposed. First, diabetes education does not necessarily lead to extensive knowledge (e.g., D. Simmons et al., 1996), so physicians and nurses should not assume that once told means always remembered. Second, even when knowledge does exist, this does not usually lead to behavior change, especially when long-established behavior patterns must be reversed. Behavioral approaches must follow diabetes knowledge acquisition. It appears that changes are best addressed gradually, with regimen components considered individually. Attempting to modify diet and exercise patterns extensively in a short time is doomed to failure, leading to reduced self-efficacy for future change. Exercise, and all other aspects of diabetes management, should be considered separately, as good adherence in one area does not imply good management in all areas. Thus, reasons for poor management will most likely vary for different areas of self-care within each individual. Health professionals are also cautioned against making normalization of metabolic control the goal of regimen adherence. Many factors affect such control, so individuals who manage their regimens effectively, but still produce elevated blood glucose readings would lose motivation, faced with this approach. The focus should be on monitoring exercise, with goals small, progressive, and in that specific domain.

Research on diabetes management is difficult to conduct. Problems include difficulty of access to samples, high costs of methods, and likely high attrition rates, whereas successful outcomes of interventions are not common, and serious ethical issues must typically be resolved. Nonetheless, more research is needed, especially on physical activity in sedentary people, as enhanced management of diabetes can improve the length and quality of their lives. Research on prevention of NIDDM, might not be so difficult to execute especially in schools. It is equally important, and there appears to be a paucity at present. Research on prevention must lead to the implementation of community-based prevention programs. Research on diabetes management and prevention must continue, but it should be acknowledged that the management of both IDDM and NIDDM is much better understood today than it was as little as 15 years ago. This offers potential for improvement in the quality of life of the large number of people who currently live with diabetes.

References

Albright, A. L. (1997). Diabetes. In American College of Sports Medicine (Ed.), *ACSM's exercise management for persons with chronic disease and disabilities* (pp. 94–100). Champaign, IL: Human Kinetics Publishers.

Allen, F. M., Stillman, E., & Fitz, R. (Eds.) (1919). *Exercise*. New York: Rockefeller Institute.

American Diabetes Association. (1986). *Diabetes facts and figures*. Alexandria, VA: Author.

American Diabetes Association. (1993). *Diabetes 1993 vital statistics*. Alexandria, VA: Author.

Anderson, J. M., Wiggins, S., Rajwani, R., Holbrook, A., Blue, C., & Ng, M. (1995). Living with a chronic illness: Chinese-Canadian and Euro-Canadian women with diabetics—exploring factors that influence management. *Social Science and Medicine, 41*, 181–195.

Artal, R. (1996). Exercise: An alternative therapy for gestational diabetes. *Physician and Sports Medicine, 24*, 54–56, 59–60, 62–63, 66.

Association for Fitness in Business. (1992). *Guidelines for employee health promotion programs*. Champaign, IL: Human Kinetics Publishers.

Ballard, D. J., Melton, L. J., Dwyer, M. S., Trautmann, J. C., Chu, C. P., O'Fallon, W. M., & Palumbo, P. J. (1986). Risk factors for diabetic retinopathy: A population-based study in Rochester, Minnesota. *Diabetes Care, 9*, 334–342.

Bandura, A. (1986). *Social foundations of thought and action: A social cognitive theory*. Englewood Cliffs, NJ: Prentice-Hall.

Bantle, J. P., Neal, L., & Frankamp, L. M. (1993). Effects of the anatomical region used for insulin injections on glycemia in type I diabetes subjects. *Diabetes Care, 16*, 1592–1597.

Barrett-Connor, E., & Orchard, T. (1985). Diabetes and heart disease. In National Diabetes Data Group (Ed.), *Diabetes in America* (NIH Publication No. 851468, pp. 1–41). Washington, DC: U.S. Department of Health and Human Services/Public Health Service.

Bauman, W. A., Schwartz, E., Rose, H. G., Eisenstein, H. N., & Johnson, D. W. (1988). Early and long-term effects of acute calorie deprivation in obese diabetic patients. *American Journal of Medicine, 85*, 38–46.

Becker, M. H., & Maiman, L. A. (1975). Sociobehavioral determinants of compliance with health and medical care recommendations. *Medical Care, 13*, 10–23.

Beeny, L. J., & Dunn, S. M. (1990). Knowledge improvement and metabolic control in diabetes education: Approaching the limits? *Patient Education and Counseling, 16*, 217–229.

Bell, D. S. (1992). Exercise for patients with diabetes. *Postgraduate Medicine, 92*, 183–198.

Berg, K. E. (1996). Guidelines for physically active diabetics. In M. B. Mellion (Ed.), *Office sports medicine* (2nd ed.). Philadelphia: Hanley & Belfus.

Bernal, H. (1986). Self-management of diabetes in a Puerto Rican population. *Public Health Nursing, 3*, 38–47.

Blair, S. N., Horton, E, Leon, A. S., Lee, I-Min, Drinkwater, B. L., Dishman, R. K., Mackey, M., & Kienholz, M. I. (1996). Physical activity, nutrition, and chronic disease. *Medicine and Science in Sports and Exercise, 28*, 335–349.

Bogardus, C., Ravussin, E., Robbins, D. C., Wolfe, R. R., Horton, E. S., & Sims, E. A. H. (1984). Effects of physical training and diet therapy on carbohydrate metabolism in patients with glucose intolerance and non-insulin-dependent diabetes mellitus. *Diabetes, 33*, 311–318.

Bond, G. G., Aiken, L. S., & Somerville, S. C. (1992). The health belief model and adolescents with insulin-dependent diabetes mellitus. *Health Psychology, 11*, 190–198.

Brown, S. A. (1988). Effects of educational interventions in diabetes care: A meta-analysis of findings. *Nursing Research, 37*, 223–230.

Brown, S. A. (1990). Studies of educational interventions and outcomes in diabetic adults: A met-analysis revisited. *Patient Education and Counseling, 16*, 189–215.

Brownlee-Duffeck, M., Peterson, L., Simonds, J. F., Goldstein, D., Kilo, C., & Hoette, S. (1987). The role of health beliefs in the regimen adherence and metabolic control of adolescents and adults with diabetes mellitus. *Journal of Consulting and Clinical Psychology, 55*, 139–144.

Cox, D. J., & Gonder-Frederick, I. (1992). Major developments in behavioral diabetes research. *Journal of Consulting and Clinical Psychology, 60*, 628–638.

Cox, D. J., Taylor, A. G., Nowacek, G., Holley-Wilcox, P., & Pohl, S. L. (1984). The relationship between psychological stress and insulin dependent diabetic blood glucose control. Preliminary investigations. *Health Psychology, 3,* 63–75.

Derksen, C. W. F., & Rorke, S. C. (1996). Diabetes prevention: A school-based model of intervention. *Canadian Association for Health, Physical Education, Recreation and Dance Journal, 62,* 4–8.

Diabetes Control and Complications Trial Research Group. (1993). The effects of intensive treatment of diabetes on the development and progression of long-term complications in insulin-dependent diabetes mellitus. *New England Medical Journal, 329,* 977–986.

Fahey, P. J., Stallkamp, E. T., & Kwatra, S. (1996). The athlete with Type I diabetes: Managing insulin, diet and exercise. *American Family Physician, 53,* 1611–1617.

Foreyt, J. P., Ramirez, A. G., & Cousins, J. H. (1991). Cuidando El Corason—a weight reduction intervention for Mexican Americans. *American Journal of Clinical Nutrition, 53,* 1639S–1641S.

Freund, A., Johnson, S. B., Silverstein, J., & Thomas, J. (1991). Assessing daily management of childhood diabetes using 24-hour recall interviews: Reliability and stability. *Health Psychology, 10,* 200–208.

Glasgow, R. E. (1994). Social-environmental factors in diabetes: Barriers to diabetes self-care. In C. Bradley (Ed.), *Handbook of psychology and diabetes: A guide to psychological measurement in diabetes research and practice* (pp. 335–350). Chur, Switzerland: Harwood Academic Publishers.

Glasgow, R. E., McCaul, K. D., & Schafer, L. C. (1986). Barriers to regimen adherence among persons with insulin-dependent diabetes. *Journal of Behavioral Medicine, 9,* 65–77.

Glasgow, R. E., McCaul, K. D., & Schafer, L. C. (1987). Self-care behaviors and glycemic control in Type I diabetes. *Journal of Chronic Disease, 40,* 399–417.

Glasgow, R. E., Toobert, D. J., Hampson, S. E., Brown, J. E., Lewinsohn, P. M., & Donnelly, J. (1992). Improving self-care among older patients with Type II diabetes: The "Sixty Something . . . " study. *Patient Education and Counseling, 19,* 61–74.

Glasgow, R. E., Toobert, D. J., Mitchell, D. L., Donnelly, J., & Calder, D. (1989). Nutrition education and social learning interventions for Type II diabetes. *Diabetes Care, 12,* 150–152.

Glasgow, R. E., Toobert, D. J., Riddle, M., Donnelly, J., Mitchell, D. L., & Calder, D. (1989). Diabetes-specific social learning variables and self-care behaviours among persons with Type II diabetes. *Health Psychology, 8,* 285–303.

Halford, W. K., Cuddihy, S., & Mortimer, R. H. (1990). Psychological stress and blood glucose regulation in Type I diabetic patients. *Health Psychology, 9,* 516–528.

Hall, M. (1997). Sport and diabetes. *British Journal of Sports Medicine, 31,* 3.

Hanson, C. L., Henggeler, S. W., & Burghen, G. A. (1987a). Model of associations between psychosocial variables and health-outcome measures of adolescents with IDDM. *Diabetes Care, 10,* 752–758.

Hanson, C. L., Henggeler, S. W., & Burghen, G. A. (1987b). Race and sex differences in metabolic control of adolescents with IDDM: A function of psychosocial variables? *Diabetes Care, 10,* 313–318.

Harris, M. (1985). The prevalence of non-insulin-dependent diabetes mellitus. In National Diabetes Data Group, *Diabetes in America: Diabetes data compiled 1984* (NIH Publication 85–1468, (pp. 1–10).

Hartwell, S. L., Kaplan, R. M., & Wallace, J. P. (1986). Comparison of behavioral interventions for control of type II diabetes mellitus. *Behavior Therapy, 17,* 447–461.

Hasson, S. M. (1994). Exercise tolerance and training for patients with genetic metabolic disorders, diabetes, and obesity. In S. M. Hasson (Ed.), *Clinical exercise physiology* (pp. 44–61). Toronto: Mosby.

Heath, G. W., Leonard, B. E., Wilson, R. H., Kendrick, J. S., & Powell, K. E. (1987). Community based exercise intervention: Zuni diabetes project. *Diabetes Care, 10,* 579–583.

Herd, J. A. (1990). Brain/body linkages in health enhancement: Effects of lifestyle change. In K. D. Craig & S. M. Weiss (Eds.), *Health enhancement, disease prevention, and early intervention: Biobehavioral perspectives* (pp. 27–45). New York: Springer.

Herman, W. H., Teutsch, S. M., & Geiss, L. S. (1987). Diabetes mellitus. In R. W. Amier & H. D. Dull (Eds.), *Closing the gap: The burden of unnecessary illness* (pp. 72–82). New York: Oxford University Press.

Horton, E. S. (1988). Exercise and diabetes mellitus. *Medical Clinician of North America, 72,* 1301–1321.

Irvine, A. A., Saunders, J. T., Blank, M., & Carter, W. (1990). Validation of scale measuring environmental barriers to diabetes regimen adherence. *Diabetes Care, 13,* 705–711.

Iverson, S. (1996). Exercise therapy for Type II diabetics. *American Fitness, 14,* 24–27.

Jarret, R. B. (1989). Epidemiology and public health aspects of non-insulin dependent diabetes mellitus. *Epidemiological Reviews, 11,* 151–171.

Johnson, S. B., Kelly, M., Henretta, J. C., Cunningham, W. R., Tomer, A., & Silverstein, J. (1992). A longitudinal analysis of adherence and health status in childhood diabetes. *Journal of Pediatric Psychology, 17,* 537–553.

Johnson, S. B., Pollak, T., Silverstein, J. H., Rosenbloom, A. L., Spillar, R., McCallum, M., & Harkavy, J. (1982). Cognitive and behavioral knowledge about insulin-dependent diabetes among children and parents. *Pediatrics, 69,* 708–713.

Johnson, S. B., Silverstein, J., Rosenbloom, A., Carter, R., & Cunningham, W. (1986). Assessing daily management in childhood diabetes. *Health Psychology, 5,* 545–564.

Johnson, S. B., Tomer, A., Cunningham, W. R., & Henretta, J. (1990). Adherence in childhood diabetes: Results of a confirmatory factor analysis. *Health Psychology, 9,* 493–501.

Kaplan, R. M., Chadwick, M. W., & Schimmel, L. E. (1985). Social learning intervention to promote metabolic control in Type I diabetes melliutis: Pilot experiment results. *Diabetes Care, 8,* 152–155.

Kaplan, R. M., Sallis, J. F., Jr., & Patterson, T. L. (1993). *Health and human behavior.* New York: McGraw-Hill.

Kemmer, F. W. (1992). Prevention of hypoglycemia during exercise in type I diabetes. *Diabetes Care, 15,* 1732–1735.

Manson, J. E., Colditz, G. A., Stampfer, M. J., Willett, W. C., Rosner, B., Monson, R. R., Speizer, F. E., & Hennekens, C. H. (1990). A prospective study of obesity and risk of coronary heart disease in women. *New England Journal of Medicine, 322,* 882–889.

Marlatt, G. A., & Gordon, J. R. (1980). Determinants of relapse: Implications for the maintenance of behavior change. In P. O. Davidson & S. M. Davidson (Eds.), *Behavioral medicine: Changing health lifestyles* (pp. 410–452). New York: Brunner Mazel.

McCaul, K. D., Glasgow, R. E., & Schafer, L. D. (1987). Diabetes regimen behaviors: Predicting adherence. *Medical Care, 25,* 868–881.

Pirart, J. (1979). Do degenerative complications differ between normal weight and obese diabetics? In J. Vague & P. H. Vague (Eds.), *Diabetes and obesity: Proceedings of the Fifth International Meeting of Endocrinology, Marseilles, June 18–21, 1978* (pp. 270–276). New York: Elsevier.

Prochaska, J. O., & DiClemente, C. C. (1983). Stages and processes of self-change of smoking: Toward an integrative model of change. *Journal of Consulting and Clinical Psychology, 51,* 390–395.

Prochaska, J. O., & Marcus, B. H. (1994). The transtheoretical model: Applications to exercise. In R. K. Dishman (Ed.), *Advances in exercise adherence* (pp. 161–180). Champaign, IL: Human Kinetics Publisher.

Puffer, J. C. (1996). Medical problems in athletes. In J. E. Zachazewski, D. J. Magee, & W. S. Quillen, (Eds.), *Athletic injuries and rehabilitation* (pp. 829–837). Philadelphia: W. B. Saunders.

Reynolds, L. A., Johnson, S. B., & Silverstein, J. (1990). Assessing daily diabetes management by 24-hour recall interview: The validity of children's reports. *Journal of Pediatric Psychology, 15,* 493–509.

Rollo, J. (1798). *Cases of diabetes mellitus with the results of the trials of certain acids and other substances in the cure of the Lues Venerea* (2nd ed.). London.

Rossini, A. A., Mordeis, J. P., & Handlar, E. S. (1989). The "tumbler hypothesis": The autoimmunity of insulin-dependent diabetes mellitus. *Diabetes Spectrum, 2,* 195–201.

Schafer, L. C., Glasgow, R. E., McCaul, K. D., & Dreher, M. (1983). Adherence to IDDM regimens: Relationship to psychosocial variables and metabolic control. *Diabetes Care, 6,* 493–498.

Schafer, L. C., McCaul, K. D., & Glasgow, R. E. (1986). Supportive and non-supportive family behaviors: Rela-

tionships to adherence and metabolic control in persons with Type I diabetes. *Diabetes Care, 9,* 179–185.

Shiffrin, A., & Parikh, S. (1985). Accommodating planned exercise in type I diabetic patients on intensive treatment. *Diabetes Care, 8,* 337–342.

Shillitoe, R., & Christie, M. (1990). Psychological approaches to the management of chronic illness: The example of diabetes mellitus. In P. Bennett, J. Weinman, & P. Spurgeon (Eds.), *Current developments in health psychology* (pp. 177–208). London, England: Harwood Academic Publishers.

Simmons, D., Fleming, C., Cameron, M., & Leakehe, L. (1996). A pilot diabetes awareness and exercise programme in a multiethnic workforce. *New Zealand Medical Journal, 109,* 373–376.

Simmons, D., Gatland, B. A., Leakehe, L., & Fleming, C. (1995). Frequency of diabetes in family members of probands with non-insulin-dependent diabetes mellitus. *Journal of Internal Medicine, 237,* 315–321.

Simmons, M. W., & Owen, N. (1992). Perspectives on the management of Type II diabetes. *Australian Psychologist, 27,* 99–102.

Simonds, J., Goldstein, D., Walker, B., & Rawlings, S. (1981). The relationship between psychological factors and blood glucose regulation in insulin-dependent diabetic adolescents. *Diabetes Care, 4,* 610–615.

Staten, M. A. (1991). Managing diabetes in older adults: How exercise can help. *Physician and Sportmedicine, 19,* 66–68, 70, 72, 74, 76–77.

Stern, M. P. (1991). Primary prevention of Type II diabetes mellitus. *Diabetes Care, 14,* 399–410.

Taylor, S. E. (1995). *Health psychology* (3rd ed.). New York: McGraw-Hill.

Thompson, K. (1996). Swimming with diabetes. *Swimming Times, 73,* 29–30.

Toobert, D. J., & Glasgow, R. E. (1991). Problem-solving and diabetes self-care. *Journal of Behavioral Medicine, 14,* 71–86.

Toobert, D. J., & Glasgow, R. E. (1994). Assessing diabetes self-management: The Summary of Diabetes Self-Care Activities questionnaire. In C. Bradley (Ed.), *Handbook of psychology and diabetes: A guide to psychological measurement in diabetes research and practice* (pp. 351–375). Chur, Switzerland: Harwood Academic Publishers.

Trousseau, A. (1882). *Glycosuria: Saccharine diabetes. Lectures delivered at the Hotel Dieu, Paris.* Philadelphia: P. Blakiston.

VanItallie, T. B. (1985). Health implications of overweight and obesity in the United States. *Annals of Internal Medicine, 103,* 983–988.

Vranic, M., Wasserman, D., & Bukowiecki, L. (1990). Metabolic implications of exercise and physical fitness in physiology and diabetes. In H. Rifkin & D. Porte, Jr. (Eds.), *Ellenberg and Rifkin's diabetes mellitus: Theory and practice* (4th ed., pp. 198–219). New York: Elsevier.

Wierenga, M. E. (1994). Life-style modification for weight

control to improve diabetes health status. *Patient Education and Counseling, 23*, 33–40.

Wierenga, M. E., & Wuethrich, K. L. (1995), Diabetes program attrition: Differences between two cultural groups. *Health Values: The Journal of Health Behavior, Education and Promotion, 19*, 12–21.

Wing, R. R. (1985). Improving dietary adherence in patients with diabetes. In L. Jovanovic & C. M. Peterson (Eds.), *Nutrition and diabetes* (pp. 161–186). New York: Alan R. Liss.

Wing, R. R. (1989). Behavioral strategies for weight reduction in obese Type II diabetes patients. *Diabetes Care, 12*, 139–144.

Wing, R. R. (1992). Very low calorie diets in the treatment of Type II diabetes: Psychological and physiological effects. In T. A. Wadden & T. B. VanItallie (Eds.), *Treatment of the seriously obese patient* (pp. 231–251). New York: Guilford Press.

Wing, R. R., Epstein, L. H., Nowalk, M. P., Koeske, R., & Hagg. S. (1985). Behavior change, weight loss and physiological improvements in Type II diabetic patients. *Journal of Consulting and Clinical Psychology, 53*, 111–122.

Wing, R. R., Epstein, L. H., Nowalk, M. P., & Scott, N. (1988). Self-regulation in the treatment of type II diabetes. *Behavior Therapy, 19*, 11–23.

Wing, R. R., Epstein, L. H., Nowalk, M. P., Scott, N., Koeske, R., & Hagg. S. (1986). Does self-monitoring of blood glucose levels improve dietary compliance for obese patients with type II diabetes? *American Journal of Medicine, 81*, 830–836.

Wing, R. R., Epstein, L. H., Paternostro-Bayles, M., Kriska, A., Nowalk, M. P., & Gooding, W. (1988). Exercise in a behavioral weight control programme for obese patients with type 2 (non-insulin-dependent) diabetes. *Diabetologia, 31*, 902–909.

Wing, R. R., & Jeffery, R. W. (1979). Outpatient treatments of obesity: A comparison of methodology and clinical results. *International Journal of Obesity, 3*, 261–279.

Wing, R. R., Koeske, R., Epstein, L. H., Nowalk, M. P., Gooding, W., & Becker, D. (1987). Long-term effects of modest weight loss in type II diabetic patients. *Archives of Internal Medicine, 147*, 1749–1753.

Wing, R. R., Marcus, M. D., Blair, E. H., & Burton, L. R. (1991). Psychological responses of obese type II diabetic subjects to very-low-calorie diet. *Diabetes Care, 14*, 596–599.

Wing, R. R., Marcus, M. D., Salata, R., Epstein, L. H., Miaskiewicz, S., & Blair, E. H. (1991). Effects of very low-calorie diet on long-term glycemic control in obese type 2 diabetic subjects. *Archives of Internal Medicine, 151*, 1334–1340.

Wing, R. R., Nowalk, M. P., & Guare, J. C. (1988). Diabetes mellitus. In E. A. Blechman & K. D. Brownell (Eds.), *Handbook of behavioral medicine for women* (pp. 236–252). Oxford, England: Pergamon Press.

Zimmerman, R. S., & Connor, C. (1989). Health promotion in context: The effects of significant others on health behavior change. *Health Education, 1989, 16*, 57–75.

Zimmet, P. (1988). Primary prevention of diabetes mellitus. *Diabetes Care, 11*, 258–262.

Zinman, B., Zuniga-Guajardo, S., & Kelly, D. (1984). Comparison of the acute and long-term effects of exercise on glucose control in type I diabetes. *Diabetes Care, 7*, 515–519.

17

The Psychology of Exercise and Immunology: Implications for HIV Infection

Frank M. Perna

Randal W. Bryner

The effect of exercise on the stress response provides the backdrop for understanding the role of exercise and immunology in health maintenance for individuals with HIV-1 infection and for people in the general population. The purposes of this chapter are to provide the reader with a basic understanding of the immune system, stressor effects on neuroendocrine release and immune function, and the rationale linking exercise and immunology.

The Physical and Psychological Paths From Exercise to Health Outcomes: An Overview

Traditionally, exercise training has been considered a somatic intervention to improve cardiovascular and skeletal muscular fitness and overall physical well-being for the general population. Exercise is also a well-established adjuvant treatment for persons with chronic illness such as cardiovascular disease, HIV-1 infection, and more recently, cancer. Engagement in regular exercise is inversely associated with morbidity and mortality, and exercise has been causally linked

to reductions in health-risk factors (e.g., obesity, hypertension) for the major causes of death in the United States (Blair & Connelly, 1996; U.S. Department of Health and Human Services [USDHHS], 1996). The physical effects of exercise have been directly related to improvements in health outcomes and quality of life. A similarly compelling argument can be made concerning the data supporting the psychological effects of exercise to reduce anxiety and depression and to improve self-esteem and coping, psychological effects that may directly and indirectly influence both quality of life and health outcomes (Biddle, 1995; Dubbert, 1992; Leith, 1994).

Psychoneuroimmunology (PNI) examines the relationship among psychological factors (e.g., stress, negative affect, coping), the nervous system, and the immune system. Because exercise is known to affect each of these areas, increasing attention has been paid to exercise and psychoneurimmunology (LaPerriere, Ironson, Antoni, et al., 1994; Perna, Schneiderman, & LaPerriere, 1997). LaPerriere and colleagues (LaPerriere et al., 1994), drawing heavily upon findings from the field of PNI, have provided the most comprehensive model of exercise and immunology (see Figures 2 and 3). Although the model was originally derived to explain the physiological effects of psychological stress and the rationale for exercise and psychological intervention to promote health among persons with HIV-1, the basic model is potentially applicable to several chronic diseases where psychological stress and immune functioning have been implicated in disease progression (Ironson, Antoni, & Lutgendorf, 1995; Kiecolt-Glaser & Glaser, 1992).

An assumption of this model is that psy-chological stressors cause an individual to initiate efforts at coping that, in turn, activate the autonomic nervous system (ANS), yielding the release of neuroendocrines, neuropeptides, and glucocorticoids. Many immune cells have receptors for neuroendocrines and glucocorticoids, and many tissues where immune cells reside are innervated by the sympathetic nervous system (SNS). Direct innervation by the SNS and hormonal action provide the mechanistic links that have been used to explain how the brain and associated cognitive-affective processes (e.g., threat appraisal of a stressor) may influence immune

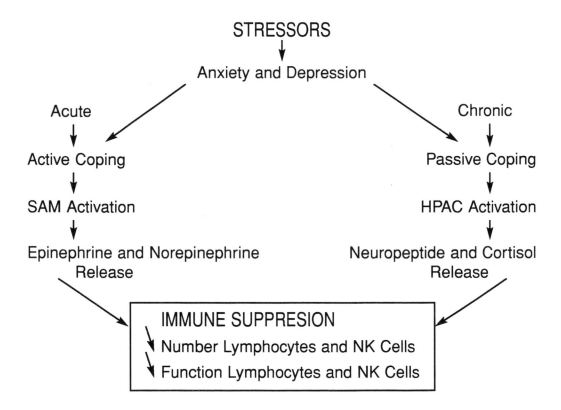

Figure 1

A psychoneuroimmunologic model for stress-related immunomodulator effects (reprinted with permission from the author from "Exercise and Health Maintenance in HIV-1" by A. LaPerriere, M. Antoni, M. A. Fletcher, et al., in Clinical Assessment and Treatment of HIV, *ed. by M. L. Galantino, Slack, Inc., 1992, p. 67.)*

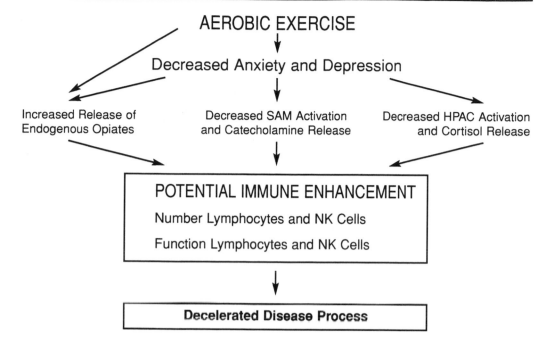

Figure 2

A heuristic of exercise and psychoneuroimmunology model demonstrating how exercise training may decelerate disease progression (reprinted with permission from the author from "Exercise and Health Maintenance in HIV-1" by A. LaPerriere, M. Antoni, M. A. Fletcher, et al., in Clinical Assessment and Treatment of HIV, *ed. by M. L. Galantino, Slack, Inc., 1992, p. 69).*

system functioning in general and immunosuppression in particular (Ader, Felten, & Cohen, 1991). As is also apparent in the model, the type and duration of a stressor (acute versus chronic) and its associated degree of negative affect as well as the individual's perceived ability to cope may all influence autonomic response, which, in turn, also influences ANS activity and immune response. Similarly, because exercise may influence both affective (depression) and cognitive processes (perceived ability to cope) associated with life stressors and the release of endogenous opiates, exercise has been hypothesized to be a particularly potent immune modulator. We shall consider each of these

model characteristics in turn, but first, let us begin with an overview of the immune system.

The Immune System: An Overview of Phenotypes and Function

A primary purpose of the immune system is to protect the body from damage caused by invading microorganisms as well as from tumor growth and allergens. The immune system is quite effective at this task as is evident by the limited duration of most infections. However, there are times when an invading microorganism (e.g., HIV-1) can overwhelm even the healthiest of individuals to the point where the immune system can no longer limit the spread of the infectious agent or tumor cell.

The immune system is divided into two primary functional units: *innate* immunity and *acquired* (adaptive) immunity. Innate, or "natural" immunity, is the first line of defense against invading microorganisms. The innate immune response does not require prior exposure to an invading pathogen and is capable of limiting most potential pathogens before they result in a full infection. If, however, the pathogen is not stopped by the innate response, the acquired response is called upon. Acquired immunity is specific for the inducing agent and is characterized by an elevated response to repeated exposures with the agent. Therefore, once an infectious agent has elicited an immune response, the acquired immune system "remembers" that particular agent and can prevent it from causing disease during a subsequent exposure. Innate and acquired immunity require a number of molecules and cells distributed throughout the body whose functions can be found in Table 1. Leukocytes are the primary cells of the immune system and are divided into two broad categories: (a) lymphocytes, which control the acquired immune response; and (b) phagocytes, including neutrophil polymorphs, monocytes, and macrophages, which form part of the innate immune system.

Lymphocytes are the primary cells controlling the immune response. They are able to recognize foreign material and distinguish it from the body's own tissue. Lymphocytes are produced in the primary lymphoid organs (thymus and adult bone marrow) at a rate of about 10^9 cells each day. The average individual has approximately 10^{12} lymphoid cells, which represent about 20% of the total white blood cells (leukocytes) present in adult circulation. Two broad classes of lymphocytes exist: the T-lymphocytes and the B-lymphocytes.

T-lymphocytes have a number of important regulatory functions such as the ability to recognize and destroy virally infected cells, to activate phagocytes to destroy pathogens, to facilitate the production of antibodies by B-cells, to inhibit certain types of immune responses, and to cause the mobilization of the inflammatory response. Invading microorganisms express antigens on their surface. Lymphocytes recognize foreign material by specific cell-surface antigen receptor molecules. Each lymphocyte has only one type of antigen receptor indicating a high degree of specificity for these cells. However, because each T-cell clone forms

Table 1. Overview of Primary Branches and Components of the Immune System

	Innate Immune Response	Acquired Immune Response
	Resistance not improved by repeated infection	Resistance improved by repeated infection
Soluble factors	lysozyme, complement, ... acute phase proteins (i.e., interferon)	antibody
Cells	phagocytes . . . . natural killer (NK) cells Monocytes/macrophages	T lymphocytes B lymphocytes
Physical barriers	skin, mucus	

different antigen receptors, the entire population of lymphocytes can recognize an enormous variety of foreign substances.

T-cells account for nearly all forms of cellular immunity, including cell-mediated lympholysis, delayed-type hypersensitivity, and transplantation reactions such as graft-versus-host disease and allograft rejection (Sprent, 1993). T-cells originate from the hematopoietic stem cell within the bone marrow, undergo differentiation in the thymus (hence the name "thymus-derived" or T-lymphocyte), and then migrate to peripheral lymphoid tissues (i.e., spleen, lymph nodes) and to the recirculating pool of lymphocytes. T-cells may be subdivided into two main classes: *T-helper/inducer* cells (T_H) and *T-cytotoxic/suppressor* cells (T_C/T_S). Recognition of these two classes of cells is based on the cell-surface receptor proteins that they express. For instance, the T_H cells express the surface receptor molecule CD4 (cluster designation 4) whereas the T_C/T_S express the CD8 protein (Bierer, Sleckman, Ratnofsky, & Burakof, 1989). CD4 cells are activated when they come into contact with antigens that are combined with major histocompatibility complex (MHC) class II molecules whereas the CD8 are activated once they recognize antigen proteins together with MHC class I molecules. These two classes of cells differ considerably with regard to their specific functions. The response of T-cells can be measured in vitro by proliferation tests (*blastogenesis*) in which a blood sample is exposed to a mitogen (e.g., concavalin-A [ConA] or phytohemagglutinin [PHA]) and the ensuing T-cell divisions are counted. Generally speaking, relatively higher counts are associated with relatively greater T-cell function.

T_H-cells are generally defined as T-cells that enhance a B-cell's ability to produce antibody responses to foreign proteins and other T-dependent antigens. T-cells must be activated in order to provide either cell contact- or lymphokine-mediated help (to be discussed later) for antibody responses. Once activated, T_H cells bind to B-cells, causing the formerly "naïve" B-cell to begin to differentiate and secrete immunoglobulins (antibodies) (Noelle & Snow, 1991). T_H cells may also facilitate the microbicidal action of monocytes and macrophages.

Other T-cells have the ability to lyse (kill) cells that express specific antigens and are collectively referred to as cytotoxic T-cells (T_C). Most cells with such cytotoxic activity are CD8 T-cells that recognize peptides derived from proteins within the target cell (Rammensee, Falk, & Rotzschke, 1993). The exact mechanism that leads to cell lysis by T_C cells is unknown. One mechanism that has been proposed is that T_C cells secrete a lytic substance (i.e., *perforin*) that forms holes on the target cell surface causing subsequent cell lysis. However, not all T_C cells contain perforin, and other cytotoxic mechanisms have been suggested, such as the activation of programmed cell death in target cells (Paul, 1993).

Just as the immune system must have the ability to activate (turn on), it is also important to have a turn-off mechanism. Cells that have such an effect are referred to as *suppressor CD8 T-cells* (T_S). The exact nature of how these cells work or whether they are truly "suppressor" cells remains controversial. The inhibition of specific immune responses by certain T-cells may simply reflect the fact that sets of T-cells with distinct lymphokine-producing phenotypes oppose one another's action. The action of one set of T-cells may be simply to redirect the immune response and not cause suppression of other cells.

B-lymphocytes (B-cells) represent approximately 5–15% of the circulating pool of lymphocytes, and they are derived from the hematopoietic stem cells (Roitt, Brostoff, & Male, 1989). B-cells are identified by the surface markers CD19, CD20, and CD22. The mechanisms that lead to B-cell maturation occur in the fetal liver and, in adult life, primarily within the bone marrow (hence the name B-cell). When stimulated, B-cells multiply and produce a variety of immunoglobulins (i.e., antibodies) that, in turn, effect a number of different functions. Antibodies secreted to the surface by a B-cell allow it to bind with antigen receptors expressed on an invading cell.

The primary immunoglobulins include IgA, IgG, IgD, IgM, and IgE [see Roitt et al., 1989 for a review]. IgA is produced primarily in mucosal fluids, and it is thought to play an important role in the prevention of upper respiratory infections. IgG is the primary blood immunoglobulin, and it provides the main antibody effect against most antigens. IgD is found in small quantities in the blood, and it acts as a cell surface receptor for many B-cells. IgM coats foreign microorganisms with proteins (*complement*) that identify them as targets for phagocytic cells. IgE mediates allergic reactions (e.g., asthma and hay fever).

A mature B-cell can become activated directly when it interacts with an antigen or indirectly after it binds to a T_H cell (Noelle & Snow, 1991). B-cell activation prepares the cell to divide and to differentiate into either an antibody-secreting cell or a memory cell. Assays using *poke weed mitogen* (PWM) test the proliferative response of B-cells.

A *memory cell* is a B-cell that has been activated by a particular antigen challenge. Upon subsequent exposure to that same antigen, the memory cell will secrete antibody that is of greater magnitude, occurs more promptly, and is of higher affinity for the antigen. For example, memory B-cell functions provide the rationale for vaccinations (e.g., measles or hepatitis B). Antibody titers to a specific virus (e.g., Epstein-Barr virus) can be used to test the ability of the immune system to keep a latent virus in check. For example, Epstein-Barr virus (the virus that causes mononucleosis) antibody titers have been found to rise during medical school examinations, which suggests that the immune system must work harder under stressful conditions to keep the virus in check (Glaser et al., 1987).

Natural killer cells (NK-cells) are responsible for the "natural cytotoxicity" observed against a variety of tumor and virus-infected cells in vitro (Berke, 1993). Unlike T-cells, NK-cells do not require a prior or prolonged exposure to kill a foreign or abnormal cell. NK-cells appear to be involved in tumor resistance, host immunity to viral and other microbial infections, and regulation of lymphoid and other hematopoietic cell populations (Berke, 1993). NK-cells normally express CD16 and CD56 cell surface markers in humans. The precise lineage of these cells is uncertain. NK-cells are normally found in association with large granular lymphocytes (LGL). The LGL comprise approximately 15% of all lymphocytes and are found in the peripheral blood, spleen, and liver. NK-cell counts and their *cytotoxic activity* (NKCA) are commonly measured through laboratory testing.

Phagocytes engulf foreign pathogens and break down their cell membranes (phagocytosis), and they clear away damaged tissue and infected host (self) cells. A number of different cell types have phagocytic capacities, and each of these cells is derived from bone marrow stem cells. The blood phagocytes include *neutrophils* and blood *monocytes*. Once stimulated, monocytes can differentiate into a tissue *macrophage*. The monocyte/macrophage cell population makes up approximately 10–15% of circulating leukocytes. These cells are somewhat large (10 to 18 μm) and are involved in the early immune response via the phagocytosis of microorganisms and the presentation of antigen to lymphocytes. Neutrophils are the most prevalent leukocyte, making up approximately 60% of circulating leukocytes. Neutrophils destroy ingested microorganisms by releasing protease from cytoplasmic granules and by generating toxic molecules such as hydrogen peroxide.

Phagocytes migrate to areas of infections by way of chemotaxis factors produced by a number of other leukocytes. Once they have arrived, they must recognize the infectious agent by the expressed antigens. Receptors on the phagocytes allow them to bind to a variety of microorganisms that express a given antigen. The binding is greatly enhanced if the microorganism has been "primed" prior to the interaction with the phagocyte. This is accomplished by coating the microorganism with complement (discussed under B-cells), a process known as *opsonization*. Both neutrophils and macrophages have receptors that specifically bind to complement, which allows the phagocytes to recognize their targets.

Phagocytosis can be summarized as follows: migrating of phagocytic cells to the site of infection; binding to the invading microorganism; engulfing and internalizing the organism; and destroying the organism. Once the degradation process has occurred, the foreign antigens are processed and displayed on the phagocyte's surface. The process of *antigen presentation* is critical for the activation of T-lymphocytes.

Antigen presentation is the term used to describe the essential cellular and biochemical events that activate lymphocytes. Antigens are protein molecules expressed on the surface of invading or abnormal cells that induce the formation of antibody. There are a variety of *antigen presenting cells* (APC) that can engulf an antigen and present it in a form that can stimulate lymphocytes. Phagocytes are the most common APCs. Antigens are presented with protein molecules encoded by *the major histocompatibility* gene complex

(MHC) that are bound to the surface of the APC. T-lymphocytes have receptors on their cell surface that bind to the antigen-MHC, ultimately resulting in activation of the T-cell. The sequence of events leading to lymphocyte activation is as follows: uptake of the protein antigen by an APC; biochemical processing of the antigen and its association with MHC molecules; expression of the molecules on the cell surface of the APC; and binding of the lymphocyte cell surface receptor with the antigen-MHC, resulting in growth and differentiation of the lymphocyte.

Cytokines

Much of the way T-cells are able to function and communicate among themselves is through a series of proteins collectively referred to as cytokines. Cytokines are protein mediators involved in cell growth, inflammation, immunity, differentiation, and repair (Howard, Miyajima, & Coffman, 1993). Cytokines are often classified by their site of origin; those produced by lymphocytes have become known as *lymphokines* whereas those produced by monocytes have collectively been referred to as *monokines*. Primary cytokines include interleukin-2 (IL-2), IL-3, IL-4, IL-5, IL-6, IL-9, IL-10, granulocyte-macrophage colony-stimulating factor (GM-CSF), interferon-gamma (IFN-γ), tumor necrosis factor alpha (TNF-α), and TNF-β.

Cytokines are not naturally produced by T-cells but are induced following receptor-mediated T-cell activation, usually caused by antigen presentation to the T-cell by APC. Two particularly striking features of this family of molecules are their extensive pleiotropy and redundancy; that is, each cytokine has multiple functions, and any one function is generally mediated by more then one cytokine (Paul, 1989).

Interleukins (IL) are lymphocyte growth factors secreted primarily by T-cells but also by macrophages, B-cells, and LGL. At present, at least 12 types of IL have been identified in the human (Mackinnon, 1992) although IL-1 through IL-6 have been the most studied and characterized of all the IL molecules.

IL-1 is primarily produced by macrophages although other cell types produce IL-1 activity. IL-1 is one of the best examples of a pleiotropic cytokine in that it can affect a large variety of immune and nonimmune cells. These actions include IL-2 production and IL-2 receptor expression on T_H cells, monocyte/macrophage production of other cytokines (i.e., IL-6 and TNF), B-cell proliferation and differentiation, and increased antibody production; and it can directly interact with T_C, NK-cells, and activated macrophages, augmenting their ability to kill neoplastic target cells (e.g., cancer cells). IL-1 can also profoundly affect the activity of nonimmune cells. An example of this is the ability of IL-1 to alter the function of cells of the central nervous system and induce fever by indirectly enhancing prostaglandin production.

IL-2 is produced predominantly by T-cells and to a lesser degree by immunocompetent thymocytes. By far the major activity of IL-2 is to act as a growth (proliferation) stimulator for T-cells. IL-2 causes growth and differentiation for both T_H and T_C, and it also enhances the biosynthesis of other T-cell-derived lymphokines, such as IFN-γ, lymphotoxin, and B-cell growth and differentiation factors. Additionally, IL-2 has been reported to induce B-cell growth and differentiation by enhancing the actions of IL-4 and B-cell growth factor. IL-2 also increases the activity of NK-cells.

IL-3 is produced by activated T_H cells, and IL-3's primary function is to stimulate the differentiation of granulocytes and monocytes. IL-4 has been identified as a B-cell stimulatory factor (Howard et al., 1982). It is also a short-term growth costimulant for both T_H and

T_C lymphocytes (Mosmann, Bond, Coffman, Ohara, & Paul, 1986). In addition, IL-4 has been shown to enhance the antigen presenting ability of bone-marrow-derived macrophages, as well as to increase class II MHC antigen expression and tumoricidal activity of peritoneal macrophages. IL-5 is a potent regulator of eosinophils, causing them to proliferate and to differentiate into mature effector cells. IL-3 may also be involved with this latter function. IL-5 can also serve as a stimulator of B-cell growth. IL-6 is involved in B-cell differentiation, enhancing the stimulation of IgG secretion and activation of T-cells.

Tumor Necrosis Factor (TNF)

TNF is produced by activated macrophages and other cells and has a broad spectrum of biological actions on many different target cells, both immune and nonimmune (Durum & Oppenheim, 1993). TNF was first discovered by its ability to induce hemorrhagic necrosis in certain tumors in vivo (Old, 1985) and is referred to as cachectin (TNF-α). TNF is considered a major inflammatory mediator. Lymphotoxin, a T-cell product, has also been called TNF-β because many of its actions are similar to those of TNF-α and because both bind to the same receptor on target tissues.

Interferons

Based on a number of characteristics, interferons are divided into three distinct classes: α, β, and γ. IFN-α and IFN-β are classic interferons that are induced as a direct result of viral infection of cells. In contrast, IFN-γ is not induced directly by viral infection, but is induced by immune stimuli only. Although it can induce antiviral activity in cells, this activity is several times less than that of IFN-α and IFN-β. However, IFN-γ is 100 to 10,000 times more active as an immunomodulator than the other two classes of interferons.

Types of Stressors and Neuroendocrine Response

In the previous sections, we suggested that psychological stressors and exercise may influence the immune system through the actions of the SNS and stress-related hormones, and we provided an overview of the immune system. Therefore, it is important to understand how stressors affect stress hormone response.

Selye (1956) postulated that the stress response is a general alarm reaction that can be elicited by any of a large number of divergent stimuli. The induced response was believed to follow a specific physiological pattern, which varies only in its particulars among eliciting events. A hallmark of the stress response was thought to be activation of the hypothalamus-pituitary-adrenocortical (HPA) axis. The notion of a single nonspecific response pattern has been challenged by others who observed differentiated hormonal profiles to diverse physical and psychological stressors (Mason, 1975).

Studies from the animal behavior laboratory showed that mammals confronted by a stressor tend to reveal one pattern of cardiorespiratory activation (*defense reaction*) if appropriate coping responses are attempted, but a different pattern (*inhibitory coping*) in highly adverse situations in which coping responses appear to be unavailable (Abrahams, Hilton, & Zbrozyna, 1960; Cannon, 1992; Hess, 1957; Perna et al., 1997). The former pattern is generally associated with movement, whereas the latter pattern is associated with an inhibition of movement (Schneiderman, 1978; Schneiderman & McCabe, 1989).

A similar dichotomy seems to exist when one examines human responses to stressors. Thus, on the one hand, relatively acute active coping activities (pattern 1) that involve physical movement (representational, anticipated, or actual) tend to elicit responses that resemble the defense reaction of temporal increases in sympathoadrenal medulla (SAM) activity. SAM activity is characterized by norepinephrine (NE) release from postganglionic sympathetic neurons, epinephrine (E) release by the adrenal medulla, and reductions in total peripheral resistance to blood flow (Perna et al., 1997). On the other hand, activities that involve inhibitory coping (pattern 2) may lead to prolonged increases in SAM activity, an increase, rather than a decrease, in total peripheral resistance, and an increase in HPA-axis activation (Hurwitz et al., 1993). Activation of the HPA-axis is associated with release of corticotropin-releasing hormone (CRH) from the hypothalamus, adrenocorticotropic hormone (ACTH) from the pituitary, and cortisol from the adrenal cortex.

Frankenhaeuser (1990) has also documented specific hormone profiles in response to stressors that depend upon the individual's perceived ability to cope with the stressor. Frankenhaeuser and others (McCabe & Schneiderman, 1985) suggest that increases in catecholamines (epinephrine and norepinephrine) reflect general SAM activation and *intensity of affect* associated with a stressor or challenge, whereas elevations in cortisol reflect *degree of distress* associated with a stressor. Frankenhaeuser has used the term *effort without distress* to describe coping associated with SAM activation but limited HPA-axis activation and *effort with distress* to describe coping associated with SAM activation and pronounced HPA-axis activation. McCabe and Schneiderman have posited a similar position, namely, that cortisol release is primarily dependent upon cognitive appraisal of a stress situation. Additionally, although an initial cortisol rise may be a necessary stress response, prolonged activation of the HPA-axis is deleterious. Hence, both pattern 1 (active coping or effort without distress) and pattern 2 (inhibitory coping or effort with distress) responses are associated with SAM activation (McCabe & Schneiderman), but HPA-axis activation is dependent upon the intensity, duration, and other characteristics of the stressor that influence affective tone and perceived ability to cope with a stressor/challenge.

Therefore, we see that in contrast to Selye's (1956) notion of a generalized stress response, specific types of stressors elicit differentiated neuroendocrine responses. The patterning of neuroendocrine responses to stressors goes far beyond an academic discussion. For example, from our description of differential stress responses, one can also see how two individuals faced with the same stressor, but with different cognitive appraisals, may have divergent neuroendocrine responses that, in turn, may influence immune response. It is also very important to note that activation of the "stress response" can be extremely useful and necessary. Activation of the stress response does prepare people for challenge situations, and performance on cognitive and physical tasks is positively associated with catecholamine levels (Dienstbier, 1989; Frankenhaeuser, 1990).

Exercise Versus Psychological Stress: Implications for Immunity and Intervention

Because exercise can present a challenge to an organism, it can operate as a stressor. As with psychological stressors, neuroendocrine patterning differs depending on characteristics of exercise (e.g., intensity); that also partially explains the different immune response to high- versus moderate-intensity exercise. Although it is a stressor, moderate-intensity exercise elicits a very different affective, cognitive, and physiological response than do psychological stressors (e.g., a negative life event). For example, unlike a stressful life

event, engaging in exercise is generally perceived as enjoyable and within a person's control rather than as an unpleasant event outside of one's control. Exercise is also associated with optimism and general feelings of self-efficacy that contrast with feelings of helplessness that one may encounter with severe life events such as the diagnoses and treatment of a chronic disease (Kavussanu & McCauley, 1995; LaPerriere, Ironson, Antoni, et al., 1994). Exercise training is also well known to decrease negative affect, particularly depression (North, McCullagh, & Tran, 1990; Petruzzello, Landers, Hatfield, Kubitz, & Salazar, 1991), which has been positively related to HPA-axis activity (Nemeroff et al., 1984).

Physiologically, exercise can be differentiated from psychological stress (Dienstbier, 1989; McCabe & Schneiderman, 1985; Schneiderman & McCabe, 1989). For example, psychological stress is known to cause a preferential release of epinephrine relative to norepinephrine (McCabe & Schneiderman). In contrast, relative to psychological stress, moderate-intensity physical exercise elicits a preferential release of norepinephrine relative to epinephrine. Exercise training has long been known to decrease resting heart rate that is a function of reduced beta-adrenergic activity and increased parasympathetic activity, a hallmark of the relaxation response (Frick, Elovainio, & Sommer, 1967; Frick, Kottinen, & Sarajas, 1963; LaPerriere, Ironson, Antoni, et al., 1994). Additionally, aerobic exercise has also been shown to reduce SAM response to mental stress (Blumenthal, et al., 1990).

Moreover, Dienstbier (1989), drawing upon animal and human models of stress reactivity, has posited that exercise training leads to "physiological toughness," which is characterized by optimal catecholamine but limited cortisol releases in the face of stressors. Because exercise can alter cognition, affect, and physiology, Dienstbier has suggested that physical exercise is one behavior that may favorably alter physiological reactivity to forthcoming psychological stressors (i.e., stress-buffering effect). Although not all researchers have found support for the psychological stress-buffering effects of exercise (Duda, Sedlock, Melby, & Thaman, 1988; Roth, 1989), many have (Brown, 1988; LaPerriere et al., 1990; Rejeski, Thompson, Brubaker, & Miller, 1992).

Because epinephrine has a much greater binding affinity than norepinephrine to beta$_2$ adrenergic receptors and many immune cells and tissues express beta$_2$ adrenergic receptors, acute psychological stressors may negatively influence the immune system (Perna et al., 1997). Considering that cortisol potentiates the actions of catecholamines as well as being generally immunosuppressive itself, prolonged or extreme psychological stress, which is characterized by cortisol release, provides another pathway by which psychological stress may influence immune functioning (Perna et al., 1997). By contrast, behaviors such as relaxation training and exercise are thought to favorably affect the immune system by altering the stress response (Kiecolt-Glaser & Glaser, 1992).

Endocrine-Immune Interaction

Because cortisol, ACTH, and beta$_2$ adrenergic receptors have been identified on lymphocytes, the hormones of the HPA-axis and SAM systems are thought to influence the immune system. For example, studies have shown that CRH can inhibit natural killer cell cytotoxic activity (NKCA) (Pawlikowski, Zelazowski, Dohler, & Stepien, 1988); ACTH impairs the responsiveness of T-lymphocytes to antigenic (CD3 antibody) and mitogenic stimuli such as concanavalin-A (Kavelaars, Ballieux, & Heijnen, 1988). Corticosteroids may also impair or modify several components of cellular immunity, including T-lymphocytes (Cupps & Fauci, 1982), macrophages (Pavlidis & Chirigos, 1980), and NKCA (Levy, Herberman, Lippman, & d'Angelo, 1987).

Similarly, increases in peripheral catecholamines influence the immune system. Sympathetic noradrenergic fibers innervate the vasculature as well as the parenchymal regions of lymphocytes and associated cells in several lymphoid organs. Nerve terminals in these organs are generally directed into zones of T-lymphocytes (Felten, Felten, Carlson, Olschawaka, & Livnat, 1985). Activation causes the release of these lymphocytes into the peripheral circulation. However, infusion studies have shown that beta-adrenergic agonists are associated with reduced NKCA (Katz, Zeytoun, & Fauci, 1982) and decreased T-lymphocyte proliferation (Plaut, 1987), which is consistent with the presence of beta-adrenergic receptors found on lymphocytes.

In general, catecholamines tend to reduce most immune functions in vitro, including NKCA (Bourne et al., 1974; Plaut, 1987). Recently, however, an in vivo study has shown that acute emotional stressors can lead to an increase in the number of NK-cells in peripheral circulation (Benschop, Oosteveen, Heijnen, & Ballieux, 1993). In the resting state, NK-cells are found along the endothelial cell layer of the arterial wall (Atherton & Born, 1972). This constitutes the vessel's marginal zone. At rest, the adhesive force between the NK-cell and the endothelium is greater than the shear forces that would free NK-cells to move into the circulating pool of lymphocytes. During acute stress (which presumably includes intense aerobic exercise), increased flow in the systemic arterial system changes the equilibrium between adhesive and shear forces, which causes NK-cells to move into circulation. In addition, beta$_2$ adrenergic receptor stimulation of lymphocytes further disrupts adhesion of

NK-cells to the endothelium (Benschop et al.). In this manner, the number of NK-cells recruited from the marginating to the circulating pool of lymphocytes is temporally increased. Lymphocytes, especially CD8 suppressor cells, may also show temporary increases during or immediately following acute stressors. Thus, although stress-induced recruitment of NK-cells and lymphocytes into the circulating pool would make an increased number of cells available for lysis (Benschop et al.), prolonged SAM activation, particularly when accompanied by HPA-axis activation, may reduce NKCA activity during the recovery from a stressor (Bourne et al.; Hellstrand & Hermodsson, 1989).

Exercise-Immune System Interaction

Acute aerobic exercise presents an active coping task, causing increased catecholamine output via SAM activation, increased cardiac output, and decreased total peripheral resistance (Landmann et al., 1984; Neiman et al., 1994; Schneiderman & McCabe, 1989). In most cases, cortisol release is dependent on exercise intensity and duration (Cashmore, Davis, & Few, 1977; Farrell, Garthwaite, & Gustafson, 1983). Cortisol, however, may initially decrease and not increase above resting levels until the participant achieves an intense exercise level approaching exhaustion (Tharp, 1975). Following high-intensity exercise (greater than 80% of functional capacity), cortisol recovery to pre-exercise levels will vary, at times remaining elevated for hours or even days (Neiman et al., 1994; Urhausen & Kinderman, 1987). However, among elite aerobic athletes, cortisol levels immediately following exhaustive exercise may decrease significantly or remain unchanged from baseline (Perna & McDowell, 1995; Snegovskaya & Viru, 1993; Tharp). These findings suggest that psychological factors in addition to phys-

iological demand may play a role in HPA-axis regulation during exercise.

Immunologic sequelae of high-intensity exercise include a general rapid increase of immune cells, particularly CD8 (suppressor/cytotoxic) and NK-cells, with a concomitant decrease in lymphocyte response to ConA and an increase in NKCA, followed by transitory decreases in NKCA and proliferation to ConA below basal levels (Field, Gougeon, & Marliss, 1991; Fry, Morton, & Keast, 1992; Neiman et al., 1994; Tvede et al., 1989). In contrast, moderate-intensity exercise elicits modest shifts in immune cell counts without either a sustained increase in cortisol or epinephrine, and in some cases, increases in NK, NKCA, or proliferative response of T-lymphocytes (Nehlsen-Cannarella et al., 1991; Neiman et al., 1994; Shepard & Shek, 1994; Tvede et al.).

Therefore, it is evident that neuroendocrine response influences the acute and recovery phase immune responses to general psychological stress and to exercise stressors. In summary, psychological stress and high-intensity or prolonged exercise produce a biphasic immune response in NK and B-cells, and a decrease in the ratio of helper T-cells (CD4 cells). Although CD4 cells rise in response to stressors, their increase is not as great as those of CD8 suppressor/cytotoxic cells. Hence, the relative percentage of circulating CD4 cells and their associated activity temporarily decrease. The cytotoxic response of NK and B-cells may rise acutely, primarily as a result of increased cell counts, but then fall below baseline during recovery when cells return from the peripheral blood to their marginating pools and neuroendocrines and cortisol impair the cytotoxic activity of the remaining individual cells on a per cell (lytic unit) basis.

The fluctuation of cell counts and cell activity could have implications for immune system function during the period after high-intensity or prolonged exercise during which the lymphocyte count dips below pre-exercise levels (Neiman et al., 1994). Mackinnon (Mackinnon, 1992; Mackinnon, Ginn, & Seymour, 1991) and others (Shepard & Shek, 1994) have referred to the biphasic immune response to high-intensity exercise as creating a *window of susceptibility* for viral infection among athletes engaged in heavy exercise training. In contrast to psychological stress and intense exercise, Nieman and colleagues (Nieman et al., 1994) have shown that the cytotoxic activity of NK-cells increases after moderate exercise but decreases after intense activity. Additionally, several studies with HIV-1 patients have documented increases in CD4 and NK-cells after moderate-intensity aerobic exercise (LaPerriere et al., 1990, 1991; Perna et al., 1999). One study has reported that moderate-intensity exercise increased NK-cell activity among recent postsurgical breast cancer patients (Lotzerich et al., 1994), whereas exercise intervention long after breast cancer surgery did not alter NK-cell count or function (Nieman et al., 1995).

Exercise, Stress, and Chronic Disease: A Focus on HIV-1

Although the "stress response" can be extremely useful and necessary, potential adverse effects tend to arise under three general circumstances:

1. Encountering many acute stressors that cause frequent activation of the SAM and possibly the HPA-axis.
2. Having an exaggerated stress response (stress reactivity) that causes some individuals to respond physiologically and psychologically to stressors to a greater degree than do people in general.
3. Having to cope with a stressor for an extended period of time (i.e., chronic stress) that, in turn, also frequently initiates its own set of acute stressors.

For example, the diagnosis of HIV-1 is a chronic stressor that may lead to many acute psychosocial, medical treatment-related, and financial stressors that may also dislodge social ties. Chronic disease, and HIV-1 in particular, by its very nature, creates the possibility for a host of acute and chronic psychological stressors that have been hypothesized to impair quality of life and possibly accelerate disease progression (Chesney & Folkman, 1994; Ironson et al., 1995). Behavioral, cognitive-affective, and psychophysiological responses have been proposed as mediating mechanisms to explain how stress may alter health outcomes, particularly those that rely on immune system involvement (Baum, Herberman, & Cohen, 1995; Ironson et al., 1985). Behavioral responses to excessive or prolonged stress may include loss of sleep or use of alcohol to emotionally numb oneself from negative emotions. These behaviors can be immunosuppressive as well as potentially detract from treatment compliance (Irwin, Smith, & Gillin, 1992). Negative affect, such as anxiety and depression, and even general negative mood state have been shown to have immunosuppressive effects (Herbert & Cohen, 1993). Additionally, although many pharmacological advances (e.g., protease inhibitors) have been made to combat HIV-1, "drug cocktail" treatments rely on strict adherence to an administration regime and, hence, high levels of self-regulatory behavior. Psychological stress is known to impair self-regulatory behavior, which may have severe consequences with respect to HIV-1 (Chesney & Folkman, 1994; Heatherton & Renn, 1995). Not only may pharmacological treatment be ineffective, but if medication protocols are not followed, drug-resistant mutations of the HIV-1 may also ensue.

Therefore, it is important to recognize the contributions of stress and stress-reduction techniques to disease outcome and quality of life. Psychological intervention has been shown to alter immunity and potentially improve HIV-1 disease progression, and psychological intervention has been espoused for other chronic diseases such as cancer (Antoni et al., 1990; Ironson et al., 1995; Kiecolt-Glaser & Glaser, 1992; Lutgendorf et al., 1997). Because exercise modulates affect, influences self-referent thought, and is itself a modifiable behavior, it has been considered a form of cognitive behavioral intervention (Dubbert, 1992). Reductions in negative affect following exercise training may also accrue in the absence of a cardiovascular fitness effect (Leith, 1994).

Pathophysiology of HIV-1 Disease

The pathogenesis of HIV-1 disease is based on the proclivity of HIV-1 to infect the immune system (Fauci, 1988). HIV-1 infection has been associated with abnormalities in cell-mediated (T-cell) and humoral (B-cell) immunity as well as decrements in NK function (Fauci, 1984, 1988). However, the primary target of HIV-1 is a subset of T-cells, the T helper/inducer cell (CD4) (Farrell et al., 1983; Fauci, Macher, & Longo, 1983; LaPerriere et al., 1997; Rosenberg & Fauci, 1990). The HIV-1 virus assimilates into the DNA of the CD4 cell by attaching itself to a surface membrane receptor (Fauci, 1984; Fauci et al., 1983). The regulatory and effector functions of the CD4 cell are then compromised (Fauci, 1984), until the cell eventually dies. Because CD4 cells are integral to the regulation of numcrous othcr immune cells, the continual decline of CD4 cells, which is a primary marker of HIV-1 progression, is of major importance to overall immune system functioning (Katz, 1987; LaPerriere, Schneiderman, Antoni, & Fletcher, 1989).

As a result of the quantitative and qualitative effects of HIV-1 on the CD4 cells, individuals infected with HIV-1 are susceptible to a variety of unusual infections and malig-

nancies that thrive in an immunosuppressed environment (Fauci, 1984, 1988; Rosenberg & Fauci, 1990). These infections are referred to as opportunistic infections, and they are a major source of morbidity and mortality in HIV-1 disease (Kaplan, Wofsky, & Volberding, 1987). Because the HIV-1 infected individual typically goes through several stages of immune suppression and clinical manifestation, disease progression occurs over an extended period of time, and HIV-1 infection is viewed as a chronic disease (Antoni et al., 1990).

The Centers for Disease Control and Prevention (CDC, 1992) and The World Health Organization (WHO, 1990) have developed criteria for HIV-1 staging based on CD4 cell count, symptoms, and presence of opportunistic infections and malignancies. It is useful to separate HIV-1 disease into three categories: asymptomatic, early symptomatic pre-AIDS, and AIDS (WHO, 1990). During the asymptomatic phase (CDC category A), which may last as long as 15 years, the individual is capable of transmitting the disease, and CD4 cell count may not be altered (Klimas et al., 1991; Munoz et al., 1990; Stevens, Taylor, & Zang, 1986; WHO, 1990). However, the individual is completely without any HIV-1 related symptomatology and is relatively healthy (Munoz et al.). The early symptomatic pre-AIDS phase (CDC category B; CDC, 1992), is characterized by the emergence of constitutional symptoms (e.g., fever and/or diarrhea persisting for more than 1 month, involuntary weight loss) and/or a diagnosis of an infectious disease associated with HIV-1 and indicative of a defect in cell-mediated immunity (e.g., oral hairy leukoplakia, multidermatomal herpes zoster). This stage of the disease may also last for several years, and CD4 cell counts typically range from 200–800 (Munoz et al.). An individual is diagnosed with AIDS when either a CD4 cell count drops below 200 or a major opportunistic infection or malignancy is diagnosed (CDC category C; CDC, 1992). Advances in the development of antiviral therapy as well as aggressive therapy for HIV-1 associated complications have made it possible to achieve several years of additional high-quality life following an AIDS diagnosis (Schooley, 1995).

Exercise and CD4 Cells

The CD4 cell count is the most widely accepted marker of disease progression, and it is routinely used as an indicator of the effectiveness of clinical trials in HIV-1 disease (LaPerriere et al., 1997). The CD4 cell also controls numerous aspects of immune system functioning. Therefore, the importance of determining the effects of exercise on the CD4 cell becomes quite clear. Just as drug therapies can have widely different effects on immunity at different stages of the disease, it is reasonable to conclude that exercise also may elicit a different immunologic effect depending on whether the individual is asymptomatic, symptomatic, or warrants an AIDS diagnosis (LaPerriere et al., 1997). Thus, obtaining homogeneous study samples, with individuals at similar stages of disease, may be important when investigating the effects of exercise on CD4 cells in HIV/AIDS (LaPerriere et al., 1997; Perna et al., 1999). Unfortunately, most exercise study samples include individuals along the entire spectrum of HIV-1 disease, so an evaluation of exercise study results according to one of the three aforementioned stages of disease is not always possible. Therefore, when reviewing those studies with heterogeneous samples, the average CD4 cell count has been used as the primary criterion to classify participants according to disease stage (LaPerriere et al., 1997).

Asymptomatic

Only one published study, to date, has reported the effects of exercise on the CD4 cell in a homogeneous sample of asymptomatic HIV-1 infected individuals (LaPerriere et al., 1991). LaPerriere and colleagues conducted a randomized controlled investigation with 16 subjects recruited exclusively from HIV-1 infected gay males to prevent against possible confounds arising from the immunologic influence of different high-risk behaviors (e.g., intravenous drug use). Each subject was administered a complete physical and medical history to ensure asymptomatic status consistent with joint CDC category A criteria (CDC, 1992) and a graded exercise test to determine cardiopulmonary fitness (VO_2 consumption). Individuals were then assigned to either the 10-week aerobic-exercise training group or the assessment-only control group. Exercise training consisted of 45 min/day, 3 days/week of stationary bicycle ergometry at 70 to 80% of maximum heart rate (HR). Following the exercise-training program, an increase in VO_2 and CD4 cells was observed in the exercise group, whereas no similar change was seen in the control group.

Using a similar 5-week protocol, a related randomized controlled study by LaPerriere and colleagues (LaPerriere et al., 1990) examined the stress-buffering effects of exercise among 50 asymptomatic gay men who were previously sedentary and whose HIV-1 serologic status was unknown. Participants were given a graded exercise test to determine fitness level (VO_2), a blood draw for immunological assay, and a mood-state measure to assess level of emotional distress at baseline, at 5 weeks postbaseline but before serostatus notification, and again at postnotification (Week 6). A similar improvement (10%) in cardiovascular fitness occurred for both seropositive and seronegative exercisers as compared to nonexercising controls. More important, following serologic notification, seropositive control participants had significantly increased anxiety and depression and

Table 2. *Recommendations for Exercise at Each Stage of HIV Infection*

General Considerations

Prior to beginning an exercise program, all persons with HIV-1 infection should
1. Have a complete physical examination.
2. Discuss exercise plans with a physician or exercise specialist who can provide an appropriate exercise prescription.
3. Discuss exercise-training adjustments upon the appearance or reappearance of symptoms.

Healthy Asymptomatic
1. Have unrestricted exercise activity.
2. Continue participation if already actively involved with competitive sports.
3. Avoid overtraining.

Symptomatic
1. Continue moderate-intensity exercise training.
2. Discontinue competition.
3. Avoid exhaustive exercise.

Diagnosed AIDS
1. Remain physically active, but continue exercise training on a symptom-limited basis.
2. Avoid strenuous exercise.
3. Avoid or curtail exercise during acute illness.

Note. Adapted from "Human Immunodeficiency Virus Infection, Exercise and Athletics," by L. H. Calabrese and A. LaPerriere, 1993, *Sports Medicine, 15,* p.10. Copyright 1993 by the American College of Sports Medicine. Adapted with permission of the author.

decreased NK-cell counts in comparison to seropositive exercisers, whose cell counts and level of distress were similar to those of the HIV-1 negative groups. Although the between-group changes in CD4 cells were not statistically significant, LaPerriere and colleagues point out that seropositive exercisers' CD4 cell counts increased an average of 56 cells whereas cell count dropped an average of 36 cells for seropositive controls. Taken together, these classic studies suggest that not only can aerobic exercise improve fitness and decrease psychological distress among asymptomatic individuals infected with HIV-1, but exercise may also favorably influence critical features of the immune system and potentially buffer the psychological and immunological effects of a powerful psychosocial stressor.

Symptomatic Pre-AIDS

Several published studies assessing the effect of aerobic-exercise training reported on changes in cardiopulmonary function, quality of life, and immune function among HIV-1 symptomatic individuals (Lox, McAuley, & Tucker, 1995; Perna et al., 1999; Rigsby, Dishman, Jackson, Maclean, & Raven, 1992; Stringer, Berezovskaya, O'Brien, Beck, & Casaburi, 1998; Wagner, Rabkin, & Rabkin, 1998). One study reported that exercise enhanced the effects of pharmacotherapy (Wagner et al.). For example, a cross-sectional study of exercising and nonexercising persons infected with HIV-1 who had progressed to either the symptomatic or AIDS stages and who were receiving testosterone therapy found that exercisers significantly increased lean body mass and decreased depression and overall distress relative to nonexercisers (Wagner et al., 1998).

A randomized controlled 6-week experimental study of HIV-1 infected persons with CD4 cells between 100 and 500 revealed nonsignificant CD4 cell changes but significant improvements in aerobic fitness and quality of life in both moderate- and high-intensity exercisers as compared to nonexercising controls (Stringer et al., 1998). However, although high-intensity exercise condition produced the largest fitness effect, only moderate-intensity exercise produced significant immunological improvement in *Candida albican* antigen skin testing and a trend towards reduced plasma HIV-1 RNA replication.

Schienzig and colleagues (cited in LaPerriere et al., 1997) conducted a randomized, controlled, prospective study of 28 HIV-1 seropositive individuals, representing the entire spectrum of HIV-1 disease. Subjects were randomly assigned to either an exercise or control group. Exercise training sessions consisted of various supervised sports games designed to improve cardiovascular endurance and were conducted 2 days/week, 1hr/day for 8 weeks. A trend toward an increase of CD4 cells was observed from pre- to postexercise training in the exercise group, but the control group also showed a similar increase.

Rigsby et al. (1992) reported the effects of a combined aerobic-exercise and strength-training program on 37 HIV-1 infected individuals, who were stratified throughout the spectrum of HIV-1 disease. The average CD4 cell count was 325 mm' at entry. Therefore, this sample could also be described as moderately immunocompromised and pre-AIDS. Subjects were randomly assigned to either the 12-week exercise program or a counseling control group. Following exercise training, significant improvements were observed in measures of cardiorespiratory fitness, strength, and flexibility. In addition, a nonsignificant trend toward increased CD4 cells was noted in the exercise group.

Preliminary results from studies by Perna and colleagues (1999) and LaPerriere and colleagues (LaPerriere, Perna, & Goldstein, 1998) provide the only evidence of aerobic-exercise training effects in a homogeneous sample of early symptomatic pre-AIDS individuals. Twenty-eight HIV-1 infected subjects classified as CDC category B (CDC, 1992; average CD4 cell count = 453) were randomly assigned to either 12 weeks of aerobic-exercise training or an assessment-only control group. Because a second aim of the study was to determine the causes of exercise nonadherence, the exercise group was further divided among compliant and noncompliant exercisers on the basis of exercise-session attendance. Exercise training consisted of stationary cycling for 45 min/day, 3 days/week. Intensity was set at 70 to 80% of maximum heart rate as determined from a graded exercise test. Participants who adhered to the exercise training protocol significantly decreased depression and improved VO_2 (12%) to a greater degree than did control participants and noncompliant exercisers. Compliant exercisers' CD4 cell counts significantly increased (13%) whereas noncompliant exercisers' CD4 cells declined (18%) significantly. Moreover, behavioral and psychosocial factors, as opposed to illness-related factors, differentiated compliant from noncompliant exercisers. It was concluded that although aerobic exercise can improve cardiopulmonary functioning, depression, and CD4 cell counts in symptomatic HIV-infected individuals with minimal health risks, attention to factors associated with exercise adherence is warranted if exercise is prescribed as an adjuvant treatment.

AIDS

Several published studies assessing the effect of aerobic-exercise training reported on changes in cardiopulmonary function, quality of life, and immune function among individuals who had progressed to AIDS. One study (MacArthur, Levine, & Birk, 1993) investigated 25 severely immunocompromised (average CD4 cell count = 144) HIV-1 infected individuals participating in a 24-week exercise program. Exercise training consisted of aerobic interval exercise for 1 hr/day, 3 days/week. Subjects were assigned to either a high-intensity (75%–85% of V02max) or low-intensity (50%–60% V02max) exercise group. Even though a significant training effect (e.g., 24% increase in V02max) was reported after 24 weeks for both groups, this was accompanied by a nonsignificant increase in CD4 cells. However, a substantial number of participants did not complete the protocol.

Finally, Florijin and Geiger (1991) assigned 42 HIV-1 seropositive individuals with an average CD4+ cell count of less than 200 to either a therapeutic sports program or a comparison control condition. The exercise program consisted of warm-up stretching, aerobic training, and sports games for 1.5 hr/day, 1 day/week. In addition, individuals assigned to the exercise condition were encouraged to exercise on their own, either at home or at a gym. An increase in CD4 cells was not shown as a result of exercise training. However, preliminary results suggest that CD4 cell counts were stabilized at 200 for up to 18 months among individuals who continued to exercise whereas a definite decline of over 100 CD4 cells was noted for individuals in the control group.

Exercise and HIV-1: Methodological and Interpretive Implications

The data clearly support the efficacy of aerobic exercise to improve aerobic fitness, particularly for asymptomatic and symptomatic HIV-1 infected persons, an improvement that potentially favorably influences the ability to meet the physical demands of everyday activities that, in turn, contribute to overall quality of life. Moreover, although few studies have examined the psychosocial benefits of exercise for persons infected with HIV-1, no study has reported undesirable psychological effects, and most find favorable effects. However, the effect of exercise on CD4 cells is less clear. For example, some studies have shown that aerobic-exercise training may increase CD4 cell counts or buffer further decline, particularly among psychologically distressed persons with HIV-1 (LaPerriere et al., 1991, 1997; Perna et al., 1999). However, other studies (MacArthur et al., 1993; Rigsby et al., 1992; Stringer et al., 1998) have not shown an increase in CD4 cells in this population.

Additionally, the benefit of exercise or the absence of a negative effect may extend only to compliant exercisers. For example, although moderate exercise, in contrast to intense exercise, is generally considered to pose no immunological threat, it may be the case that even moderate aerobic exercise exerts an immunosuppressive effect among noncompliant individuals who are already manifesting symptoms of immunological compromise (Perna et al., 1999). That is, rather than achieving a physiological adaptation to exercise, symptomatic persons with HIV-1 who exercise irregularly may fail to immunologically adapt to exercise.

The absence of a control group, sampling irregularities, or a lack of exercise-relapse data in prior studies present further difficulties in the evaluation of aerobic-exercise benefits for symptomatic individuals. For example, Rigsby et al.'s (1992) and MacArthur et al.'s (1993) samples included primarily participants who met current CDC (1992) diagnostic criteria for AIDS based on CD4 lymphocyte count. Other studies have included heterogeneous patient samples with respect to stage of HIV-1 disease (Lox et al., 1995; Stringer et al., 1998). Additionally, with few exceptions, exercise dropout rates have typically not been reported, or studies have not included a control group. When exercise relapse rates are provided, the reasons for noncompliance, such as illness, were not typically stated. Lacking a uniform sample and adequate relapse information, it is difficult to assess the effects of exercise on patients at different disease stages or to determine whether illness occurring during the exercise protocol is associated with relapse rate. Sampling and exercise noncompliance issues are especially of concern considering that in one study relatively few patients (less than 25%) completed the entire 25-week program and less than half of the patients were compliant through 12 weeks (MacArthur et al.). The most recent and well-controlled studies with symptomatic patients reported a 23% dropout rate over 6 weeks (Stringer et al.) and a 39% dropout rate over 12 weeks (Perna et al., 1999). Although these latter studies concluded that dropout was not due to illness, one study (Stringer et al.) was quite brief and contained a heterogeneous patient sample with respect to CD4 cell count.

Practical Applications

Exercise training can provide a variety of benefits to individuals at all stages of HIV-1 infection (Calabrese & LaPerriere, 1993; LaPerriere, Klimas, Major, & Perry, 1997). For example, engaging in regular exercise and remaining physically active have been attributed by long-term survivors of HIV/AIDS to be a significant reason for their longevity (LaPerriere et al., 1997; Solomon, Temoshok, O'Leary, & Zich, 1987). However, sufficient scientific evidence is not yet available that directly associates exercise training with a decrease in morbidity or mortality in HIV-1

disease. Little is also known regarding exercise adherence factors and possible negative effects associated with exercise noncompliance. Nevertheless, the few studies that have been conducted provide some suggestive data that exercise may not only decrease negative affect and improve fitness, but it may also benefit the immune system, especially among those who are immunocompromised and psychologically distressed.

To facilitate the practical application, LaPerriere and colleagues have written guidelines for exercise testing and training for persons with HIV-1 disease (Calabrese & LaPerriere, 1993; LaPerriere et al., 1997; see Table 2). These guidelines urge a comprehensive assessment of aerobic capacity, strength, neuromuscular function, and flexibility prior to initiating an exercise program. They also suggest that the individual nature of the exercise prescription take into account stage of disease, level of immunocompromise, and symptomatology. Furthermore, exercise training should be viewed as an adjuvant therapeutic technique incorporated within an overall medical treatment regime. Within this framework, exercise training may play an important role in the management of HIV-1 disease.

Lastly, although aerobic-exercise programs have been shown to yield short-term cardiovascular and possible immune benefits for HIV-1 infected individuals (LaPerriere, Antoni, Ironson, Perry, et al., 1994; LaPerriere et al., 1990, 1991, 1997; Perna et al., 1999; Stringer et al., 1998), promoting the adoption and maintenance of exercise among the general population and among persons with chronic disease appears to be influenced more by behavioral, social, and psychological factors than by a lack of participant information regarding exercise prescription (Dubbert, 1992; USDHHS, 1996). A review of behavioral and psychological considerations identified substance abuse, fear of treatment side effects, practical inconvenience, and especially depression as primary factors related to treatment noncompliance among persons with HIV-1, findings that also have relevance for exercise intervention (Chesney & Folkman, 1994). It has been suggested that targeting depression and other risk-reduction areas, especially smoking cessation and weight loss, in conjunction with an exercise program and the use of home-based intervention may be necessary to maintain exercise adherence (King et al., 1992; King, Haskell, Young, Oka, & Stefanick, 1995; LaPerriere, Antoni, Fletcher, & Schneiderman, 1992; Perna et al., 1999).

References

Abrahams, V. C., Hilton, S. M., & Zbrozyna, A. (1960). Active muscle vasodilation produced by stimulation of the brain stem: Its significance in the defense reaction. *Journal of Physiotherapy, 154*, 491–513.

Ader, R., Felten, D. L., & Cohen, N. (1991). *Psychoneuroimmunology* (2nd ed.). San Diego, CA: Academic Press, Inc.

Antoni, M. H., Schneiderman, N., Fletcher, M. A., Goldstein, D., Ironson, G., & LaPerriere, A. (1990). Psychoneuroimmunology and HIV. *Journal of Consulting Clinical Psychology, 58*, 1–12.

Atherton, A., & Born, G. V. (1972). Quantitative investigations of the adhesiveness of circulating polymorphonuclearleucocytes to blood vessel walls. *Journal of Physiotherapy, 222*, 474–474.

Baum, A., Herberman, H., & Cohen, L. (1995). Managing stress, managing illness: Survival and quality of life in chronic disease. *Journal of Clinical Psychology in Medical Settings, 2*(4), 309–333.

Benschop, R. J., Oosteveen, F. G., Heijnen, C. J., & Ballieux, R. E. (1993). Adrenergic stimulation causes detachment of natural killer cells from cultured endothelium. *European Journal of Immunology, 23*, 3242–3247.

Berke, G. (1993). The functions and mechanisms of action of cytolytic lymphocytes. In W. E. Paul (Ed.), *Fundamental immunology* (3rd ed.) (pp. 965–1014). New York: Raven Press.

Biddle, S. (1995). Exercise and psychological health. *Research Quarterly for Exercise and Sport, 66*(4), 292–297.

Bierer, B. E., Sleckman, B. P., Ratnofsky, S. E., & Burakof, S. J. (1989). The biologic roles of CD2, CD4, and CD8 in T-cell activation. *Annual Review of Immunology, 7*, 579–599.

Blair, S. N., & Connelly, J. C. (1996). How much physi-cal activity should we do? A case for moderate amounts and intensities of physical activity. *Research Quarterly for Exercise and Sport, 67*(2), 193–205.

Blumenthal, J., Fredickson, M., Kuhn, C., Ulmer, R., Walsh-Riddle, M., & Applebaum, M. (1990). Aerobic exercise reduces levels of sympathoadrenal responses to mental stress in subjects without prior evidence of myocardial ischemia. *American Journal of Cardiology, 65*, 93–98.

Bourne, H. R., Lichtenstein, L. M., Melmon, K. L., Henney, C. S., Weinstein, Y., & Shearer, G. M. (1974). Modulation of inflammation and immunity by cyclic AMP. *Science, 184*, 19–28.

Brown, J. D. S., J. M. (1988). Exercise as a buffer of life stress: A prospective study of adolescent health. *Health Psychology, 7*(4), 341–353.

Calabrese, L. H., & LaPerriere, A. (1993). Human immunodeficiency virus infection, exercise and athletics. *Sports Medicine, 15*(1), 6–13.

Cannon, W. R. (1992). *Bodily changes in pain, hunger, fear and rage* (2nd ed.). New York: Appleton.

Cashmore, C. G., Davis, C. T., & Few, J. D. (1977). Relationship between increase in plasma cortisol concentration and rate of cortisol secretion during exercise in man. *Journal of Endocrinology, 72*, 109–110.

Chesney, M. A., & Folkman, S. (1994). Psychological impact of HIV disease and implications for intervention. *Psychiatric Clinics of North America, 17*(1), 163–182.

Centers for Disease Control. (1992). *Revised classification system for HIV infection and expanded surveillance case definition for AIDS among adolescents and adults* [Morbidity and Mortality Weekly Report 41]. Atlanta, GA: U.S. Department of Health and Human Services, Public Health Service.

Cupps, T., & Fauci, A. (1982). Corticosteroid-mediated immunoregulation in man. *Immunological Review, 65*, 133–155.

Dienstbier, R. A. (1989). Arousal and physiological toughness: Implications for mental and physical health. *Psychological Review, 64*, 35–41.

Dubbert, P. M. (1992). Exercise in behavioral medicine. *Journal of Consulting and Clinical Psychology, 60*(4), 613–618.

Duda, J. L., Sedlock, D. A., Melby, C. L., & Thaman, C. (1988). The effects of physical activity level and acute exercise on heart rate and subjective response to a psychological stressor. *International Journal of Sport Psychology, 19*, 119–133.

Durum, S. K., & Oppenheim, J. J., (1993). Proinflammatory cytokines and immunity. In W. E. Paul (Ed.), *Fundamental immunology* (3rd ed., pp. 801–836). New York: Raven Press.

Farrell, P. A., Garthwaite, T. L., & Gustafson, B. (1983). Plasma adenocorticotropin and cortisol response to submaxinial and exhaustive exercise. *Journal of Applied Physiology, 55*, 1441–1444.

Fauci, A. S. (1984). Immunologic abnormalities in the

acquired immunodeficiency syndrome (AIDS). *Clinical Research, 32*, 491–499.

Fauci, A. S. (1988). The human immunodeficiency virus: Infectivity and mechanisms of pathogenesis. *Science, 239*, 617–622.

Fauci, A. S., Macher, A. M., & Longo, D. L. (1983). Acquired immundeficiency syndrome: Epidemiologic, clinical, immunologic, and therapeutic considerations. *Annals of Internal Medicine, 100*(92).

Felten, D., Felten, S., Carlson, S., Olschawaka, J., & Livnat, S. (1985). Noradrenergic and peptidergic innervation of lymptioid tissue. *Journal of Immunology* (Suppl. 2), 755s–765s.

Field, C. J., Gougeon, R., & Marliss, E. B. (1991). Circulating mononuclear cell numbers and function during intense exercise and recovery. *Journal of Applied Physiology, 71*, 1089–1097.

Florijin, Y., & Geiger, A. (1991, September). *Community based physical activity program for HIV-1 infected persons*. Paper presented at the Biological Aspects of HIV Conference, Amsterdam, Netherlands.

Frankenhaeuser, M. (1990). *A psychobiological framework for human stress and coping*. New York: Plenum.

Frick, M. Elovainio, R., & Sommer, T. (1967). The mechanism of bradycardia evoked by physical training. *Cardiolgia, 51*, 46–54.

Frick, M., Kottinen, A., & Sarajas, S. (1963). Effects of physical training on circulation at rest and during exercise. *American Journal of Cardiology, 12*, 142–147.

Fry, R. W., Morton, A. R., & Keast, D. (1992). Acute intensive interval training and T-lymphocyte function. *Medicine Science Sports Exercise, 24*, 339–345.

Glaser, R., Rice, J., Sheridan, J., Fertel, R., Stout, J., Speicher, C., Pinsky, D., Kotour, M., Post, A., Beck, M., & Kiecolt-Glaser, J. (1987). Stress related immune suppression: Health implications. *Brain, Behavior, and Immunity, 1*, 7–20.

Heatherton, T. F., & Renn, R. J. (1995). Stress and the disinhibition of behavior. *Mind/Body Medicine, 1*, 72–81.

Hellstrand, K., & Hermodsson, S. (1989). An immunopharmacological analysis of adrenaline induced suppression of human natural killer cell cytotoxicity. *International Archives of Allergy Applied Immunology, 89*, 334–341.

Herbert, T., & Cohen, S. (1993a). Depression and immunity: A meta-analytic review. *Psychological Bulletin, 113*(3), 472–486.

Herbert, T. B., & Cohen, S. (1993b). Stress and immunity in humans: A meta-analytic review. *Psychosomatic Medicine, 55*, 364–379.

Hess, W. R. (1957). *Functional organization of the diencephalon*. New York: Grune & Stratton.

Howard, M. C., Farrar, J., Hilfiker, M., Johnson, B., Takatsu, K., Hamaoka, T., & Paul, W. E. (1982). Identification of a T cell derived B cell growth factor distinct from interleukin 2. *Journal of Experimental Medicine, 155*, 914–917.

Howard, M. C., Miyajima, A ., & Coffman, R. (1993). T-Cell-derived cytokines and their receptors. In W. E. Paul

(Ed.), *Fundamentals of immunology* (3rd ed., p. 763). New York: Raven Press.

Hurwitz, B. E., Neloesen, R. A., Saab, P. G., Nagel, J. H., Spitzer, S. B., Gellman, M. D., McCabe, P. M., Phillips, D. J., & Schneiderman, N. (1993). Differential patterns of dynamic cardiovascular regulation as a function of task. *Biological Psychology, 36*, 75–79.

Ironson, G., Antoni, M. H., & Lutgendorf, S. (1995). Can psychological interventions affect immunity and survival? Present findings and suggested targets with a focus on cancer and human immunodeficiency virus. *Mind/Body Medicine, 1*(2), 85–110.

Irwin, M., Smith, T. L., & Gillin, J. C. (1992). Electroencephalographic sleep and natural killer activity in depressed patients and control subjects. *Psychosomatic Medicine, 54*, 10–21.

Kaplan, L. D., Wofsky, C. B., & Volberding, P. A. (1987). Treatment of patients with acquired immunodeficiency syndrome and associated manifestations. *Journal of the American Medical Association, 257*, 1367–1376.

Katz, H. (1987). *The immune system*. Los Altos, CA: Lange Medical Publications.

Katz, P., Zeytoun, A., & Fauci, A. (1982). Mechanisms of human cell-mediated cytotoxicity. Modulation of natural killer cell activity by cyclic nucleotides. *Journal of Immunology, 129*, 287–296.

Kavelaars, A., Ballieux, R. E., & Heijnen, C. (1988). Modulation of the immune response by proopiomelanocortin derived peptides. II. Influence of adrenocorticotropic hormone on the rise in intracellular free calcium concentration after T cell activation. *British Journal of Behavior Immunology, 2*, 57–66.

Kavussanu, M., & McAuley, E. (1995). Exercise and optimism: Are highly active individuals more optimistic? *Journal of Sport & Exercise Psychology, 17*, 246–258.

Kiecolt-Glaser, J. K., & Glaser, R. (1992). Psychoneuroimmunology: Can psychological interventions modulate immunity? *Journal of Consulting and Clinical Psychology, 60*, 569–575.

King, A. C., Blair, S. N., Bild, D. E., Dishman, R. K., Duppert, P. M., Marcus, B. H., Oldridge, N. B., Paffenbarger, R. S., Powell, K. E., & Yeager, K. K. (1992). Determinants of physical activity and interventions in adults. *Medicine and Science in Sports and Exercise, 141*(6), S221–S236.

King, A. C., Haskell, W. L., Young, D. R., Oka, R. K., & Stefanick, M. L. (1995). Long term effects of varying intensities and formats of physical activity on participation rates, fitness, and lipoproteins in men and women aged 50 to 65 years. *Circulation, 91*, 2596–2604.

Klimas, N. G., Caralis, P., LaPerriere, A., Antoni, M. H., Ironson, G., Simoneau, J., Schneiderman, N., & Fletcher, M. A. (1991). Immunologic function in a cohort of human immunodeficiency virus type 1-seropositive and -negative healthy homosexual men. *Journal of Clinical Microbiology, 29*, 1413–1421.

Landmann, P. M., Muller, F. B., Perini, C. H., Wesp, M., Eme, P., & Buhler, F. R. (1984). Changes of immunoregulatory cells induced by psychological and physical stress: Relationship to catecholamines. *Clinical Experimental Immunology, 58*, 127–135.

LaPerriere, A., Antoni, M., Fletcher, M. A., & Schneiderman, N. (1992). Exercise and health maintenance in HIV-1. In M. L. Galatino (Ed.), *Clinical assessment and treatment of HIV* (pp. 65–76). Newark, NJ: Slack, Inc.

LaPerriere, A., Antoni, M. H., Ironson, G., Perry, A., McCabe, P., Klimas, N., Helder, L., Schneiderman, N., & Fletcher, M. A. (1994a). Effects of aerobic exercise training on lymphocyte subpopulations. *International Journal of Sports Medicine, 15*, S127–S130.

LaPerriere, A., Antoni, M. H., Schneiderman, N., Ironson, G., Klimas, N., Caralis, P., & Fletcher, M. A. (1990). Exercise intervention attenuates emotional distress and natural killer cell decrements following notification of positive serologic status for HIV. *Biofeedback Self Regulation, 15*, 229–242.

LaPerriere, A., Fletcher, M. A., Antoni, M. H., Klimas, N., Ironson, G., & Schneiderman, N. (1991). Aerobic exercise training in an AIDS risk group. *International Journal of Sports Medicine, 12*, S53–S57.

LaPerriere, A., Ironson, G., Antoni, M. H., Schneiderman, N., Klimas, N., & Fletcher, M. A. (1994c). Exercise and psychoneuroimmunology. *Medical Science Sports Exercise, 26*, 182–190.

LaPerriere, A., Klimas, N., Fletcher, M. A., Perry, A., Ironson, G., Perna, F., & Schneiderman, N. (1997). Change in CD4+ cell enumeration following aerobic-exercise training in HIV-1 disease: Possible mechanisms and practical applications. *International Journal of Sports Medicine, 18* (Suppl. 1), S56–S61.

LaPerriere, A., Klimas, N., Major, P., & Perry, A. (1997). Acquired immune deficiency syndrome (AIDS). In L. Durstine (Ed.), *A CSM's Exercise management for persons with chronic diseases and disabilities* (pp. 132–136). Champaign, IL: Human Kinetics.

LaPerriere, A., Perna, F., & Goldstein, A. (1998, August). *Exercise and psychoneuroimmunology in HIV/AIDS*. Paper presented at the meeting of the American Psychological Association, San Francisco, CA.

LaPerriere, A., Schneiderman, N., Antoni, M. H., & Fletcher, M. A. (1989). *Aerobic exercise training and psychoneuroimmunology in AIDS research*. Hillsdale, NJ: Erlbaum.

Leith, L. M. (1994). *Foundations of exercise and mental health*. Morgantown, WV: Fitness Information Technology.

Levy, S., Herberman, R., Lippman, M., & d'Angelo, T. (1987). Correlation of stress factors with sustained depression of natural killer cell activity and predicted prognosis in patients with breast cancer. *Journal of Clinical Oncology, 5*, 348–353.

Lotzerich, H., Peters, C., Niemeier, B., Schule, K., Hoff, H. G., & Uhlenbruck, G. (1994). Influence of endurance training on natural cytotoxicity and behaviour in cancer patients. *Psychologische-Beitrage, 36*, 47–52.

Lox, C. L., McAuley, E., & Tucker, R. S. (1995). Exercise as an intervention for enhancing subjective wellbeing in an HIV-1 population. *Journal of Sport and Exercise Psychology, 17*(4), 345–362.

Lutgendorf, S. K., Antoni, M., Ironson, G., Klimas, N., Kumar, M., Starr, K., McCabe, P., Cleven, K., Fletcher, M. A., & Schneiderman, N. (1997). Cognitive-behavioral stress management decreases dysphoric mood and herpes simplex virus-type 2 antibody titers in symptomatic HIV-1 seropositive gay men. *Journal of Consulting and Clinical Psychology, 65*, 31–43.

MacArthur, R. D., Levine, S. D., & Birk, T. J. (1993). Supervised exercise training improves cardiopulmonary fitness in HIV-infected persons. *Medical Science Sports Exercise, 25*, 684–688.

Mackinnon, L. T. (1992). *Exercise and immunology: Current issues in exercise science*. Champaign, IL: Human Kinetics.

Mackinnon, L. T., Ginn, E., & Seymour, G. (1991). *Effects of exercise during sports training and competition on salivary IgA levels*. Boca Raton, FL: CRC Press.

Mason, J. W. (1975). A historical view of the stress field. *Part II Journal of Human Stress, 1*, 22–36.

McCabe, P. M., & Schneiderman, N. (1985). *Psychophysiologic reactions to stress*. Hillsdale, NJ: Erlbaum.

Mosmann, T., Bond, M., Coffman, R., Ohara, J., & Paul, W. E. (1986). T-cell and mast cell lines respond to B-cell stimulatory factor 1. *Proceedings of the National Academy of Science, USA, 83*(15), 5654–5658.

Munoz, A., Wang, M. C., Good, R., Detels, H., Ginsberg, L., & Phair, J. (1990). *The natural history of HIV infection, in Sande, Volberding*. Philadelphia, PA: Sanders Co.

Nehlsen-Cannarella, S. L., Neiman, D. C., Jessen, J., Chang, L., Gusewitch, G., Blix, G. G., & Ashley, E. (1991). Effects of acute moderate exercise on lymphocyte function and serum immunoglobulin levels. *International Journal of Sports Medicine, 12*, 391–398.

Nemeroff, C. B., Widerlov, E., Bissette, G., Walleus, H., Karlsson, I., Kilts, C. D., Vale, W., & Loosen, P. T. (1984). Elevated concentrations of CSF cortotropin-releasing factor-like immunoreactivity in depressed patients. *Science, 226*, 1342–1344.

Nieman, D. C., Cook, V. D., Henson, D. A., Suttles, J., Rejeski, W. J., Ribisi, P. M., Fagoaga, O. R., & Nehlsen-Cannarella, S. (1995). Moderate exercise training and natural killer cell cytotoxic activity in breast cancer patients. *International Journal of Sports Medicine, 16*, 334–337.

Nieman, D. C., Miller, A. R., Henson, D. A., Warren, B. J., Gusewitch, G., Johnson, R. L., Davis, J. M., Butterworth, D. E., Herring, J. L., & Nehlsen-Cannarelia, S. L. (1994). Effects of high-versus moderate-intensity exercise on lymphocyte subpopulations and proliferative response. *International Journal of Sports Exercise, 26*, 128–139.

Noelle, R. J., & Snow, E. C. (1991). T helper cell-dependent B cell activation. *Federation of American Society for Experimental Biology Journal, 5*, 2770–2776.

North, T. C., McCullagh, P., & Tran, Z. V. (1990). Effects

of exercise on depression. *Exercise and Sport Science Reviews, 18*, 379–415.

Old, L. J. (1995). Tumor necrosis factor (TNF). *Science, 230*, 630–632.

Paul, W. E. (1989). Pleiotropy and redundancy: T cell-derived lymphokines in the immune response. *Cell, 57*, 521.

Paul, W. E. (1993). The immune system; An introduction. In W. E. Paul (Ed.), *Fundamentals of immunology* (3rd ed., pp. 1–20). New York: Raven Press.

Pavlidis, N., & Chirigos, M. (1980). Stress-induced impairment of macrophage tumoricidal function. *Psychosomatic Medicine, 42*, 47–54.

Pawlikowski, M., Zelazowski, P., Dohler, K., & Stepien, H. (1988). Effects of two neuropeptides, somatoliberin (GRF), on human lymphocyte natural killer activity. *British Journal of Behavioral Immunology, 2*, 50–56.

Perna, F. M., LaPerriere, A., Ironson, G., Klimas, N., Perry, A., Majors, P., Pavone, J., Goldstein, A., Makemson, D., Fletcher, M. A., Koppes, L., Meijer, O. G., & Schneiderman, N. (1999). Cardiopulmonary and CD4 cell changes in response to exercise training in early symptomatic HIV infection. *Medicine and Science in Sport and Exercise, 31*, 973–939.

Perna, F. M., & McDowell, S. L. (1995). Role of psychological stress in cortisol recovery from exhaustive exercise among elite athletes. *International Journal of Behavioral Medicine, 2*, 13–26.

Perna, F. M., Schneiderman, N., & LaPerriere, A. (1997). Psychological stress, exercise, and immunity. *International Journal of Sports Medicine, 18* (Suppl. 1), S78–S83.

Petruzzello, S. J., Landers, D. M., Hatfield, B. D., Kubitz, K. A., & Salazar, W. (1991). A meta-analysis on the anxiety-reducing effects of acute and chronic exercise: Outcomes and mechanisms. *Sports Medicine, 11*, 143–182.

Plaut, M. (1987). Lymphocyte hormone receptors. *Annual Review of Immunology, 5*, 621–669.

Rammensee, H. G., Falk, K., & Rotzschke, O. (1993). Peptides naturally presented by MHC class I molecules. *Annual Review of Immunology, 11*, 213–244.

Rejeski, W. J., Thompson, A, Brubaker, P., H., & Miller, H. S. (1992). Acute exercise: Buffering effects of psychosocial stress responses in women. *Health Psychology, 11*(6), 355–362.

Rigsby, L. W., Dishman, R. K., Jackson, A. W., Maclean, G. S., & Raven, P. B. (1992). Effects of exercise training on men seropositive for the human immunodeficiency virus-1. *Medicine and Science in Sports and Exercise, 24*, 6–12.

Roitt, I., Brostoff, J., & Male, D. (1989). *Immunology.* London: Gower Medical.

Rosenberg, Z. F., & Fauci, A. S. (1990). Immunopathogenic mechanisms of HIV infection. *Immunology Today, 11*, 176–180.

Roth, D. L. (1989). Acute emotional and psychophysiological effects of aerobic exercise. *Psychophysiology, 26*(5), 593–602.

Schneiderman, N. (1978). *Animal models relating to behavioral stress and cardiovascular pathology.* New York: Springer.

Schneiderman, N., & McCabe, P. M. (1989). *Psychophysiologic strategies in laboratory research.* New York: Plenum.

Schooley, R. (1995). Correlation between viral load measurements and outcome in clinical trials of antiviral drugs. *AIDS, 9*, S15–S19.

Selye, H. A. (1956). *The stress of life.* New York: McGraw-Hill.

Shepard, R. J., & Shek, P. N. (1994). Infectious disease in athletes: New interest for an old problem. *The Journal of Sports Medicine Physical Fitness, 34*, 11–22.

Snegovskaya, V., & Viru, A. (1993). Elevation of cortisol and growth hormone levels in the course of further improvement of performance capacity in trained rowers. *International Journal of Sports Medicine, 14*, 202–206.

Solomon, G. F., Temoshok, L., O'Leary, A., & Zich, J. (1987). An intensive psychoimmunologic study of long-surviving persons with AIDS: Pilot work, background studies, hypotheses and methods. *Annals of the New York Academy of Science, 496*, 647–655.

Sprent, J. (1993). T lymphocytes and the thymus. In W. E. Paul (Ed.), *Fundamentals immunology* (3rd ed., pp. 75–110). New York: Raven Press.

Stevens, C. E., Taylor, P. E., & Zang, E. A. (1986). Human T-cell lymphotropic virus Type III in a cohort of homosexual men in New York City. *Journal of the American Medical Association, 225*, 2167–2171.

Stringer, W. W., Berezovskaya, M., O'Brien, W. A., Beck, C. K., & Casaburi, R. (1998). The effect of exercise training on aerobic fitness, immune indices, and quality of life in HIV+ patients. *Medicine and Science in Sports and Exercise, 30*, 11–16.

Tharp, G. D. (1975). The role of glucocorticoids in exercise. *Medical Science Sports, 7*, 6–11.

Tvede, N., Pedersen, B. K., Hansen, F. R., Bendix, T., Christensen, L. D., Galbo, H., & Halkjaer-Kristensen, J. (1989). Effect of physical exercise on blood mononuclear cell subpopulations and in vitro proliferative responses. *Scandinavian Journal of Immunology, 29*, 383–389.

Urhausen, A., & Kinderman, W. (1987). Behavior of testosterone, sex hormone binding globulin, and cortisol before and after a triathalon competition. *International Journal of Sports Medicine, 8*, 305–308.

U.S. Department of Health & Human Services. (1996). *Surgeon General's report on physical activity and health.* Washington, DC: Author.

Wagner, G., Rabkin, J., & Rabkin, R. (1998). Exercise as a mediator of psychological and nutritional effects of testosterone therapy in HIV+ men. *Medicine and Science in Sports and Exercise, 30*, 811–817.

World Health Organization. (1990). Interim proposal for a WHO staging system for HIV infection and disease. *Weekly Epidemiological Record, Report 29*, 65, 121–124.

18
Cancer Prevention

Anne McTiernan

Introduction

Cancer is the second leading cause of death in the United States. The American Cancer Society estimated that in 2000 more than 1.2 million Americans were diagnosed with a new cancer, and over 550,000 persons would die from this disease (Greenlee, 2000). It also estimated that over their lifetimes, one in two men and one in three women in this country will develop an invasive cancer.

Tobacco use accounts for approximately 76% of all lung cancers and from 19 to 61% of cancers of the mouth, pharynx, larynx, esophagus, pancreas, and bladder (World Cancer Research Fund Panel, 1997). Excessive radiation and some chemical exposures are known strong carcinogens, but the number of persons with significant exposure to these agents is small. Inherited predisposition to cancer accounts for at most 10–15% of cancers. Thus, environmental or lifestyle factor(s) must be responsible for the development of the majority of cancers. That environment and lifestyle are important in cancer etiology is supported by observations of international variations in cancer rates. As shown in Figure 1, there is a wide difference in occurrence of several cancers between the United States and Japan, two highly developed counties.

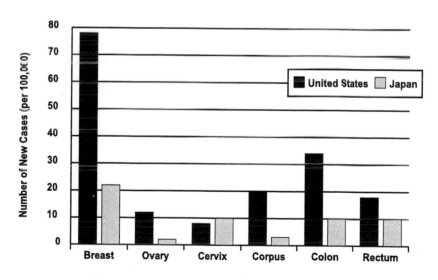

Figure 1

Age-standardized incidence rates for cancer of selected sites in women in the United States and Japan, 1980. From International Agency for Research on Cancer: Patterns of cancer in five continents. Lyon: IARC, 1990 (IARC Scl Publ. 102).

Further support comes from observations of populations migrating from countries with low cancer incidence to countries with high cancer incidence. Such populations tend to take on the cancer risk patterns of their adoptive countries, even while keeping their gene pool constant by marrying within their own population.

The incidence and mortality of cancer have risen dramatically over the past 100 years. Prior to the middle of the twentieth century, cancer was a rare disease; a 1909 U.S. Census report noted that cancer accounted for only 4% of all deaths (World Cancer Research Fund Panel, 1997). The rise in lung cancer incidence and mortality in this century is almost entirely due to the widespread use of tobacco that began after World War II and increased in prevalence until the 1980s. The increased incidences of breast, colon, and prostate cancers in this century are in part due to increased screening for early disease. Most of the increases in occurrence of these common cancers, however, reflect real increases in tumor development and likely reflect changes in lifestyle or environment.

Cancer Development

The United States has undergone marked environmental and economic changes during this period of change in cancer incidence. With the increase in industrialization, modern conveniences, and prepared-food availability has come a change in body habitus of almost an entire population. American adults and children are becoming more sedentary, are eating more calories, and are becoming more overweight and obese. Thus, there are three global routes through which physical activity could affect cancer risk: (a) a direct

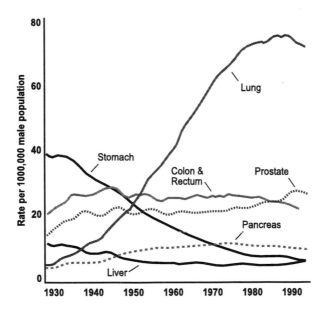

Figure 2

Age-adjusted cancer death rates in males by site, United States, 1930–1990. *
Source: American Cancer Society, Surveillance Research, 1998, and Vital Statistics of the United States, 1997.

*Rates are per 100,000 and are age-adjusted to the 1970 U.S. standard population.

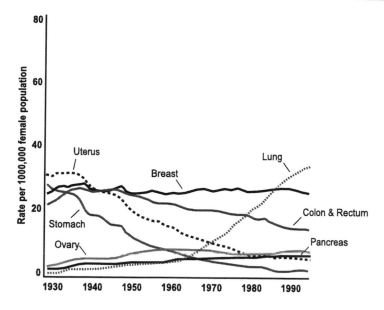

Figure 3

Age-adjusted cancer death rates in females by site, United States, 1930–1994. *
Source: American Cancer Society, Surveillance Research, 1998, and Vital Statistics of the United States, 1997.

*Rates are per 100,000 and are age-adjusted to the 1970 U.S. standard population. Uterine cancer deaths are for cervix and endometrium combined.

effect of physical activity itself, (b) a beneficial effect on body habitus, or (c) an indirect role by influencing dietary changes.

The development of cancer is generally thought to be a two-step process. In cancer initiation, a factor causes a structural or functional change in cellular DNA that is not severe enough to cause cell death but that, if stimulated, can cause abnormal growth. Cancer promotion occurs when some factor or factors cause an initiated cancer cell to multiply and grow exponentially without internal or external controls. Carcinogens can be initiators, promoters, or both. Physical activity could work at either level in its effects on cancer development, but likely has its major effects in reducing tumor promotion.

Several small-animal experiments have been conducted, with some showing decreased tumors developing in animals forced to exercise and some showing increased tu-

mors developing with similar exercise exposures. Significant elevations in immune cell activity and a trend toward lower numbers of breast tumors developing have been observed in physically active vs. sedentary mice (Hoffman-Goetz et al., 1998). Clearance of radio-labeled tumor cells has been observed to be higher in trained mice compared with sedentary control mice. It has been difficult in animal experiments to determine the exact effects of exercise, however, as with forced exercise there is a concomitant stress response that has physiologic effects that can influence tumor development and growth.

Epidemiologic Evidence

The scientific knowledge linking exercise to cancer risk in humans is limited to observational epidemiologic data. One observational study design is the cohort study, in which measurements are made of physical activity levels of a group of individuals, and then the individuals are followed in time until they develop cancer or die from cancer. The analysis of this type of study involves dividing persons on level of physical activity (for example, into quartiles) and comparing the proportion of persons developing cancer among the categories of physical activity. A second type of observational study is the case-control study in which persons with cancer (usually identified from a cancer registry or hospital records) and comparable individuals without cancer are interviewed regarding their current and past physical activity habits. A comparison between the physical activity experiences of the case group and the control group is made. Either type of observational study can yield an estimate of relative risk,

which is an estimate of the risk of cancer development in one group compared with that of another group (for example, in heavy exercisers vs. sedentary persons).

International variation in cancer incidence might give some support to a link between physical activity and cancer occurrence. Certainly, individuals in developed countries with access to many modern conveniences might expend less energy as part of their daily activities of living. Figure 4 shows the association between the annual incidence of breast cancer in individual countries that collect such data and per capita automobile ownership. The latter factor could be seen as a marker of level of development in the country and of likely level of physical activity expended in daily life. Individuals without access to automobiles must use means of

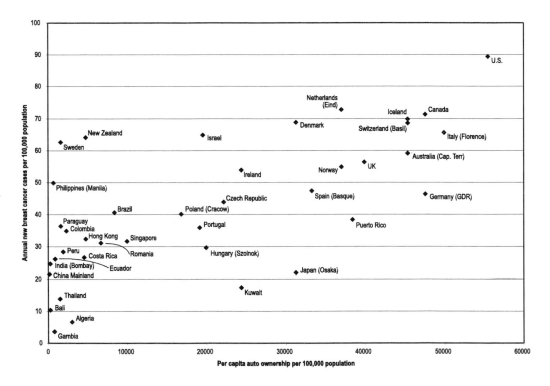

Figure 4

International association between incidence of breast cancer and per capita automobile ownership.

transportation with greater individual expenditure of energy. As seen in the graph, there is a direct, positive association between average per capita automobile ownership and the annual incidence of breast cancer. A similar association has been observed for per capita average dietary fat intake and incidence of breast cancer. Associations such as these, therefore, do not prove cause and effect, but may give clues to etiology.

The association between exercise and cancer has been studied in human populations for cancers of the colon, rectum, breast, endometrium, ovary, prostate, testicle, and lung. Of these, the greatest amount of information is available about colon, rectum, breast, and prostate cancers; fewer data have been published on physical activity and other cancers.

Colorectal Cancer

Numerous epidemiologic studies, including over 13,000 colon cancer cases and a greater number of control subjects, have found an inverse association between physical activity and risk of colon cancer (G. A. Colditz, Cannuscio, & Frazier, 1997). This relationship has been observed in both sexes and in various racial and ethnic groups in diverse geographic areas around the globe.

In all but a few epidemiologic studies, the risk for colon cancer was decreased in persons in the highest category of activity compared with persons in the lowest category for at least one measure of activity, with reduction in risk ranging from 10% to 60%. (G. A. Colditz et al.; McTiernan, Ulrich, Slate, & Potter, 1998; Thune & Lund, 1996). The Nurses' Health Study of over 120,000 U.S. nurses found that the most active women (those in the highest quintile of a measured index of current physical activity) had half the risk of developing colorectal cancer compared with sedentary women (Martinez et al., 1997). In several studies, a dose-response effect of decreasing risk of colon cancer with

increasing levels of recreational physical activity was observed. The association between physical activity and colon cancer incidence has been consistent across studies with widely differing methods of measuring exercise exposure. Accounting for factors such as age, diet, and obesity has not diminished the observed associations between physical activity and colon cancer occurrence. In the Nurses' Health Study, physical activity, body mass index (weight in kg/[height in meters]^2), and waist-to-hip ratio were independently associated with risk of colon cancer, indicating that a combination of energy intake, output, and metabolism may be key in the etiology of this disease (Martinez et al.). In support of this concept, Slattery, Edwards, Ma, Friedman, and Potter (1997) found an interaction between body mass index and activity such that the highest risk for colon cancer was observed in those with the highest body mass index and the lowest level of physical activity. In most studies, the greatest reduction in risk was seen in individuals who had exercised throughout much of their lifetime; less protection was seen with only recent exercise.

The evidence for an association between physical activity and risk of rectal cancer is substantially weaker than that for colon cancer. Physical activity was associated with a significantly reduced rectal cancer risk in only a small number of the studies that have specifically examined the association whereas in others the association was neutral (McTiernan, Ulrich, et al., 1998).

Breast Cancer

There is a quickly growing body of epidemiologic data on the association between exercise and breast cancer (Friedenreich, Thune, Brinton, & Albanes, 1998; Gammon, John, & Britton, 1998). Some studies compared women according to participation in college sports, some looked at occupational physical activity only, several examined recreational exercise only, and others studied both occupational and recreational physical activity (McTiernan, Ulrich, et al., 1998). Seventeen of the 23 studies found an inverse association between physical activity and risk of breast cancer, ranging from a risk reduction of 10 to 80% for participation in the highest level of activity as compared with a sedentary lifestyle. Three cohort studies and four case-control studies did not support an inverse association between exercise and breast cancer risk. In a study of over 25,000 Norwegian women, statistically significant trends toward decreasing risk for breast cancer with increasing levels of leisure-time physical activity and physical activity at work were observed (Thune, Brenn, Lund, & Gaard, 1997). The Nurses' Health Study of more than 116,000 U.S. nurses followed for 6 years, however, showed no association between late adolescent or recent nonoccupational physi-

cal activity and reduced risk for breast cancer in pre- and perimenopausal women (Rockhill et al., 1998), although a re-analysis with followup data did show a benefit from exercise (Rockhill, et al., 1999).

Most epidemiologic studies have included breast cancer cases of all ages, which may lead to difficulties in interpretation as some known risk factors differ in degree or direction between premenopausal and postmenopausal breast cancers (e.g., body mass index, lactation, family history). Nevertheless, reduced risks have been observed in some studies for pre-, peri-, and postmenopausal women (McTiernan, Standford, Weiss, Daling, & Voigt, 1996).

The age at which physical activity occurred did not appear to affect risk in most studies. In a case-control study of 545 breast cancer cases under age 41 and 545 control women of similar age, lifetime leisure-time physical activity was ascertained from menar-

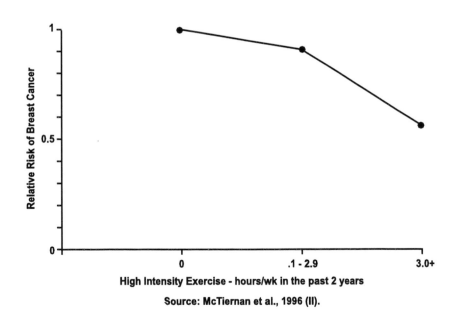

Source: McTiernan et al., 1996 (II).

Figure 5

Risk of breast cancer occurrence in women aged 50–64 years, by level of recent high intensity physical activity (Seattle, Washington).

che to one year prior to the case patient's date of diagnosis (or similar date for controls); lifetime activity was found to be inversely associated with risk (Bernstein, Henderson, Hanisch, Sullivan-Halley, & Ross, 1994). Three studies compared college athletes with nonathletes; relative risks for activity levels beyond this were not ascertained, so it is not clear if the effect of physical activity levels in young adulthood carried over to later adulthood (Gammon et al., 1998; McTiernan, Ulrich, et al., 1998). Two of the three studies found a reduced risk for breast cancer among college athletes compared with nonathletes. The association between physical activity and reduced risk of breast cancer occurrence was not affected by factors such as age, reproductive history, diet, and body mass index in those studies that accounted for these factors.

Endometrial Cancer

Three case-control studies of physical activity and endometrial cancer risk reported an inverse association between physical activity and endometrial cancer occurrence with a risk reduction for active vs. sedentary lifestyle of about 30 to 60% (McTiernan, Ulrich, et al., 1998). In most of the analyses, adjusting for body mass index and caloric intake did not attenuate the effect of physical activity on cancer risk. One study found an inverse association only with occupational activity, but no association with recreational activity. Another study reported that combined recreational and nonrecreational activity was protective.

Ovarian Cancer

There are few data assessing the association between physical activity and risk of ovarian cancer. A few cohort studies of cancer and physical activity in women have included ovarian cancer as an outcome, but numbers of cases have been small, and results have been inconsistent. Findings for an association between ovarian cancer and a physical activity have ranged from a slight increased risk to moderate decreased risk in active vs. sedentary women (McTiernan, Ulrich, et al., 1998). In a cohort of 31,396 postmenopausal Iowan women in which 97 women developed ovarian cancer, women with "high" levels of physical activity compared with those with "low" physical activity had almost a doubling of risk of developing ovarian cancer, after adjustments for reproductive and demographic factors (Mink, Folsom, Sellers, & Kushi, 1996).

Testicular Cancer

A population-based case-control study of testicular cancer in Canada observed that men who were at the highest level of recreational activity had a statistically significant 30% decreased risk of cancer occurrence, whereas occupational activity was unrelated to testicular cancer risk. A similar-design study of testicular cancer in the United Kingdom found an increasing risk of cancer of the testes with an increasing number of hours spent sitting down. Furthermore, increasing amount of time spent in exercise was associated with increasingly lower risks. A Norwegian cohort of 53,000 men failed to show any association of physical activity with risk for testicular cancer, although the age at which the men entered the cohort (in their 30s and 40s) is past the age at highest risk for this cancer (Thune & Lund, 1994). A small hospital-based case-control study in British Columbia observed an increased risk of testicular cancer with bicycle riding and horseback riding, two activities associated with increased heat and trauma to the testes (McTiernan, Ulrich, et al., 1998).

Prostate Cancer

Inconsistent findings have been observed in the 11 cohort, nine case-control, and two linkage studies that have examined the effect of physical activity and prostate cancer (Mc-Tiernan, Ulrich, et al., 1998; Thune & Lund, 1994). Three studies examined activity in college or adolescence, and several looked at only occupational activity. Some studies explored recreational activity only, others studied both occupational and recreational activity, and one study did not indicate the type of activity measured. Methods of ascertainment of physical activity varied widely across studies. In general, estimates of relative risk observed in all of these studies are distributed almost evenly around 1.0 and indicate little or no effect of physical activity on prostate cancer risk (Oliveria & Lee, 1997).

Other Cancers

Very little information is available on the relationship between exercise and other types of cancers (McTiernan, Ulrich, et al., 1998). A small number of studies have evaluated the effect of physical activity on lung cancer risk in men. Increased levels of physical activity were associated with a 30–50% decreased risk for lung cancer, both before and after adjusting for the effects of smoking in two studies. In the Norwegian cohort study of 53,242 men and 28,274 women aged 20–49 years at baseline, leisure-time physical activity was associated with decreased lung cancer occurrence in men but not in women (Thune & Lund, 1997). Men who exercised 4 or more hours per week had a 29% reduced risk of lung cancer occurrence over 13 to 19 years of followup. Risk reduction was especially marked for small-cell carcinoma of the lung. These results were adjusted for smoking, body mass index, age, and geographic region, but protection was observed even among smokers. In the few cohort studies that have included other cancer endpoints, no significant associations between occupational activity or college athletics and cancers of the stomach, bladder, or pancreas were observed.

Mechanisms for a Role of Exercise in Cancer Prevention

Physical activity could affect cancer risk either indirectly through other, correlated factors (confounding) or through real biological mechanisms. Individuals who choose to exercise are different from sedentary persons in several ways. They enjoy a generally higher health status, are more likely to adopt and maintain other health habits such as a low-fat diet, avoidance of alcohol and smoking, and use of preventive medical care (McTiernan, Stanford, Daling, & Voigt, 1998). Several factors that are correlated with activity are also independently related to cancer occurrence, setting up the potential for a confounded relationship between physical activity and cancer. Nevertheless, physical activity has profound effects on many organs and physiological functions, and could affect cancer occurrence through several different biological mechanisms (Hoffman-Goetz et al., 1998).

A putative relationship between physical activity and cancer occurrence could be due to a mutual relationship with obesity. There is considerable evidence that increased body weight increases the risk for postmenopausal breast cancer, endometrial cancer, and colorectal cancer (McTiernan, Ulrich, et al., 1998). Obese individuals generally exhibit a lower level of habitual physical activity than that of nonobese controls. Most importantly, regular exercise is a powerful predictor of long-term maintenance of weight loss in obese individuals.

Exercise may prevent cancer development through a reduction in the highly metabolic abdominal fat mass. Abdominal fat, particularly visceral (intra-abdominal) fat, appears to be the most metabolically active of fat depots. Clinical trials have shown that changes in visceral fat of as little as 3 to 4 pounds can have profound effects on glucose tolerance, fasting insulin, and lipids. Aerobic exercise

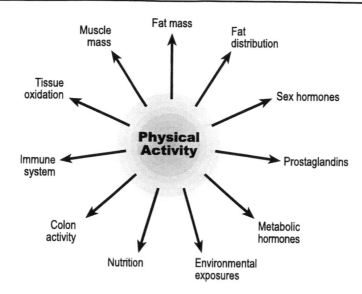

Figure 6

Factors affected by physical activity that might explain the observed associations between level of physical activity and risk of developing cancer.

preferentially causes reduction in visceral fat in men and in women. That abdominal fat may be important in cancer risk is supported by the observation of increased risk of breast and colon cancers in women with increased waist circumference or increased waist-to-hip ratio (Hoffman-Goertz et al., 1998; Martinez et al., 1997). Visceral obesity is associated with increased insulin resistance and lower concentrations of sex hormone-binding globulin. This protein binds estrogen and androgen and, if present at lower levels, allows more free (active) sex hormone to circulate. High levels of free estrogens and androgens may be important in the development of breast, endometrial, ovarian, prostate, and other cancers (Hoffman-Goertz et al., 1998; McTiernan, Ulrich, et al., 1998).

Weight patterns and fluctuations throughout adulthood may be important in the etiology of some cancers. A high body mass index at age 18 reduces risk of breast cancer. Large amounts of weight gain (> 20 kg) do not affect risk of breast cancer before menopause, but significantly increases risk of breast cancer in postmenopausal women (Huang et al., 1997). These disparate associations depending on age at cancer diagnosis may be explained by varying effects of obesity on endogenous sex hormone production at different life stages in women. Obesity-associated anovulation in young women might be protective against breast cancer development, but obesity-related increases in postmenopausal estrogen production in fat tissues (see below) may increase breast cancer risk.

Events of early and late menstrual and reproductive life may be important in the induction or promotion of hormonally related cancers such as breast and endometrium. Early menarche (before age 12), increased numbers of ovulatory menstrual cycles, late age at first full-term pregnancy (after age 30), nulliparity, lack of lactation, and late menopause (after age 55) have each been found to increase risk of breast cancer from 20% to more than 100% (McTiernan, Ulrich, et al., 1998). Exercise can affect several of these menstrual and reproductive factors. Girls participating in vigorous sports such as ballet dancing and running experience a high incidence of primary and secondary amenorrhea, delayed menarche, and more irregular cycles, compared with nonathlete girls. A high-intensity exercise intervention in untrained college women with normal ovulation and luteal adequacy also results in reversible abnormal luteal function and loss of luteinizing hormone surge in some women. The most marked disturbances have been observed during the periods of most intense training and in those women who have lost weight.

Another plausible mechanism for an exercise effect on breast and endometrial cancer risk is through the effect of exercise on circulating sex hormones in postmenopausal women (McTiernan, Ulrich, et al., 1998). Postmenopausal women may continue to produce estrogen through the peripheral conversion (mainly in fat cells) of adrenal andro-

gens to estrogens. Elevated circulating estrogen levels in postmenopausal women have been found in several recent studies to increase risk of breast cancer (G. Colditz, 1998). Increased bone mineral density, a marker for lifetime increased estrogen exposure, doubles or triples risk for breast cancer occurrence (G. Colditz).

Absolute and relative levels of estrogens and androgens may predict risk of developing prostate cancer. In the Physicians Health Study, men in the top half of plasma testosterone level had more than double the risk for prostate cancer development compared with men in the bottom half (Gann, Hennekens, Ma, Longcope, & Stampfer, 1996). An inverse trend in risk for prostate cancer with increasing levels of sex hormone-binding globulin was observed, which indicates that lower amounts of bioavailable testosterone were associated with decreased risk for prostate cancer.

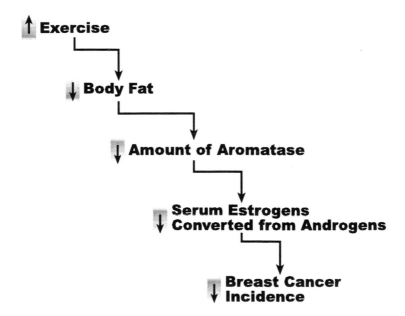

Figure 7
One hypothesized mechanism through which increased level of physical activity might protect against breast cancer development.

Increased physical activity measured through self-report and by movement monitors has been found to be associated with decreased serum concentrations of estradiol, estrone, and androgens in postmenopausal women (McTiernan, Ulrich, et al., 1998). This significant association persists after adjustment for body mass index.

Individuals with colon cancer have been noted to have a higher than expected prevalence of the syndrome of hyperinsulinemia, hyperglycemia, hypertriglyceridemia, and low HDL cholesterol—Syndrome X. Elevated blood insulin concentrations have been associated with breast cancer risk. Exercise significantly lowers insulin, glucose, and triglycerides, and raises HDL cholesterol; thus, physical activity could exert a protective effect against cancer through a metabolic pathway.

Insulin-like growth factors (IGFs) stimulate cell turnover in most body tissues, and have been associated with increased risk of prostate and breast cancers. IGF is downregulated by increased production of its binding protein (IGFBP-3), which can result from increased exercise, decreased caloric intake, and decreased body weight. Decreased IGF activity may increase the hepatic synthesis of sex hormone-binding globulin, resulting in diminished availability of free sex hormones. Thus, increased exercise could result in lowered biologically available endogenous sex hormones via a cascade of metabolic events and, thus, a lowered risk of hormone-related cancers such as breast, endometrium, and prostate.

Another possible mechanism of the exercise-cancer relationship may be via immunological effects (Hoffman-Goetz et al., 1998). The increased risk of some cancers in immune-suppressed individuals (e.g., lymphoma and Kaposi's sarcoma in AIDS patients and various tumors in organ-transplant patients) and the role of immune function in maintaining cancer remission support a role of the immune function in cancer etiology. The immune system is capable of recognizing and eliminating neoplastic cells through lymphokine-activated killer cells, tumor-infiltrating macrophages, and activated natural killer cells, and their by products—cytokines and eicosanoids. The direction of exercise-induced immune modulation is unclear, however, and is dependent upon exercise type, intensity, duration, and the immune parameters examined. Exercise and physical training affect a variety of immune parameters, reflecting hemodynamic changes, migration of immune cells from tissue reservoirs, and endocrine effects such as release of glucocorticoids, catecholamines, and opioid hormones. The association between physical activity, immune function, and etiology of some cancers may be, in part, due to a sex hormone effect, as natural killer cell activity may be influenced by endogenous estrogen. Experimental conditions have shown varying effects of training on immune function or cell number in humans, however.

An intriguing hypothesis for a mechanism through which exercise might protect against colon cancer is that the decreased bowel transit time induced by physical activity, possibly through increased vagal tone and subsequent increased peristalsis, may lead to less opportunity for carcinogens to have contact with the bowel mucosa, thereby allowing less opportunity for the initiation or promotion of carcinogenesis (McTiernan, Ulrich, et al., 1998). Although stool bulk is a good correlate of colorectal cancer risk, however, transit time is much less well established, despite its prime facie plausibility. Other exercise effects that might explain a reduced risk of colon cancer in active persons include exercise-induced reduction in bile acids or prostaglandins.

Increased heat or trauma to the testes, as might occur with prolonged sitting or with such sports as horseback or bicycle riding, has been postulated to increase risk for testicular cancer (McTiernan, Ulrich, et al., 1998).

Clinical Recommendations

Cancer is a preventable disease. For those cancers that can be diagnosed at a premalignant stage, prevention includes regular screening and treatment of cancer precursor lesions. For the average-risk adult, this includes mammography and breast examination for breast cancer, pap smears for cervical cancer, flexible sigmoidoscopy and fecal occult blood testing for colorectal cancer, prostate specific antigen and digital rectal examination for prostate cancer, pelvic examination for ovarian cancer, and visual inspection for skin cancer. New screening modalities are being tested for many cancers. Cancer prevention also includes avoidance of known carcinogens such as tobacco smoking, excess radiation, and certain chemical exposures.

New pharmaceutical interventions to prevent cancer are being tested such as selective estrogen-receptor modulators (for example, tamoxifen and raloxifene) for breast cancer prevention, calcium and salicylates for colorectal cancer prevention, and finasteride for prostate cancer prevention. The risks and benefits of these medications must be placed in the context of risk of cancer incidence and mortality. If a medication has a high incidence of adverse effects, it may be appropriate only for individuals who have a high likelihood of developing advanced cancer or dying from cancer. Such "high-risk" persons might include those with an inherited predisposition (e.g., BRCA1 or BRCA2 for breast cancer or ovarian cancer), history of cancer precursor (e.g., adenomatous colon polyps), or exposure to known carcinogens (e.g., smokers).

Although the role of diet and nutrition in cancer prevention has not been clearly defined, experts recommend a diet that is rich in fruits and vegetable (five or more per day),

high in fiber, and low in total fats (less than 30% of total caloric intake; World Cancer Research Fund Panel, 1997). A number of individual nutrients have been or are being tested as cancer preventive agents. Several large-scale clinical trials of vitamin A and beta carotene compounds found that these agents afforded no cancer protection and may in fact increase risk of cancer development. In preliminary studies, selenium, calcium, vitamin D, and vitamin E have shown some promise in reducing risk of particular cancers or cancer-precursors. The effect of a low fat dietary pattern on the incidence of breast and colorectal cancers is being tested in the Women's Health Initiative clinical trial, but the results will not be known until 2005 or later (Women's Health Initiative Study Group, 1998).

The role of exercise in cancer prevention has received less attention than these other modalities. The evidence in humans supports an association between high activity levels and reduced risk for colon, and possibly breast, cancer. There are more questions than answers, however. If there is a cause and effect relationship between exercise and cancer development, the amount, type, intensity, frequency, and timing of exercise needed to protect against cancer are unknown.

More research studies, particularly randomized controlled clinical trials of exercise interventions, are needed to answer these questions. Until the scientific evidence is established, it is prudent to recommend to all adult patients that they exercise at a moderate or greater aerobic intensity level for at least 30 minutes per day on most days of the week. Weight training two to three times per week may aid in achieving the aerobic-exercise goals and in controlling amount of fat mass, by building muscle, improving strength and balance, and increasing metabolism.

To minimize adult gain of fat mass and the risk of childhood and adult-onset obesity, programs to encourage sports and physical activity in children, adolescents, and young adults are needed. Care must be taken, however, to minimize associated risks of sports. For example, the delay in menses and reduction in ovulation seen in some athletic girls may increase risk of early-onset osteoporosis.

Exercise goals and prescriptions for individual patients will vary by patient age, sex, conditioning, and lifestyle. The knowledge that increased activity might be protective against cancer will be an additional incentive for individuals to incorporate physical activity into their lives.

Conclusion

There are consistent observational data in humans suggesting a role of physical activity in reducing risk for some cancers. There are several biologically plausible mechanisms that might explain the observed associations. It is also plausible that the links between physical activity and cancer are the result of bias, due partly or entirely to some other factor or factors correlated with activity such as diet or exposure to carcinogens (McTiernan, Stanford, Daling, et al., 1998; McTiernan, Ulrich, et al., 1998). More research is needed to fully explore these associations, develop a biological model or models, and provide information that could be used to develop individual exercise prescriptions for cancer prevention.

References

Bernstein, I., Henderson, B. E., Hanisch, R., Sullivan-Halley, J., & Ross, R. K. (1994). Physical exercise and reduced risk of breast cancer in young women [see comments]. *Journal of the National Cancer Institute, 86*, 1403–1408.

Colditz, G. (1998). Relationship between estrogen levels, use of hormone replacement therapy, and breast cancer. *Journal of the National Cancer Institute, 90*, 814–823.

Colditz, G. A., Cannuscio, C. C., & Frazier, A. L. (1997). Physical activity and reduced risk of colon cancer: Implications for prevention. *Cancer Causes & Control, 8*, 649–667.

Freidenreich, C. M., Thune, I., Brinton, L. A., & Albanes, D. (1998). Epidemiologic issues related to the association between physical activity and breast cancer. *Cancer, 83*, 600–610.

Gammon, M. D., John, E. M., & Britton, J. A. (1998). Recreational and occupational physical activities and risk of breast cancer. *Journal of the National Cancer Institute, 90*, 100–117.

Gann, P. H., Hennekens, C. H., Ma, J., Longcope, C., & Stampfer, M. J. (1996). Prospective study of sex hormone levels and risk of prostate cancer [see comments]. *Journal of the National Cancer Institute, 88*, 1118–1126.

Greenlee, R. T., Murray, T., Bolden, S., & Wingo, P. A. (2000). Cancer statistics. *Cancer Journal for Clinicians, 50*, 7–33.

Hoffman-Goetz, L., Apter, D., Demark-Wahnefried, W., Goran M. I., McTiernan A., & Reichman M. E. (1998). Possible mechanisms mediating an association between physical activity and breast cancer. *Cancer, 83*, 621–628.

Huang, Z., Hankinson, S. E., & Colditz, G. A., Stampler, M. J., Hunter, D. J., Manson, J. E., Hennekens, C. H., Rosner, B., Speizer, F. E., & Willett, W. C. (1997). Dual effects of weight and weight gain on breast cancer risk. *Journal of the American Medical Association, 278*, 1407–1411.

Martinez M. E., Giovannucci, E., Speigelman, D., et al. (1997). Leisure-time, physical activity, body size, and colon cancer in women. *Journal of the National Cancer Institute, 89*, 948–955.

McTiernan, A., Stanford, J., Daling, J., & Voigt, L. (1998). Prevalence and correlates of recreational physical activity in women aged 50–64 years. *Menopause, 5*, 95–101.

McTiernan, A., Stanford, J. L., Weiss, N. S., Daling, J. R., & Voigt, L. F. (1996). Occurrence of breast cancer in relation to recreational exercise in women age 50–64 years. *Epidemiology, 7*, 598–604.

McTiernan, A., Ulrich, C., Slate, S., & Potter, J. (1998). Physical activity and cancer etiology: Associations and mechanisms. *Cancer causes and control, 9*(5), 487–509.

Mink, P. J., Folsom, A. R., Sellers, T. A., & Kushi, L. H. (1996). Physical activity, waist-to-hip ratio, and other risk factors for ovarian cancer: A followup study of older women. *Epidemiology, 7*, 38–45.

Oliveria, S. A., & Lee, I. M. (1997). Is exercise beneficial in the prevention of prostate cancer? *Sports Medicine, 23*, 271–278.

Rockhill, B., Willett, W. C., Hunter, D. J., Manson, J. E., Hankinson, S. E., Spiegelman, D., & Colditz, G. (1998). A. Physical activity and breast cancer risk in a cohort of young women. *New England Journal of Medicine, 90*(15), 1155–1160.

Rockhill, B., Willett, W. C., Hunter, D. J., Manson, J. E., Hankinson, S. E., & Colditz, G. A. (1999). A prospective study of recreational physical activity and breast cancer risk. *Archives of Internal Medicine, 159*, 2290–2296.

Slattery, M. L., Edwards, S. L., Ma, K. N., Friedman, G. D., & Potter, J. D. (1997). Physical activity and colon cancer: A public health perspective. *Annals of Epidemiology, 7*, 137–145.

Thune, I., Brenn, T., Lund, E., & Gaard, M. (1997). Physical activity and the risk of breast cancer. *New England Journal of Medicine, 336*, 1269–1275.

Thune, I., & Lund, E. (1994). Physical activity and the risk of prostate and testicular cancer: a cohort study of 53,000 Norwegian men. *Cancer Causes & Control, 5*, 549–556.

Thune, I., & Lund, E. (1996). Physical activity and risk of colorectal cancer in men and women. *British Journal of Cancer, 73*, 1134–1140.

Thune, I., & Lund, E. (1997). The influence of physical activity on lung-cancer risk: A prospective study of 81,516 men and women. *International Journal of Cancer, 70*, 57–62.

Women's Health Initiative Study Group. (1998). *Design of the Women's Health Initiative Clinical Trial and Observational Study.* Controlled Clinical Trials 1998, *19*, 61–109.

World Cancer Research Fund Panel (Potter, J. D., Chair). (1997). *Food, nutrition and the prevention of cancer: A global perspective.* Washington, DC: American Institute for Cancer Research.

The Editors

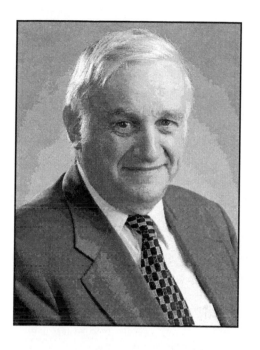

David I. Mostofsky is a professor of psychology at Boston University and holds associate appointments at several major medical institutions in the Boston area. A Charter Fellow of the Academy for Behavioral Medicine Research, he has been active in behavioral medicine for many years and has published numerous articles and books on a variety of topics in this area. He has been the recipient of many awards, including a Marshal Fund Award, an Einstein Award, an NIH/Fogarty Fellowship, and a Fulbright Fellowship.

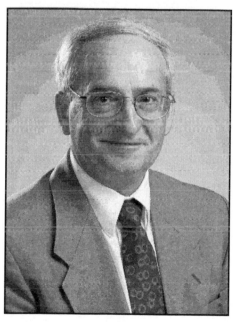

Leonard D. Zaichkowsky is professor of education at Boston University and head of the graduate program in sport and exercise psychology. He is both past president and a Fellow of the Association for the Advancement of Applied Sport Psychology (AAASP), a member of the United States Olympic Committee Sport Psychology Registry, and a certified consultant AAASP. Len has published numerous articles and books on sport psychology and research design. In addition to his scholarly work he is a staff psychologist at New England Baptist Hospital and a consulting psychologist for the Boston Celtics.

Contributing Authors

Mark B. Andersen is a registered psychologist and associate professor at Victoria University in Melbourne, Australia. He is the chair of the Division of Research in the School of Human Movement, Recreation, and Performance and coordinates the master of applied psychology degree (sport and exercise psychology emphasis) in the Department of Psychology. He received his doctorate from the University of Arizona in 1988 and immigrated to Australia in 1994. His teaching includes statistics, research design, psychology of rehabilitation, and the professional practice of psychology. His areas of research interest include the psychology of injury and rehabilitation; the role of exercise in mental health, well being, and quality of life; the training and supervision of graduate students; and the practice of sport psychology service delivery.

J. David Branch is an associate professor of exercise science and coordinator of the undergraduate program at Old Dominion University in Norfolk, Virginia. He is a Fellow in the American College of Sports Medicine. His research interests include the effects of creatine and ginseng supplementation on performance. He has coauthored peer-reviewed research on the effects of creatine and ginseng supplementation, as well as the book *Creatine: The Power Supplement* and other book chapters on supplementation. He is a recreational runner. David and his wife, Carol, live in Norfolk, Virginia, with his two stepchildren, David and Anne, and their dog, Kelly.

Glenn S. Brassington is a postdoctoral Fellow at the Stanford Center for Research in Disease Prevention (Stanford University School of Medicine). He has a doctorate in clinical psychology. His research and clinical work focuses on the role of behavior in health promotion and disease prevention.

Britton W. Brewer is an associate professor of psychology at Springfield College in Springfield, Massachusetts, where he teaches undergraduate and graduate psychology courses, conducts research on psychological aspects of sport injury, and coaches the men's cross country team. He is listed in the United States Olympic Committee Sport Psychology Registry, 20002004, and is a Certified Consultant, Association for the Advancement of Applied Sport Psychology.

Randall W. Bryner is an associate professor in the Division of Exercise Physiology in the School of Medicine at West Virginia University. Dr. Bryner's research interests include exploration of exercise effects on prostate cancer development, metabolic changes with weight loss, and ergogenic aids and exercise. Dr. Bryner enjoys cycling and running (slowly), and serves as youth basketball coach.

Bjørn Ellertsen is professor in clinical neuropsychology at the Department of Biological and Medical Psychology at the University of Bergen, Norway. He graduated as a psychologist from the University of Bergen in 1975 and received his Ph.D. from the Faculty of Psychology at the University of Bergen in 1987. He is a specialist in clinical psychology and clinical neuropsychology. His current research interest covers clinical neuropsychology and electroencephalographic methods and work with personality testing like MMPI2 and MMPIA.

Hege R. Eriksen is a postdoctoral Fellow at the Department of Biological and Medical Psychology at the University of Bergen, Norway. She is also a research coordinator for the Norwegian Back Pain Network. Her basic training is from the Norwegian University of Sport and Physical Education, where she wrote her master's thesis on the effects of physical exercise on women with epilepsy. She has studied the psychophysiology of psychological defense mechanisms at the Department of Anatomy and Cell Biology, UCLA. She received her Ph.D. from the Faculty of Psychology at the University of Bergen in 1998. Her doctoral thesis was on stress, coping, and subjective health complaints.

Avery D. Faigenbaum, is an assistant professor of human performance and fitness at the University of Massachusetts in Boston. He received an Ed.D., and is an NSCA Certified Strength and Conditioning Specialist and an ACSM-Certified Health/Fitness Director. He has authored two books on youth fitness, including *Strength and Power for Young Athletes*, and serves on the editorial boards of several fitness journals.

Steve Fuchs was awarded his Ed.D. at Boston University and developed numerous clinical and research activities while on staff at the Cambridge Health Alliance, Behavioral Medicine Program, and at Harvard Medical School in the Department of Psychiatry.

Michael Gaudette, MS, PT, OCS, is trained in sports medicine rehabilitation and has worked with professional, Olympic, collegiate, and high school athletes. He has lectured nationally on orthopedic and sports medicine topics, including functional rehabilitation. Mike has successfully applied sports medicine techniques and concepts to the treatment of all patients, including the "industrial athletes."

Knut Hestad graduated as a psychologist from the University of Oslo in 1982. He is a specialist in clinical psychology and clinical neuropsychology. He received his Ph.D. from the Faculty of Psychology at the University of Bergen in 1996. His doctoral thesis was on HIV dementia. He is currently working as a clinical neuropsychologist and is an associate professor at Department of Biological and Medical Psychology at the University of Bergen, Norway.

Fred Kantrowitz, M.D. is a practicing rheumatologist and a clinical assistant professor at Harvard Medical School. He is also a team physician (internal medicine) for the Boston Celtics basketball team.

Urho M. Kujala, is the chief physician at the Unit for Sports and Exercise Medicine, University of Helsinki, and at The Finnish Foundation of Sports Medicine, Helsinki, Finland. He completed his M.D. and Ph.D., and has worked as a clinical specialist physician in sports and exercise medicine since 1991 and as a senior lecturer in sports and exercise medicine at the University of Helsinki since 1994. His scientific work includes more than 100 original research articles in international scientific journals. The main focus of his scientific work has been the associations between physical activity and health, including studies of twins and athletics.

Kim Larsson is a registered nurse and the Director of Biofeedback Services at Harvard Vanguard Medical Associates in Boston and a doctoral candidate in nursing at Boston College. Kim has been involved with behavioral medicine for over 14 years, including directing mind/body programs for pain and other chronic symptom management. Her clinical research explores the dynamics of somatization; the role, expression, and meaning of pain; and the treatment of diabetes.

Egil W. Martinsen is a psychiatrist and Research Director at Modum Bad, a private psychiatric clinic in Norway. During the last 20 years, he has been involved in research and clinical practice utilizing exercise as a treatment intervention for patients with various psychiatric disorders.

Anne McTiernan earned both an M.D. and a Ph.D., and holds an appointment with the Fred Hutchinson Cancer Research Center, Cancer Prevention Research Program, in Seattle, Washington, where she is Director of the Exercise Testing and Training Laboratory and the Prevention Studies Clinic. She serves as Principal Investigator for several clinical trials with exercise and diet interventions and is the lead physician in the Women's Health Initiative Clinical Coordinating Center. Her main focus of research is on testing the effect of exercise on biomarkers of cancer risk, although she participates in drug testing trials, risk counseling trials, and cohort studies in healthy persons and in breast cancer patients. She is lead author of *Breast Fitness: An Optimal Exercise and Health Plan for Reducing Your Risk of Breast Casncer* (St. Martin's Press, 2000).

Tony Morris is a professor of sport and exercise psychology at Victoria University in Melbourne, Australia. Tony has extensive experience of teaching, research, and service in this field in the UK and Australia. He has written and edited several books on sport and exercise psychology, and has a substantial number of research publications. Tony is President of the Asian South Pacific Association of Sport Psychology and a member of the Managing Council of the International Society of Sport Psychology.

Lyle Joseph Micheli a leading authority on sports and dance medicine, with a concentration on pediatric and adolescent care. He received his undergraduate and medical degrees from Harvard University. Director of the USA's first sports medicine clinic for young athletes, which he founded in 1974, he is a past president of the American College of Sports Medicine, Chairman of the Massachusetts Governor's Council on Fitness and Sports, Chairman of the Education Commission of the International Federation of Sports Medicine, and a member of the Board of Directors of the United States Rugby Football Foundation. Dr. Micheli is also the attending physician for the Boston Ballet and a medical consultant to the Boston Ballet School.

Frank M. Perna, Ed.D., Ph.D., is an associate professor in the Division of Psychiatry in the School of Medicine at Boston University and an adjunct appointment in the Department of Anatomy and Clinical Neuroscience. Dr. Perna, an avid runner, is a licensed psychologist specializing in clinical health psychology, behavioral medicine, and sport psychology. He listed on the sport psychology registry of the United States Olympic Committee and serves as an AAASP-certified consultant. Dr. Perna's work emphasizes psychoneuroimmunology, exercise, and cognitive-behavioral intervention with chronic disease and athletic populations.

Daniel S. Rooks, Sc.D., is Director of the Be Well! Tanger Center for Health Management and a member of the Divisions of Rheumatology and Gerontology (Department of Medicine) and the Department of Orthopedic Surgery at Beth Israel Deaconess Medical Center. He is an instructor in medicine at Harvard Medical School

Roy J. Shephard, M.D. [Lond.], Ph.D. is former Director of the School of Physical Education and Health and the Graduate Programme in Exercise Sciences at the University of Toronto. A former President of the Canadian Association of Exercise Sciences and the American College of Sports Medicine, he holds the Honor Award of both of these organizations. He has also received honorary degrees from the Universities of Ghent and Montreal.

Mara D. H. Smith is a certified birth educator and doula (professional birth coach). Her work utilizing sport psychology principles includes childbirth, positive parenting in sport, and working with teams and individual athletes. Mara lives in the Olympic village of Lake Placid, New York, with her favorite team—her husband and four young children.

Georgina Sutherland completed her doctoral studies in the School of Human Movement, Recreation and Performance at Victoria University in Melbourne, Australia. Her dissertation, in the health psychology field, investigated the effects of exercise and autogenic training on the psychological well being of people with multiple sclerosis. Dr. Sutherland is particularly interested in health-related quality of life and health promotion for people with disabilities. She is currently involved in a number of research projects with people with intellectual disabilities at the Centre for Developmental Disability Health Victoria, Monash University, Melbourne, Australia.

William K. Thierfelder, is a former Olympian, National Champion, two-time All-American, and NCAA Division I coach. An Ed.D., DABPS, ACSM, CSCS, he is the Executive Director of ProSportDoc, a sports performance services company. He provides comprehensive year-round training and support to professional athletes in all major sports. He received his master's and doctoral degrees in sports psychology and human movement from Boston University. He is a licensed psychologist and member of the 2000–2004 United States Olympic Committee Sport Psychology Registry.

Toshihiko Tsutsumi is an associate professor in the Department of Social Work at Kinki Welfare University, Japan. After receiving his doctorate in sport psychology, he continued research in the psychological aspects of strength training in older adults.

Judy L. Van Raalte, Ph.D., is an associate professor of psychology at Springfield College in Springfield, Massachusetts, where she teaches undergraduate and graduate psychology courses and conducts research on cognitive factors and sport performance. She served as coach of the women's tennis team for five years and is an associate editor of the *Journal of Applied Sport Psychology*. She is listed in the United States Olympic Committee Sport Psychology Registry, 20002004 and is a Certified Consultant, Association for the Advancement of Applied Sport Psychology.

Debra Wein, holds a bachelor's degree in nutritional sciences from Cornell University and a master's in nutrition and applied physiology from Columbia University. She is an adjunct faculty member at the University of Massachusetts, Simmons College, and The Boston Conservatory. With over ten years of experience managing leading university fitness centers in New York and Boston, she is President of The Sensible Nutrition Connection, Inc., a consulting firm providing nutrition services to universities, corporate wellness programs, health clubs across Massachusetts, and nonprofit groups, and is the author of *SNaC Pack: The Health Professional's Guide to Nutrition.*

Index